D1326225

Mac Keith Press
30 Furnival Street
London
EC4A 1JQ
UK
Telephone +44 (0) 20 7405 5355
Fax +44 (0) 20 7405 5365
E-Mail allat@mackeith.co.uk

ERRATUM

The Clinical Management of Craniosynostosis   Hayward et al.
Mac Keith Press   ISBN1 898683 36 0

On page 366, first line of the paragraph headed 'Pain Management', the dosage of fentanyl is incorrect. It should read:

5–10 µg/kg

We recommend that the correct dose is written onto the page in case this erratum slip is lost.

We offer our apologies for this error.

Clinics in Developmental Medicine No. 163
THE CLINICAL MANAGEMENT OF
CRANIOSYNOSTOSIS

© 2004 Mac Keith Press
30 Furnival Street, London EC4A 1JQ

Senior Editor: Martin C.O. Bax
Editor: Hilary M. Hart
Managing Editor: Michael Pountney
Project Manager: Sarah Pearsall

First published in this edition 2004

British Library Cataloguing-in-Publication data
A catalogue record for this book is available from the British Library

ISSN: 0069 4835
ISBN: 1 898683 36 0

Typeset by Keystroke, Jacaranda Lodge, Wolverhampton
Printed by The Lavenham Press Ltd, Water Street, Lavenham, Suffolk
Mac Keith Press is supported by Scope

Clinics in Developmental Medicine No. 163

The Clinical Management of Craniosynostosis

Edited by

RICHARD HAYWARD Consultant Neurosurgeon
BARRY JONES Consultant Plastic and Craniofacial Surgeon
DAVID DUNAWAY Consultant Plastic and Craniofacial Surgeon
ROBERT EVANS Consultant Orthodontist

Great Ormond Street Hospital for Children
London

Preface by
PAUL TESSIER

2004
Mac Keith Press

Distributed by 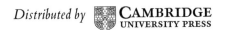 CAMBRIDGE
UNIVERSITY PRESS

CONTENTS

AUTHORS' APPOINTMENTS

D. Armstrong	Neuroradiologist, Hospital for Sick Children, Toronto
R.I. Aviv	Fellow in Neuroradiology, Hospital for Sick Children, Toronto
R. Bingham	Consultant Anaesthetist, Great Ormond Street Hospital for Children, London
Rachel Bradford	Research Fellow, Great Ormond Street Hospital for Children, London
Jonathan Britto	Craniofacial Fellow, Department of Plastic Surgery, Hospital for Sick Children, Toronto, Canada
Lucinda J. Carr	Consultant Paediatric Neurologist, Great Ormond Street Hospital for Children, London
Lyn S. Chitty	Senior Lecturer in Genetics and Fetal Medicine, Institute of Child Health and University College London Hospital, London, and Consultant in Fetal Medicine, Elizabeth Garrett Anderson Hospital, London
W.K. Chong	Consultant Paediatric Neuroradiologist, Great Ormond Street Hospital for Children, London
David Dunaway	Consultant Plastic and Craniofacial Surgeon, Great Ormond Street Hospital for Children, London
Robert D. Evans	Consultant Orthodontist/Senior Lecturer in Orthodontics, Great Ormond Street Hospital for Children, London
Richard Hayward	Consultant Neurosurgeon, Great Ormond Street Hospital for Children, London
Daniela Hearst	Consultant Clinical Psychologist, Great Ormond Street Hospital for Children, London
Barry Jones	Consultant Plastic and Craniofacial Surgeon, Great Ormond Street Hospital for Children, London
Roderick Lane	Consultant Clinical Scientist and Head of Sleep and Respiratory Services, Institute of Child Health, London, and Senior Lecturer in Respiratory Medicine, Institute of Child Health, London
Susanna Leighton	Consultant Paediatric Otolaryngologist, Great Ormond Street Hospital for Children, London

S. Mallory	Consultant Anaesthetist, Great Ormond Street Hospital for Children, London
Ken K. Nischal	Consultant Ophthalmologist, Great Ormond Street Hospital for Children, London, and Honorary Senior Lecturer, the Institute of Child Health, London
Valerie Pereira	Speech and Language Therapist, Great Ormond Street Hospital for Children, London
Olav B. Petersen	Consultant in Fetal Medicine, Skejby University Hospital, Aarhus, Denmark
Willie Reardon	Consultant Clinical Geneticist, National Centre for Medical Genetics, Our Lady's Hospital for Sick Children, Dublin, Ireland
Caroleen Shipster	Senior Specialist Speech Therapist, Great Ormond Street Hospital for Children, London
Tony Sirimanna	Consultant Audiological Physician, Great Ormond Street Hospital for Children, London
D.N.P. Thompson	Consultant Paediatric Neurosurgeon, Great Ormond Street Hospital for Children, London
Andrea White	Clinical Nurse Specialist, Craniofacial Unit, Great Ormond Street Hospital for Children, London
Louise C. Wilson	Consultant Clinical Geneticist, Great Ormond Street Hospital for Children, London

PREFACE

Paul Tessier

There are few men who have had only a single love in their life. I can proudly claim to have had three successive surgical 'love affairs' on the opposite side of the channel covering three generations of surgeons.

The story began after the Second World War when, despite the deprivations of food rationing, I discovered in and around London a banquet of surgical talent in the persons of four New Zealanders – Sir Harold Gillies, Sir Archibald McIndoe, Rainsford Mowlem and John Barron. For four years the channel was my highway as I spent my vacations observing them in Basingstoke, London, East Grinstead, St Albans and Northwood. As adopted Englishmen, naturally they travelled by Bentley, an experience that I enjoyed sharing. This was the first 'affair'.

In 1970, when craniofacial surgery was in its adolescence, David Mathews, the senior plastic surgeon at London's Great Ormond Street Hospital, arrived at the Hôpital Foch in Paris (where I was working) and made plans for me to come to London to help develop craniofacial surgery there. This heralded several trips back and forth to London to train the two surgical teams to work together. Again, transport on the north side of the channel was by a not always functional, but thoroughly English, Bentley. 'Affair' number two.

A generation later, Barry Jones appeared in my operating room. Presumably he enjoyed the experience, since he returned and eventually invited me to Great Ormond Street to operate and see patients with him and Richard Hayward. What could have been more attractive for someone who had been seeing malformed children in his clinic in Paris over a period of thirty years? So the third 'affair' began. During several visits we saw many patients together and operated on two particularly challenging syndromic problems. Although by this time daily transport for British doctors was no longer provided by Bentley Motors I thought it no accident that on one occasion Barry collected me from the Eurotunnel terminal at *Waterloo* Station and took me to the *Wellington* Hospital via *Trafalgar* Square. I pointed out to him that while in Paris I had not insisted that he operate at the Napoleon hospital!! Affair number three.

This book will fill a gap in the practice of craniofacial surgery for children, providing information for parents, paediatricians and other medical professionals involved in their initial and long-term care.

Craniofacial surgery for malformation is a strange and esoteric world. While so-called 'simple' synostoses have been treated for forty years or more (initially by neurosurgeons working in isolation), the treatment of syndromic craniofacial dysostoses is relatively recent and much controversy continues to surround fundamental issues such as the timing of surgical intervention and the preferred type of procedure, e.g. the place of distraction osteogenesis compared with more traditional surgical approaches. Many difficult and unsolved problems remain in the treatment of complex facial clefts and aplastic conditions such as arrhinia, Franchisetti (Treacher Collins) syndrome, Goldenhar syndrome and anophthalmia, which will challenge the imagination and resource of future surgical generations. This is not surgery for the occasional practitioner but for committed specialists.

In 1985 I wrote a foreword for the proceedings of the first meeting of the International Society of Craniofacial Surgeons. In it I outlined several concerns, which even twenty years later remain worthy of consideration.

We do not operate for syndromes but we treat patients with particular dysfunctions and dysmorphias. Treatment can consist in a radical one-stage procedure or be staged over several years, depending on the clinical form, age, previous operative procedures, associated malformations, and the strategy adopted by a given team.

What does the word 'craniofacial' cover? Most of us agree that there are only two correct uses for the word 'craniofacial'! One refers to the anatomy and it includes all the facial malformations, injuries and tumours that have a major orbitocranial component. The other refers to surgical practice and includes all procedures in which the intracranial approach to the midfacial segment is used. These two empiric categories mean that the craniofacial field is sufficiently wide and also sufficiently restrictive to be a separate speciality in its own right.

Is the paramount importance given to Craniosynostosis justified? Craniosynostosis is a dominant factor in craniofacial malformations. But this does not mean that the procedures and timing appropriate for craniosynostosis are also valid for other categories of malformations, or that releasing fused sutures will necessarily promote better development within the midfacial segment or the mandible.

In the hierarchy of importance, the brain and the respiratory and ocular functions always prevail. Speech and the relationship between the jaws follow, and some of these goals overlap. When a surgical procedure is performed on a child, the main goals are to improve the vital functions and to give the cranium, midface and mandible a better chance for development, but this is not always achieved. What might be successful at 15 years of age may not be so at 3 years. Conversely a procedure that needs to be done before the age of 3 will no longer be indicated at 15. Any attempt to apply a ready formulated treatment, such as midfacial advancement or frontofacial bipartition, to patients regardless of their individual needs is nonsense.

Uncertainties remain. Now, 30 years after what Sam Pruzansky called 'our experiments on nature's experiments', we know that satisfactory results can be provided by the fundamental major procedures that had by then already been described. But after four generations of life, we also know that a simple closure of the lip and palate does not solve all the problems of speech, breathing, jaw function and facial morphology. Many people still believe that, whatever the age of the patient, a Le Fort III type midfacial advancement solves all the problems of Crouzon syndrome, that frontofacial bipartition is the definitive solution for all hyperteloric children, or that calvarial bone grafts, mandibular lengthening, and chin implants will make handsome a child with Treacher–Collins syndrome. These assumptions are very naïve, because technical enthusiasm masks some striking facts. These are:

First, the initially displaced facial segments are not normal. They are abnormal in shape, volume, and growth potential. Consequently, the abnormal position of abnormal segments is changed into a normal position of abnormal segments.

Second, in complex malformations such as hemi-facial microsomia, Treacher–Collins syndrome, or orbitofacial clefts, where abnormal segments are either lacking or deformed, the relationship between the facial segments can be changed and normality is after achieved. However, because of the uneven distribution of the deformity over the upper face, midface and lower face, no one can predict how growth will proceed.

Third, the position of the midfacial segment or the mandible is generally changed with reference to the dental occlusion. However, orthognatic is not craniofacial. The relative position of the jaws is only one component of facial morphology, serving more as a landmark than as a facial standard. Moreover, the growth of the maxilla and mandible does not proceed in response to the same stimuli or follow the same timing.

Fourth, changing the position of the midfacial segment or the mandible always changes the dynamic action of muscles that may be normal (Crouzon and Apert), or hypoplastic or non-existent, either unilaterally (hemi-facial microsomia) or bilaterally (Treacher–Collins). The secondary changes resulting from the dynamic action of such muscles are still unpredictable.

The advisability of 'early' surgery in craniofacial malformation is a frequent topic of debate. There is no longer any doubt about the desirability of releasing active craniosynostosis, e.g. unilateral coronal synostosis (plagiocephaly), complete coronal synostosis (brachycephaly), multiple sutural synostosis (Crouzon's or trilobar deformity), during infancy. Early intervention has been clearly documented as preventing major brain damage and often ocular dysfunction. However, at present, no one can pretend that early craniectomy, frontal advancement, or even frontofacial advancement will provide for long-term facial growth.

Some operations must be done at 6 months, while others are better performed at 3 or 4 years of age; for some malformations, the age of 7–10 years is a better choice. Any procedures that are carried out prematurely will have to be repeated, with increasing difficulties.

'The earlier the better' is a sound maxim for severe craniostenosis, but is nonsense for most other craniofacial malformations.

What makes a craniofacial unit? A unit where craniofacial procedures are performed does not automatically become a craniofacial centre because of the plate on the door. There are few departments devoted exclusively to craniofacial malformation as delineated above. One reason for this is that the relative scarcity of such malformations prevents any individual surgeon from performing only major craniofacial procedures. At what point does a caseload reach a 'critical mass'? It is my belief that a caseload of several major procedures a week is a minimum. No activity means no experience, no safety, and no progression.

Unfortunately and paradoxically, fewer and fewer craniofacial malformations will be seen primarily in the future, because increasing numbers of children with craniosynostosis are being operated on by neurosurgeons alone. It must also be foreseen that therapeutic abortion will drastically reduce the number of major malformations presented for consultation.

I am convinced that major reconstructive procedures for the treatment of oribitocranial injuries and tumours in adults can, because of their frequency, be sufficiently well performed by a surgeon well trained in osteoplastic techniques. However, on the other hand, I am also convinced that these surgeons should avoid malformations since by virtue of their nature, rarity, complexity and association with age and growth, they belong in a completely different and strange world. Beware of plunging from malformation to deformity.

Craniofacial surgery is a lonely field for the main actor. The appearance of the patient is never a vague idea at the back of the surgeon's mind, but at the front of the stage all the time. There is no prescribed way of providing a pleasing shape for a patient with Apert or Treacher–Collins syndrome. It is completely different from changing a cardiac valve or completing a jejuno-ureteroplasty. In these procedures, 25 to 75 per cent of the operation can be performed by a well-trained senior resident. In orthomorphic craniofacial procedures, the expert has to run along the whole of the rough track, especially in the asymmetric cases. Dissection becomes a step-by-step exploration, which reveals the landmark and the general view, the details and proportion, the direction and perspective. Paradoxically, the 'osteotomy', which is pure mechanics, can be delegated to assistants. But the construction, segment by segment, stone by stone, nail by nail, canthus by canthus, is endless. Even the levelling of the eyebrows, cheeks, lips and chin, and the dressing must be handled by the expert up to the very last.

Warning: there is an exciting challenge in most human endeavours, but there is no challenge at all in grappling with the worst malformations until a long step-by-step personal experience has demonstrated that all the wheels and traps in the simpler cases have been mastered. Disappointing as it may be, many must realise that there is no room for them in the strange world of craniofacial malformations. If they have a conscience they will relinquish their dreams and give up before they become disheartened by numerous pitfalls. Would they be willing to have their own cataracts extracted or a coronary bypass performed by their best friend if he treated only two cases a year? This is the acid test.

INTRODUCTION

Richard Hayward, David Dunaway, Robert D. Evans and Barry Jones

It is not surprising that the stimulus to take on the management of conditions that have previously been avoided or overlooked often comes from the passionate advocacy of a lone pioneer working, by definition, within a single specialty. For children with craniosynostosis – not to mention craniofacial surgery as a whole – their tireless advocate has been Paul Tessier, a man whose boundless energy, supreme technical skills and restless imagination have made him a true contemporary hero. We are most grateful to him for the eloquent introduction he has provided for us. But as interest and knowledge grow, a single specialty approach – surgical in this instance – to a complex disorder can lead to particular disadvantages, prime amongst which is the tendency to limit the perspective of possibilities to what can be dealt with by that specialty alone, leaving overlooked other potentially vital aspects of a patient's care. To say that such a state of affairs exists in the management of craniosynostosis would be too strong, but there is no doubt that we have reached a stage now when the full breadth of the complexity of the problems suffered by these children needs to be appreciated if they are to receive proper care.

Which brings us again to the purpose of this volume: to present the care of children with craniosynostosis '*in the round*'.

What does this mean? First, it means that those looking for a textbook of surgical techniques – those whose view of the subject is still essentially a surgical one – may be disappointed. The operations most commonly employed in the treatment of these children are indeed described – but only briefly and with the intention of providing those who are not craniofacial surgeons with some idea of the various techniques we employ, their scale and their rationale.

Instead, we have tried to present the management of the child with craniosynostosis as these children and their families will find themselves being cared for if they are referred to a unit that has, like ourselves, embraced the management philosophy that sees the child as a whole rather than an assembly of surgical challenges.

To this end a total of 16 specialists – the majority non-surgical, but each with a large experience and a particular interest in craniosynostosis – have contributed to this book. Not only does this demonstrate our commitment to the holistic management of these children, it also allows those specialists not working within a unit such as ours but who have contact with children with craniosynostosis on a more occasional basis to bring themselves up to date with present-day thinking on all aspects of their management.

Fortunately the numbers of affected children are few and therefore the number of multi-specialty units needed to care for them need not be great. But this means that by definition many children will live far from their craniofacial unit, and the major part of their everyday care will be in the hands of local paediatricians and family doctors. We hope that this book will be useful to them also in explaining the ideas, both general and specific, that govern our management policies.

At Great Ormond Street Hospital for Children we are fortunate in having been able to put together a team of specialists who have now been working together for 15 years or more. This has enabled us to audit our work and carry out both the clinical and laboratory-based research that has guided us towards the general philosophy of treatment that we describe in Chapter 7. It also accounts for our ability to put together a multi-author text whose contributors all come from the same institution. Each author has contributed to the management protocols we have modified and refined over the years and can describe their firsthand experience of a large caseload.

A word of caution. What we describe in these pages is our practice now. But does it represent contemporary practice universally, or indeed will we be making the same recommendations in, say, five years from now? To both questions the answer is no. The management of craniosynostosis (and its allied disorders) is both too young a subject and one that has advanced too rapidly for there to be any single 'correct' school. We hope, however, that we have succeeded here in presenting a convincing case for the policies we have, through personal experience, developed and refined over the years. And these policies will change in the years to come. There is no area of clinical practice, medical or surgical, that cannot be improved upon and our aim will always be to discover new ways of helping the children referred to us.

To this end we have tried to follow the Great Ormond Street Hospital for Children's motto, *'The child first and always'*, in our approach to these complex conditions, and hope that this book, reflecting our long experience here, will be a useful contribution to the many specialists with responsibility – frequent or occasional – for the care of affected children.

ACKNOWLEDGEMENTS

The editors would like to pay particular thanks to Michael Pountney and Martin Bax and their team at Mac Keith Press for all their help during the preparation of this volume.

As we have stated in Chapter 7 ('Principles of management of the child with craniosynostosis'), no amount of specialist care on the part of the most dedicated craniofacial unit for our children would be properly effective if it were not for the care that they receive locally from their community and acute paediatric services. We would therefore like to thank particularly Drs Paul Munyard, M. Ward Platt, Deirdre Walsh, Karen Whiting and Maryam Zahir for the many suggestions they provided during the preparation of this book.

We are fortunate in having a distinguished plastic surgeon provide the illustrations for Chapter 19 – on the operations most commonly employed in the treatment of children with craniosynostosis. He is Michael J. Earley M.ch., FRCSI, FRCS plast (Consultant Plastic Surgeon, Dublin). We are most grateful for his contribution.

We must also express our gratitude to the Department of Health which, recognising the importance of concentrating the care of patients with rare conditions requiring extensive multidisciplinary care into specialised centres, has since 1987 provided the craniofacial unit at Great Ormond Street Hospital for Children (together with colleague units in Birmingham, Oxford and Liverpool) with supra-regional funding through the National Specialist Commissioning Advisory Group (NSCAG).

1
CRANIOFACIAL GROWTH AND DEVELOPMENT: A CLINICAL PERSPECTIVE

David Dunaway

An understanding of craniofacial growth and development is important to the understanding of the management of craniosynostosis. Disordered growth caused by craniosynostosis results in deformity which in turn is responsible for many of the functional problems associated with the condition. Disordered growth associated with simple (single suture) synostosis affects mainly (but not exclusively) the skull vault and occurs principally *in utero* and infancy. In complex (syndromic and multi-suture) synostosis, abnormalities of growth and development continue into childhood and adolescence.

These abnormal growth patterns create dilemmas in the timing of reconstructive surgery – a topic dealt with also in Chapters 8 and 19. Early surgery is clearly desirable to correct deformity and prevent functional problems. However, continuing disordered growth subsequent to early surgery may result in relapse and reversion towards the original phenotype. Early operations, particularly in the midfacial region, may also disrupt growth potential still further. It is for these reasons that definitive reconstructive procedures in syndromic craniosynostosis are often best delayed until the end of growth. This is not a rule, however. Functional problems occurring in infancy and childhood and the emergence of psychological problems in childhood and adolescence due to the patient's abnormal appearance often demand intervention before the ideal time for definitive reconstructive surgery. If surgery is undertaken at an early age, though, secondary procedures are often needed later for a definitive correction of the deformity. These secondary – or repeat – operations can be more difficult to perform than primary procedures and may be associated with increased complication rates.

An appreciation of the events that occur at different times in craniofacial development should therefore guide decisions on the timing and type of surgical intervention undertaken for children with all manifestations of craniosynostosis but particularly those with the syndromic forms now known to be associated with specific genetic mutations (see Chapter 3).

This chapter will describe the relevant aspects of growth and development in craniofacial morphology. The pathogenesis of craniosynostosis is discussed elsewhere. Before considering growth in craniosynostosis, the processes occurring in normal craniofacial development will be discussed.

Normal craniofacial growth and development

Craniofacial growth occurs at varying rates and for differing periods of time in the various regions of the craniofacial skeleton. At birth the brain is relatively well developed and so the skull vault (neurocranium) protecting the brain is necessarily much larger in comparison to the more diminutive facial skeleton (viscerocranium). With subsequent development the neurocranium grows at a slower rate, while the facial skeleton must grow significantly throughout childhood and adolescence to accommodate the developing dentition, orbits and airways. It is these changing functional demands which dictate the patterns of differential growth between the various components of the craniofacial skeleton (Fig. 1.1).

The various processes involved in normal growth of the craniofacial skeleton include:

- Endochondral ossification
- Intramembranous ossification and sutural growth
- Remodelling
- Displacement

ENDOCHONDRAL OSSIFICATION

This is the process by which new bone is formed by the replacement of endochondral cartilage within bone. It is important in long bone growth, but has a relatively limited role in craniofacial growth. Endochondral growth occurs at the synchondroses at the skull base, but the degree to which it contributes to craniofacial development is a matter of controversy.

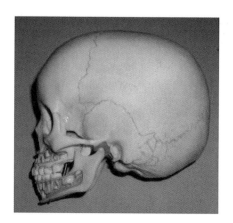 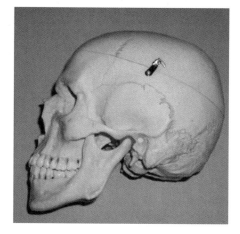

Fig. 1.1 Models of infant and adult skulls demonstrating the relative difference in size of the neurocranium and facial skeleton. When compared to the dimensions of the adult skull, the infant skull has a large neurocranium to accommodate the brain, which reaches near adult size early in life. The facial skeleton is diminutive in size and much of it is taken up by the orbits protecting the orbital contents, which also reach near adult size early. The mandible and lower part of the maxilla remain underdeveloped and will only increase significantly in size with the development of the secondary dentition and growth of the masticatory musculature.

In more primitive mammals, growth at these basal synchondroses is the major mechanism by which cranial base growth occurs. However, in the human skull the number and extent of these sutures are insufficient to allow for growth to accommodate the enlarging brain. Sutural growth and remodelling therefore play the most important role.

INTRAMEMBRANOUS OSSIFICATION AND SUTURAL GROWTH

Most of the bones of the skull are membranous bones. Growth of these bones occurs as a result of a positive balance between deposition (osteoblastic activity) and resorption (osteoclastic activity) by the surrounding periosteum externally and the outer layer of the dura internally, and the process is particularly active at the sutural interfaces between the bones of the skull vault. This type of growth is driven by the development of the soft tissues with which the bones are associated. Thus development of the brain, orbital contents and facial musculature are all important factors in driving this process. If an eye fails to develop normally, for example, there will be a small orbit and if the brain fails to grow to normal size the calvarium will be small (microcephaly).

The skull sutures are thought not to be growth centres in themselves, but areas in which ossification is occurring in response to external forces such as those described above. Premature sutural fusion occurring in craniosynostosis interferes with growth by preventing this process.

REMODELLING

Remodelling is the process by which the shape of a bone is altered by selective deposition and resorption of bone in different parts of its structure. An example of this process is the enlargement of the maxillary and frontal sinuses. The sinuses enlarge by a process of resorption of bone at the internal periosteal membrane and simultaneous deposition of bone at the outer surface.

As the craniofacial skeleton grows, the morphology of individual bones alters as different areas of the bone are selectively resorbed or added to by the periosteum. The process has an important role in most parts of the craniofacial skeleton. It is most simply demonstrated by the change in curvature that occurs in the calvarial bones as the skull vault enlarges.

DISPLACEMENT

Apparent growth can occur by displacement of bones. An example of this process is the anterior displacement of the body of the mandible by growth of the condylar neck. The process is also important in calvarial growth. In early life calvarial enlargement occurs by outward displacement of the calvarial bones by the enlarging brain. The bones enlarge by deposition at the sutural interfaces and remodelling alters their curvature.

The complexity of craniofacial growth can best be considered by dividing the head into five anatomically distinct regions, whose growth patterns may differ in their rates and timing, although they are of course interrelated:

1   Cranial vault (calvarium)
2   Cranial base

3   Orbits
4   Naso-maxillary complex
5   Mandible

THE NEUROCRANIUM (CRANIAL VAULT AND SKULL BASE)
The flat intramembranous bones of the calvarium are sandwiched between the dura internally and the pericranial membrane externally. With growth of the underlying brain, the
calvarial bones become separated at the sutures and bone growth occurs here to maintain
the integrity of the calvarium. A limited amount of remodelling is required to adjust the
curvatures of the calvarial bones.

The basicranium (skull base) is a more complicated structure than the calvarium
and requires extensive remodelling throughout growth. The shape of the skull base has to
accommodate (support) the enlarging cerebral hemispheres and maintain the relationships
of numerous foramina for the passage of cranial nerves and major blood vessels. Growth
at the spheno-occipital synchondrosis along with sutural growth plays a limited role in skull
base growth, but remodelling is the most important mechanism.

GROWTH AND DEVELOPMENT OF THE FACE
The facial bones are effectively suspended from the skull base. Changes and abnormalities
in the skull base will therefore affect facial morphology. The depth of the orbits and
anterior–posterior dimensions of the upper airway are determined in part by the anterior–
posterior dimensions of the anterior and middle cranial fossae to which they are attached.
In many craniodysostotic syndromes these dimensions are short, leading to deformity and
contributing to functional problems such as exorbitism and airway obstruction. Exorbitism
in this context is the result of restriction of the depth of the orbit because of failure of the
anterior fossa to elongate, leaving it with insufficient volume to contain the orbital contents.
Similarly failure of forward growth of the anterior skull base in the midline reduces the
anterior–posterior length of the nasopharynx and contributes to airway obstruction. The
angle of the cranial base (between the anterior fossa floor and the clivus) will also affect these
structures.

Growth and development of the face are affected by many factors, which guide
development to correspond to functional demands. Theses changes are described but not
necessarily explained by Moss's functional matrix theory. This states that osteogenic
membranes (such as periosteum) react to the sum of functional and morphogenic processes
(the functional matrix) acting upon them. We have already discussed the way in which
the calvarial bones respond to the enlarging brain, and this represents one of the matrices
influencing craniofacial development. In the same way, the face grows as a reaction to
similar forces (the development of the eye, for example), rather than as a result of growth
centres acting autonomously.

Other components of the functional matrix include the action of the muscles of
mastication and the developing dentition. If the pterygo-masseteric sling of muscles is
poorly developed, the angle of the mandible to which they are attached fails to develop
fully. Similarly, if the teeth fail to grow for some reason (perhaps they have been affected

4

by trauma, infection or injudicious surgery), the alveolar processes of the maxilla and mandible fail to develop to a normal size. Facial growth must also accommodate the need for a larger upper airway, and this structure also forms part of the functional matrix.

There are also a number of active cartilaginous (endochondral) growth centres within the face (for example, within the mandibular condyles or nasal septum) which may play an important role in growth. Although Moss's theory does not explain the mechanism by which development is controlled at a cellular or molecular level (see Chapter 3), it is useful in predicting and explaining the changing interrelationships that occur during growth.

The processes of intramembranous ossification, sutural growth, remodelling, displacement and possibly endochondral ossification (nasal septal cartilage) are all important in facial development. Where particularly relevant to the effects of craniosynostosis, they will be discussed below.

CRANIOFACIAL GROWTH PATTERNS

Craniofacial morphology changes very significantly during infancy and childhood to reflect the changing functional demands placed on the craniofacial skeleton. In infancy, the cranium and orbits are large in relation to the diminutive size of the face (Fig. 1.1), because the brain and eye undergo their most rapid period of growth during the first year or two of life. In contrast, the development of facial function is much slower; facial growth is driven by the development of the teeth and the muscles of mastication, and the need to enlarge the upper airway. The teeth and paranasal sinuses are poorly developed at birth and the secondary dentition is not fully established until well into adolescence (see Chapter 11). Facial growth therefore continues over a much longer period of time than the calvarium and, as it does so, the face enlarges in relation to the cranium.

If this process is considered in terms of the functional matrices described above, it can be seen how they dictate the rate of growth of different parts of the craniofacial skeleton and determine the timing of completion of growth. Growth of the calvarium is very rapid during the first year of life, and then dramatically slows. In contrast, upper midfacial and orbital growth is less dramatic in the first year of life but continues into much later childhood. Growth of the lower midface (the alveolar process of the maxilla, for example), which is largely driven by the developing dentition and masticatory apparatus, continues for longer than the upper midface (the infraorbital and malar regions). Mandibular growth continues for the longest of all, and in males is not normally complete until around the age of 20.

Growth potential is often reduced in craniosynostosis and so surgery to provide a definitive correction of deformity should ideally be delayed until the completion of growth of the affected region. An understanding of the timing of growth is therefore very important in planning the timing of surgery.

Large amounts of normative data have been collected on craniofacial development. The analysis of axial computerised tomographic (CT) scan data by Waitzman et al has clearly demonstrated differing rates of growth in the upper craniofacial region. At birth the infant's head circumference is 74 per cent of adult size. At 1 year this rises to 84 per cent and by 2 this figure has risen to 87 per cent. In contrast, the upper midfacial skeleton grows relatively slowly in the first year of life, but continues later into childhood. Midfacial

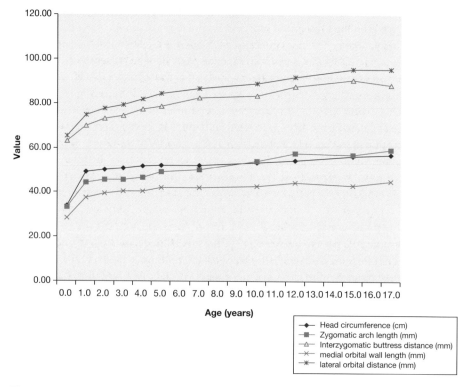

Fig. 1.2 Normal craniofacial growth. Plotting the increase in size of different regions of the craniofacial skeleton against time reveals varying rates and duration of growth. Head circumference increases rapidly in the first year of life and then relatively slowly. Zygomatic arch length, and the distance between the zygomas and lateral orbital walls are all measures of facial growth, and show a much more sustained growth pattern throughout childhood and adolescence.

Source: Data from Farkas (1994) and Posnick (2000).

projection measured by interzygomatic arch length is approximately 60 per cent of adult dimensions at birth, 77 per cent by 2 years, and 88 per cent by the age of 6. Growth in midfacial width measured by interzygomatic buttress distance follows a similar pattern to midfacial projection (Fig. 1.2).

Orbital growth patterns vary according to the dimensions measured. This is because the orbit enlarges both in response to growth of the eye and to growth of surrounding structures. The depth of the orbits measured by orbital wall length follows cranial growth patterns, as it is largely dependent on the increase in size of the anterior cranial fossa floor which forms the orbital roof. Orbital depth therefore increases significantly in size during the first year of life and relatively little after that. The width of the craniofacial skeleton in the orbital region follows upper midfacial growth and thus continues to increase in size significantly until the age of 6 or 7.

Growth of the lower midface and mandible is related to dental development and therefore continues well into adolescence. Dental occlusal relationships are not fully established until adulthood (see Chapter 11).

These findings have great implications for the timing of craniofacial surgery designed to correct deformity. Definitive surgery (defined as what the surgeon hopes will be a result free from the risk of subsequent reversion towards the original deformity) is ideally delayed until growth in the relevant part of the craniofacial skeleton is nearing completion. Definitive surgery limited to the calvarium can therefore be considered early, while that dealing with the mandible and maxilla needs to be delayed until towards the end of facial growth.

The growth patterns of surrounding areas also need to be taken into account when considering the timing of surgery. For example, the correction of hypertelorism (the excessive horizontal separation of the orbits) by a box osteotomy (see Chapter 19) cannot be considered until after the permanent canines have descended sufficiently to make space for the osteotomy cuts that would otherwise disrupt the maxillary region containing the developing permanent teeth. Similarly, maxillary and mandibular osteotomies to correct dental occlusion will not produce a result free from the risk of further displacement (reversion) until forward growth of the mandible is complete.

The earliest times that surgery to definitively correct deformity can be considered in the various regions of the craniofacial skeleton are as follows:

Cranium	1 year (6 months for sagittal synostosis)
Orbits	5 years +
Upper maxilla	9–12 years +
Lower maxilla	17 years +
Mandible	17 years +

These constraints greatly influence craniofacial management, a situation summarised in Chapter 7. Some form of active intervention, however, is often needed in the craniofacial dysostoses (effectively the syndromic forms of craniosynostosis) before the completion of growth, for functional or psychological reasons, and other strategies may need to be considered while completion of growth is awaited. For example, continuous positive airway pressure (CPAP), a nasal prong or even a tracheostomy may be required in childhood to treat airway problems arising from midfacial retrusion, while definitive surgery (perhaps a Le Fort III maxillary advance – see Chapter 19) is delayed for as long as possible – and preferably until timing is optimal.

Although our own management policy is designed to facilitate the correction of deformity with the minimum number of major surgical interventions (see Chapter 7), it must be noted that, particularly in the syndromic forms of synostosis, functional problems often dictate the need for surgery at times which are undesirable in respect to growth. When such conflicts occur, it may be necessary to operate early and accept that further surgery will be needed at a later date to correct the deformity that will result from further disordered growth (reversion towards the original phenotype).

Surgery can however often be staged to manage different functional problems in children with syndromic craniosynostosis, in whom the growth of both the cranium and midface is abnormal, and does not all need to be delayed until the completion of all growth. A frontal advancement can be undertaken early in life to address raised intracranial pressure, and advancement of orbits and midface can be performed around the age of 9 to treat exorbitism. Surgery at the completion of facial growth may then be limited to correcting the morphology of the lower midface and mandible and correcting dental occlusal relationships.

Disordered craniofacial growth in cranial synostosis

The mechanisms by which cranial synostosis occurs and interferes with growth are discussed in Chapters 2 and 3. From a simplistic point of view growth can be considered as being prevented by the synostosed suture – a mechanistic view that until comparatively recently provided the surgical rationale for the management of all forms of craniosynostosis and which can be summarised as 'Surgery that establishes a gap between the previously fused bones (effectively a suturectomy) will allow normal growth to be restored.' It was once even thought that an operation that opened up the base of skull sutures in children with, say, Crouzon syndrome, would lead to subsequent normal development of the face. It did not take too long, however, for it to become apparent that, perhaps with the exception of some children with sagittal synostosis who were operated upon early, normal growth of either face or skull was not restored by merely opening up the sutures, and surgeons began to add reconstructions of variable complexity to their suturectomies.

Craniosynostosis in its various forms, simple (single suture) and complex (syndromic and multiple suture), is better thought of as a disorder of growth, one manifestation of which is premature closure (fusion) of one or more skull sutures. This is not to say that such suture closures have no mechanical influence upon subsequent growth, but instead to point out how too great a dependence upon a mechanical view of how growth in craniosynostosis is affected will lead to less effective management strategies.

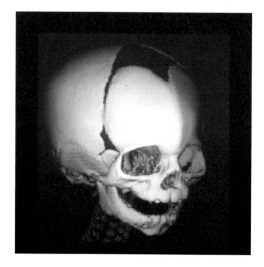

Fig. 1.3 Metopic synostosis. Early fusion of the metopic suture has resulted in trigonocephaly. There is an associated pronounced central forehead ridge. This condition is often associated with mild degrees of hypotelorism.

In the various forms of syndromic craniosynostosis the sutures of the skull vault and the skull base as well as growth centres within the midface are often severely affected. This interferes with facial growth and results in maxillary hypoplasia, midfacial retrusion and exorbitism. Understanding of such growth abnormalities and of the timing of maximal growth and its completion in the affected parts of the craniofacial skeleton is therefore most important in planning surgery for aesthetic and functional reasons.

SINGLE SUTURE SYNOSTOSIS

The effects on skull and facial growth associated with premature fusion of a single skull vault suture are described in Chapter 2. Suffice it to say at this point, however, that the complex asymmetries of facial development seen in 'simple' unicoronal and metopic synostosis provide good examples of the complexities of the growth disorders that underlie them.

COMPLEX (SYNDROMIC AND/OR MULTIPLE SUTURE) SYNOSTOSIS

Midfacial underdevelopment is usually a feature of the craniofacial dysostoses and is seen in its severest forms in Crouzon, Apert and Pfeiffer syndromes (see Chapters 2 and 3). The reduced antero-posterior length of the anterior skull base from which the midfacial skeleton is suspended contributes to the midfacial retrusion and shallow orbits.

A further contribution (probably the major component) comes from the significantly decreased growth potential within the midface itself. The face is generally not only retruded, it is also reduced in its vertical dimensions. This underdevelopment of the midfacial structures results in exorbitism, a decrease in size of the upper airways and an abnormal dental arch relationship. The antero-posterior abnormalities give rise to a class III occlusion,

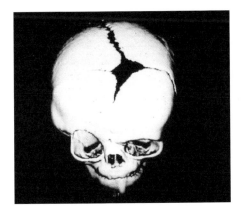

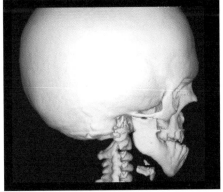

Fig. 1.4 Unicoronal synostosis. Premature fusion of a single coronal suture produces a craniofacial asymmetry consisting of ipsilateral frontal flattening and contralateral frontal bossing. Other cranial and facial asymmetries associated with this condition are discussed in the text.

Fig. 1.5 Three-dimensional CT scan of a patient with Crouzon syndrome. There is a multisutural synostosis (note the absence of suture markings). The midface is underdeveloped, resulting in a severe class III malocclusion. Midfacial retrusion may cause upper airway obstruction, and the shallow orbits result in exorbitism.

often with a very significantly reversed overjet, while failure of vertical growth in the anterior part of the maxilla leads to an anterior open bite. The width of the maxilla in the dental region is also often restricted, which significantly narrows the dental arch and may cause severe crowding of the maxillary teeth (see Chapter 11).

These anatomical abnormalities may cause pressing ophthalmological problems, as well as severe restriction of the upper airways, and in turn give rise to significant dilemmas when deciding optimum management. For example, functional issues may dictate that surgery is performed early, although any attempt at a definitive correction of the responsible deformity should ideally be delayed until craniofacial growth of the affected area is virtually complete. An example of the variable growth patterns to be seen in these children is demonstrated by Fig. 1.6, which shows serial photographs taken throughout growth in a child with Crouzon syndrome. It can be seen that early on there is relatively little evidence of midfacial retrusion. However, as growth continues, the midfacial retrusion and exorbitism become progressively more pronounced. Any beneficial effects of an operation performed early in childhood on such a patient (and particularly one involving facial structures) are therefore likely to be undone by subsequent abnormal growth, which is dependent upon the 'drive' of the gene mutation responsible for the syndrome in the first place, and which will not of course have been affected by surgery.

Another difficulty with surgery on the facial bones of a young child is the position of the developing dentition. Until approximately the age of 9 years the maxilla is packed

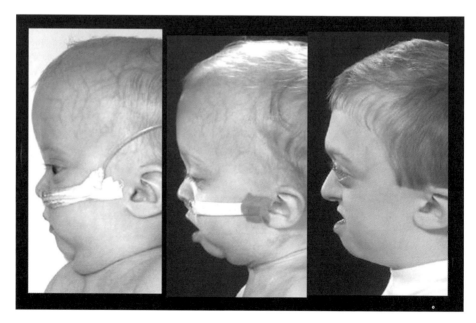

Fig. 1.6 Serial photographs of a child with Crouzon syndrome. Disordered growth continues throughout childhood. Note the progressive exorbitism and midfacial retrusion. (Note: this child undergoing midface distraction is also illustrated in Chapter 19 – see Fig. 19.14.)

10

with the developing secondary dentition. This means that it is very difficult to perform osteotomies in the upper maxillary and infraorbital region without damaging secondary dentition. As well as creating problems with the establishment of proper dentition, damage to the teeth may further retard growth potential of the midface. In general, therefore, definitive surgery is best delayed if possible until the end of facial growth.

However, if functional problems are severe, then early midfacial advancement needs to be considered, although if performed at this age it must be accepted that repeat osteotomies are likely to be required later – towards the end of craniofacial growth. As discussed later (see Chapters 7 and 19), many children with craniofacial dysostoses require either monobloc or Le Fort III advancements. From a growth point of view it is ideal to delay these operations until at least the age of 10–12, when orbital growth is complete. The greater part of subsequent development takes place in the lower midface, and therefore delaying midface surgery until this age will at least reduce the scale of future craniofacial operations from a repetition of the original procedure to one restricted to a lower level of the face – a Le Fort I osteotomy – a relatively less major operation and one which does not involve previously operated tissues.

Summary

An understanding of craniofacial growth is important to the understanding and management of craniosynostosis. It guides the planning of correction of deformity in the growing child and contributes to the understanding of many functional problems that occur. Growth of the craniofacial skeleton dictates the ideal timing of surgery to correct deformity. It must be remembered however that functional and psychological factors often dictate that surgical intervention takes place at times that adversely affect facial growth. A thorough understanding of craniofacial growth can allow these interventions to be planned to minimise their effects on facial development.

REFERENCES

Farkas LG (1994) *Anthropemetry of the Head and Face.* New York: Raven Press.
Posnick LG (2000) *Craniofacial and Maxillofacial Surgery in Children and Young Adults.* London: WB Saunders.

2
CLASSIFICATION AND CLINICAL DIAGNOSIS

D.N.P. Thompson and Jonathan Britto

While advances in molecular genetics have revolutionised our understanding of syndrome delineation in craniosynostosis and improved techniques of imaging have allowed us to see not only the calvarial changes in detail but also the extensive effects on the basicranium and viscerocranium, the initial diagnosis or at least suspicion of craniosynostosis rests on the clinical appearance. The aims of this chapter are to provide a simple classification of craniosynostosis and to describe the salient clinical features of the more common non-syndromic and syndromic varieties of craniosynostosis that may present to the clinician.

Terminology

The terminology of craniosynostosis not infrequently leads to confusion since the conditions are variously described, by the suture involved, the resulting head shape, the person responsible for the initial description, and more recently according to the underlying genetic mutation. The result is an array of synonyms and pseudonyms; some of the more commonly encountered descriptions are listed in Table 2.1. No attempt is made here to compound this state of affairs by trying to provide a new all-encompassing nomenclature; rather it has been the intention to bring together existing terms within a simple classification.

TABLE 2.1
Common descriptive terms for abnormal head shape and causative fused suture

Clinical description	Suture involvement	Head shape
Scaphocephaly syn dolichocephaly	Sagittal	Elongated
Plagiocephaly	Unicoronal	Asymmetric forehead flattening
Trigonocephaly	Metopic	Pointed, triangular forehead
Posterior plagiocephaly	Lambdoid*	Asymmetric occipital flattening
Brachycephaly	Bicoronal	Spherical
Acrocephaly syn, oxycephaly**	Bicoronal/multiple	Pointed, tower

* See text regarding positional moulding.
** The term turricephaly is also sometimes used to describe the tower-shaped deformity.

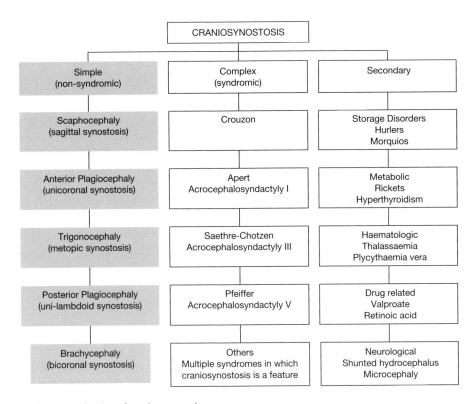

Fig. 2.1 Classification of craniosynostosis.

Broadly speaking there are three subgroups of craniosynostosis (Fig. 2.1). The non-syndromic and syndromic varieties of craniosynostosis are those where there is a congenital abnormality of sutural biology (the underlying genetic abnormalities responsible for this are discussed in Chapter 3), and it is these which are the primary concern of the craniofacial surgeon. Some idea of the relative frequency of each of the craniosynostosis phenotypes can be gained from Fig. 2.2, which summarises by diagnosis our recent series of craniosynostosis patients undergoing cranial vault surgery.

A third subgroup exists in which the premature fusion of one (or more usually multiple) cranial sutures occurs as a consequence of some other condition; these may be termed secondary craniosynostosis. Secondary craniosynostosis does not usually result in significant cosmetic deformity; the main functional concern in cases of secondary craniosynostosis is the development of raised intracranial pressure and its effects on vision, and in such circumstances treatment is guided by the same principles that govern the treatment of congenital craniosynostosis.

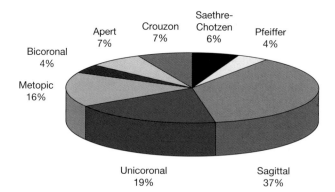

Bicoronal 4%

Apert 7%

Crouzon 7%

Saethre-Chotzen 6%

Pfeiffer 4%

Metopic 16%

Unicoronal 19%

Sagittal 37%

Fig. 2.2 Distribution of diagnosis amongst 425 children undergoing cranial vault surgery (GOS 1994–2002).

Non-syndromic craniosynostosis

Sometimes referred to as simple or single suture synostosis, this group of conditions results from premature fusion of one (occasionally two in the case of non-syndromic bicoronal synostosis) of the major cranial sutures. The consequences are for the most part cosmetic, resulting in a misshapen skull; there are limited effects on the facial skeleton, and the functional implications with respect to vision, breathing and feeding that are so frequent amongst the syndromic forms are not generally seen. The non-syndromic forms of craniosynostosis are more common than their syndromic counterparts.

SAGITTAL CRANIOSYNOSTOSIS

Premature closure of the sagittal suture is the most frequent form of craniosynostosis and leads to the characteristic dolichocephalic or scaphocephalic deformity of the calvarium. A prevalence of approximately 1 in 5000 children has been estimated and the condition is more frequently seen in boys (Lajeunie et al 1996). Familial cases comprise 6 per cent. Transmission follows an autosomal dominant pattern with a penetrance rate of 38 per cent.

The clinical diagnosis is usually straightforward and is commonly recognised at the time of birth. The skull has a boat-shaped deformity in which the antero-posterior dimension is increased and the bi-parietal diameter reduced (Fig. 2.3). The ratio of these two measurements, the cephalic index, may serve as a semi-quantitative estimate of severity; such measurements have limited clinical application but may be of use as an indicator of the effect of surgical correction. A bony ridge is frequently palpable along the line of the prematurely fused sagittal suture. On plain skull radiographs this is seen as a line of sclerosis and bone thickening. The synostotic process does not always involve the entire suture and sometimes both on X-ray and subsequently at surgery the anterior part of the sagittal suture can appear quite normal.

In addition to the skull elongation there are compensatory changes that occur in the skull vault and adjacent sutures which may accentuate the deformity. These changes include frontal bossing with prominence of the forehead and hollowing in the temporal regions; in addition the occipital region may become unduly prominent and pointed. These

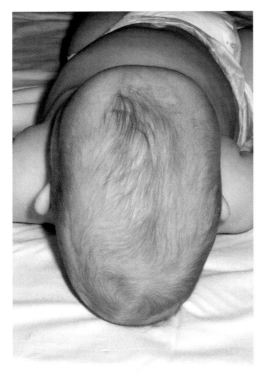

Fig. 2.3 Scaphocephaly.

features may become increasingly obvious as the child grows, and so any surgical procedure undertaken to correct the deformity must take into account these secondary changes, or, ideally, the correction should be performed prior to the onset of these changes.

While intracranial abnormalities are occasionally revealed on CT or MR imaging (Boop et al 1996) these are rarely of neurosurgical or obvious prognostic significance. The subarachnoid spaces are sometimes prominent, particularly over the frontal and occipital poles (Chadduck et al 1992); however, in contrast to the syndromic varieties of cranio-synostosis, overt hydrocephalus is distinctly unusual (Golabi et al 1987). Abnormalities of intracranial pressure too, although more commonly seen in the context of multisutural and syndromic craniosynostosis, are well recognised in single suture craniosynostosis (Renier et al 1982, Thompson et al 1995a), in particular when the midline sutures, sagittal and metopic, are involved (Thompson et al 1995c). The precise significance of these, often borderline, elevations of intracranial pressure remain unclear, although it may be pertinent to note that it is also in these two groups of single suture craniosynostosis that the incidence of neurocognitive deficits is most evident (Sidoti et al 1996, Virtanen et al 1999, Magge et al 2002).

The scaphocephalic skull shape is commonly seen in pre-term infants. This situation is analogous to posterior positional moulding (see below). The child will lie with the head to one side for long periods and the soft cartilaginous cranium will deform easily in response

15

to the external pressure. This process may be accentuated in the shunted premature infant where the additional factors of parenchymal brain loss and reduced intracranial tension increase the susceptibility to these deforming external forces. In these children the sagittal suture is rarely fused and this deformity does not require surgical correction and indeed is likely to improve as the child grows and develops an upright posture (Baum and Searls 1971).

METOPIC CRANIOSYNOSTOSIS
The metopic suture is the first of the major calvarial sutures to close, this process beginning in the second year. Some mild ridging along the line of the suture may be seen in normal infants; in this situation the overall skull shape, in particular the supraorbital ridges, is normal; this appearance does not progress and does not require intervention. True synostosis of the metopic suture produces a keel-like prominence of the forehead; the supraorbital ridges are flattened on either side giving rise to the triangular, trigonocephalic deformity of the skull vault (Fig. 2.4). The deformity is often best appreciated when viewed from above. The narrowing of the entire anterior cranial vault results in hypotelorism. The anterior cranial fossa is of small volume due more to the reduced interpterional distance and frontal height than foreshortening of the floor of the anterior cranial fossa. The severity of the deformity may vary quite markedly, and, as in plagiocephaly, it has been postulated that this is a consequence of the variable involvement of other anterior cranial fossa sutures (fronto-ethmoid, pre-sphenoid, meso-ethmoid and ecto-ethmoid sutures).

In a large study of metopic craniosynostosis, Lajeunie et al estimated a prevalence of 1 in 15,000; 5.6 per cent of cases were familial. As with sagittal synostosis there is a male preponderance of approximately three to one (Lajeunie et al 1998).

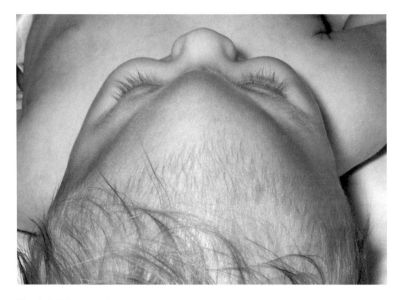

Fig. 2.4 Trigonocephaly.

Although the term trigonocephaly is inclusive of cases of simple, single suture metopic craniosynostosis, it is important to appreciate that this is a quite heterogeneous group in which there is a higher incidence of primary brain malformations and other syndromic diagnoses. Midline brain anomalies such as holoprosencephaly, meningocele and corpus callosum dysgenesis are well described in association with trigonocephaly. In Lajeunie's series of 237 patients with trigonocephaly there were 184 cases of non-syndromal trigonocephaly; in the remaining 53 patients additional malformations were identified and in 13 of this latter group a recognisable syndrome was diagnosed (Lajeunie et al 1998).

Syndromes in which the trigonocephalic head shape is apparent include Opitz trigono-cephaly (C syndrome), a rare disorder, where in addition to the trigonocephalic deformity there is learning disability, hypotonia, a characteristic facial appearance and widespread visceral and skeletal anomalies. The prognosis is extremely poor, approximately half the cases not surviving beyond infancy (Opitz 1969). Other such syndromes that have been reported in which metopic craniosynostosis is a significant feature of the phenotype include: Frydman syndrome (Frydman et al 1984), an autosomal dominant condition consisting of metopic craniosynostosis, omphalocele, large phallus, lumbar hemivertebra and normal intellectual development; and the Say–Meyer trigonocephaly syndrome (Say and Meyer 1981), an incompletely defined syndrome in which there is developmental delay and short stature, as well as a cranosynostosis of the metopic and possibly other sutures; it is thought to be inherited as an X-linked recessive disorder. Maternal exposure to sodium valproate is also a risk factor in the development of metopic craniosynostosis (Lajeunie et al 2001).

Abnormalities of intracranial pressure have been reported in metopic craniosynostosis (Renier et al 1982, Thompson et al 1995a, 1995c), although in common with scaphocephaly the clinical significance of this is currently not fully understood and raised intracranial pressure is rarely an indication in itself for surgical intervention.

UNICORONAL CRANIOSYNOSTOSIS

'Non-syndromic' coronal synostosis is associated with a variety of cranial phenotypes that are distinct from the eponymous syndromes associated with mutations in FGFR2 and FGFR1. The common cranial phenotypes are plagiocephaly associated with a unicoronal synostosis, and brachycephaly, associated with bicoronal synostosis. The combined inci-dence of these phenotypes is calculated as 1 in 2100–2500 (Lajeunie et al 1995). Unicoronal craniosynostosis accounts for 18 per cent of our surgical series. It is now well recognised that a proportion of so-called non-syndromic unicoronal craniosynostosis patients have the FGFR3 mutation described by Muenke et al (Muenke et al 1997) and so would now be classified as Muenke syndrome (see below).

Craniosynostosis of a single coronal suture produces a characteristic asymmetry of the forehead, frontal plagiocephaly. The supraorbital ridge on the affected side is recessed (Fig. 2.5). Although the primary pathology is unilateral, the resulting skull shape abnormality frequently affects both sides. On the ipsilateral side the supraorbital ridge and forehead are flattened, and when viewed from above the upper eyelid and eyelashes can be seen. On the contralateral side the frontal region may be bossed, accentuating the asymmetry, and when viewed from above the eyelid and eyelashes are obscured. There may be palpable ridging along the line of the fused coronal suture, which is somewhat more anterior than its normal counterpart. In the young infant the resulting asymmetry of the anterior fontanelle can be felt. The anterior cranial fossa is shortened on the affected side, the ipsilateral orbit is shallow and, in addition to the cranial deformity, facial asymmetry is commonly seen in association with unicoronal synostosis, and comprises a facial scoliosis centred around the nasion and concave to the side of the synostosed suture. The margins of the orbit are distorted in frontal plagiocephaly, the supraorbital region being drawn upwards and backwards toward the elevated lateral wing of the sphenoid bone, which is usually markedly thickened in the region of the pterion. This gives rise to the characteristic harlequin eye appearance on the AP skull radiograph. The deformation of the orbits results in malposition of the extraocular muscle origins, and the clinical picture is frequently accompanied by strabismus and a secondary compensatory head tilt (Gosain et al 1996b).

Although traditionally considered a single suture condition, it is now well recognised that the adjacent anterior cranial fossa sutures – in particular the frontosphenoidal, frontoethmoidal and sphenoethmoidal sutures – are frequently involved. Indeed it has been suggested that the sutures of the anterior cranial fossa behave as a functional unit, the coronal ring. This explains the variable pattern of associated vault changes that accompany unicoronal synostosis (Cohen 1993b). Failure to appreciate the complexity and heterogeneity within this condition has been advanced as a reason for the variable surgical outcome reported in some series (Di Rocco and Velardi 1988, McCarthy et al 1995).

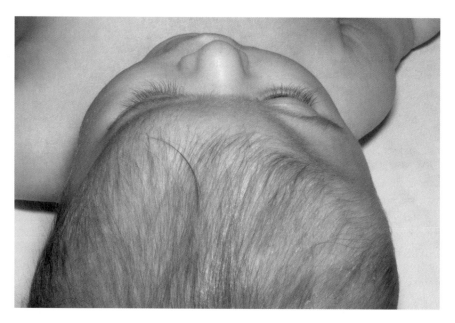

Fig. 2.5 Right frontal plagiocephaly.

BICORONAL SYNOSTOSIS

Involvement of the coronal sutures is a characteristic feature of the craniosynostosis syndromes. The term non-syndromic bicoronal synostosis has been applied to those children who have the premature fusion of the coronal sutures but who lack the additional clinical features that typify the syndromes (see below). Recent studies have however shown that these cases are much more commonly familial than hitherto supposed (Lajeunie et al 1995).

Bicoronal craniosynostosis results in the brachycephalic deformity; the head assumes a more spherical shape, widened in the coronal plane, and in addition the height of the cranium is frequently exaggerated (turricephaly). The forehead is wide and flattened; recession of the supraorbital ridges is often present but less severe than in the syndromic groups. There is no dystopia and the midface is not recessed as seen in the 'Crouzon–Pfeiffer' group of FGFR2-related syndromes. There are no specifically related dental problems and the incidence of intracranial abnormality is very low.

LAMBDOIDAL SYNOSTOSIS

This is a condition that has provoked considerable interest and indeed controversy in recent years. Lambdoidal craniosynostosis is a rare condition; it accounted for only 2.3 per cent of Shillito and Matson's series of 519 cases (Shillito and Matson 1968), and subsequent surgical series report a similar incidence. During the course of the last decade surgical series were published in which the incidence of lambdoidal craniosynostosis was significantly greater than this – epidemics of this condition were reported in the media. Lambdoidal craniosynostosis produces an asymmetric flattening of the occipital region, posterior plagio-cephaly. A not dissimilar appearance is also seen in the condition of posterior positional deformation.

Posterior positional deformation, also known as positional plagiocephaly or positional moulding, is a much more commonly encountered condition than lambdoidal craniosynos-tosis and it accounts for a number of referrals to the craniofacial unit. The cartilaginous cranium of the infant is soft and malleable and will deform in response to external pressure (this feature is exploited in some cultures for cosmetic benefit). Children will commonly show a preference to lie on one side, with the result that the occiput moulds against the relatively flat surface, analogous to resting a bag of water on a table. The whole head may develop a parallelogram shape in cross-section. The greater the deformity the greater the tendency for the child to assume this preferred resting position. It was noted that the apparent epidemic in this condition occurred soon after the introduction of guidelines recommending supine positioning in the infant in order to reduce the risk of Sudden Infant Death Syndrome (SIDS) (Kane et al 1996).

It is frequently possible to distinguish between true lambdoidal synostosis and positional deformation on clinical grounds (Huang et al 1998). In positional moulding there is commonly a history of preferential head positioning and occasionally torticollis with tight sternomastoid; neurodevelopmental delay is also more frequent than in children with true lambdoidal craniosynostosis. Where there is synostosis the growth of the posterior fossa is restricted on the involved side and the ipsilateral ear is drawn backward relative to the

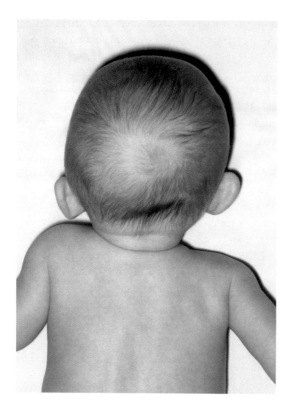

Fig. 2.6 Right posterior positional plagiocephaly.

opposite side; by contrast the occipital flattening of positional deformation tends to push the ipsilateral ear forward (Fig. 2.6). In cross-section the head shape of positional deformation is a parallelogram, with ipsilateral frontal bossing, whereas in lambdoidal synostosis the cross-sectional shape is more trapezoid, the frontal bossing if present being contralateral to the occipital flattening.

In positional plagiocephaly the lambdoid suture is patent and functionally normal. No surgical intervention is indicated; the condition will often correct spontaneously as the child develops an upright posture and the ossification of the skull proceeds. Alternating the child's sleeping position is recommended to parents, and in some institutions the use of helmets to mould the skull back into position has been shown to be effective (Littlefield et al 1998). Even in the case of true lambdoidal craniosynostosis surgical intervention is not commonly indicated. The surgery is not without morbidity and mortality and is reserved for situations in which there is severe cosmetic deformity with secondary deformity in the rest of the craniofacial skeleton.

NON-SYNDROMIC MULTIPLE SUTURE CRANIOSYNOSTOSIS

There are some cases of craniosynostosis in which the pattern of sutural fusion does not lend itself to classification within the scheme proposed here. Two or sometimes more sutures are involved yet there are none of the associated features which permit a syndromic diagnosis.

Such cases comprise 5 per cent of our surgical series; this is comparable with other large series. This is a heterogeneous group and may contain cases of secondary craniosynostosis. The principles of assessment and surgical treatment for these patients are similar to other cases of craniosynostosis, although individualised modifications of technique may be required for those with many sutures involved. The functional and cosmetic outcomes seem to be somewhat worse in these patients, with increased rates of re-operation compared with other non-syndromic cases (Chumas et al 1997).

Syndromic craniosynostosis

A characteristic feature of the craniosynostosis syndromes is the involvement, not only of the skull vault or neurocranium, but also of the facial skeleton or viscerocranium, and in many cases the axial and appendicular skeleton as well. It is the deformity of the viscerocranium that is responsible for many of the functional disabilities that are so common in this group of patients: proptosis, upper airway obstruction, feeding difficulties and so on.

While there are facial characteristics typical to each of these syndromes, diagnosis is often aided by the extracranial anomalies, for example in the hands and feet. Indeed, the term acrocephalosyndactyly was coined by Apert to describe the condition which now bears his name; the use of the term was later expanded to encompass other craniosynostosis syndromes with unique digital features: Saethre–Chotzen (type III) and Pfeiffer (type V), Apert syndrome being acrocephalosyndactyly type I. Crouzon syndrome which has no obvious extracranial phenotypic features is therefore not included in this sub-classification. The phenotypic features of each of the more common syndromes are addressed below.

CROUZON SYNDROME

In 1912 Crouzon described a condition featuring craniosynostosis, maxillary hypoplasia with exorbitism and class III malocclusion, and hypertelorism (Crouzon 1912). The Crouzon phenotype lacks the obvious extracranial skeletal manifestations of the related Apert and Pfeiffer phenotypes. However, a reappraisal of limb radiographs in a series of Crouzon patients indicates that while the limbs in many cases may be clinically silent of obvious abnormality, subtle anomalies occur (Anderson et al 1997a, 1997b).

Cohen and Kreiborg estimated that Crouzon syndrome represents approximately 4.8 per cent of cases of craniosynostosis at birth, compared to Apert syndrome, estimated at 4.5 per cent of cases (Cohen and Kreiborg 1992a, Cohen et al 1992). The birth prevalence was estimated to be 16.5 per million births. There is a relatively high rate of vertical transmission (familial cases = 44 per cent; sporadic cases = 56 per cent) and a significant influence of paternal age amongst new sporadic cases (Glaser et al 2000).

Phenotypic variability between generations is a common observation. The craniofacial variability includes the severity of the midface retrusion and exorbitism, and variable features such as supraorbital recession. Craniosynostosis may be absent or delayed (Reddy et al 1990, Pulleyn et al 1996). Cohen reported the insidious and late onset of familial non-syndromic craniosynostosis, which may have been labelled Crouzon syndrome. A mother, son and daughter were described in whom serial photographs documented an insidious and late onset of exorbitism and midfacial retrusion. Intracranial hypertension in the absence of a severe craniofacial phenotype was also observed, and if unchecked this may progress to optic nerve damage, retinal damage and visual loss (Cohen et al 1993).

The craniofacial phenotype

The craniofacial manifestations of the 'Crouzon–Pfeiffer' group of syndromes are comparatively variable with respect to the more consistent Apert craniofacial phenotype. At the most severe end of the spectrum, cloverleaf skull has been reported (Hall et al 1972), and a wide range of less severe craniosynostosis phenotypes commonly occurs. The most useful published data relate to work done on Crouzon patients in comparison to the Apert phenotype (Kreiborg et al 1993). Reports of phenotype variability include cases of Crouzon syndrome without an apparent craniosynostosis, but a marked midfacial retrusion and the secondary ocular and occlusal problems thereof. Early closure of the basicranial synchondroses, contrasting with later closure in Apert syndrome, is a commonly reported feature (Kreiborg et al 1993), and is thought to contribute to the shallow posterior fossa, cerebellar tonsillar herniation (Cinalli et al 1995), and raised intracranial pressure (Thompson et al 1997) observed in these patients.

The commonest cranial phenotype of this group is brachycephaly from a bicoronal synostosis, and combinations of sutural fusion invariably include the coronal suture. The

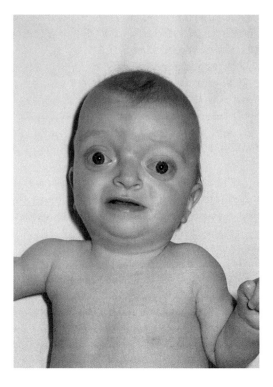

Fig. 2.7 Exorbitism in Crouzon syndrome.

sagittal and lambdoid sutures are also commonly involved. Median time to closure of various sutures in a series of Apert (n=65) and Crouzon (n=68) patients, as measured by plain radiography using uniform criteria, has been reported (Cinalli et al 1995). Despite the inaccuracies inherent in using plain radiography as a measure, the trends are for similar time to closure of the coronal suture (Apert: 5 months, Crouzon: 8 months). However, accelerated closure of both sagittal and lambdoid sutures correlates with Crouzon syndrome (sagittal suture – Crouzon: 6 months, Apert by default ossification: 51 months; lambdoid suture – Crouzon: 20 months, Apert: 60 months). Comparison of the cranial features of the Crouzon-type syndromes and Apert phenotype is given above.

Midface retrusion in the 'Crouzon–Pfeiffer' group is not accompanied by a gross hypertelorism or the laterally down-slanting palpebral cant of Apert syndrome (Cohen et al 1993). The midfacial retrusion is accompanied by the dental and ocular problems encountered in other craniofacial dysostosis syndromes of the group. Ocular problems include strabismus and problems of exposure keratitis secondary to lagophthalmos. Visual loss secondary to unrecognised raised intracranial pressure is a constant clinical concern (Thompson et al 1995a, Taylor et al 2001). There is also evidence for the primary involvement of FGFR2 in the development of the anterior chamber of the ocular globe. The FGFR2 Ser351Cys (1231C to G) mutation in association with Crouzon and Pfeiffer syndrome causes ocular anomaly, including opaque corneae, thickened irides and ciliary bodies, and shallow anterior chambers with occluded angles (Okajima et al 1999).

Cleft lip and/or palate are not commonly associated, though in Kreiborg's series rates of 2 per cent and 3 per cent were reported respectively (n=61), and these may have been unrelated chance occurrences (Kreiborg and Cohen 1992). The palate is high-arched and short, reflecting the maxillary hypoplasia and short cranial base (Peterson and Pruzansky 1974). In 3/13 Crouzon palates, the short, high-arched palatal morphology with lateral soft-tissue swelling of the upper arch mucosa was indistinguishable from the Apert palate; but in the majority of cases the palatal morphology is nearer normal. Nasopharyngeal volume is restricted, and both the anterior and posterior cranial bases are short – features which worsen with age (Peterson-Falzone et al 1981).

Intellectual performance: the CNS phenotype
The Crouzon population generally has normal intelligence. Marked intellectual compromise was manifest in only 3 per cent of Kreiborg's series (n=61) (Kreiborg 1981). Central nervous system anomalies are not as common as in the Pfeiffer or Apert group. Agenesis of the corpus callosum has been reported in single cases, but the commonest malformation is herniation of the cerebellar tonsils (CTH) from the posterior fossa via the foramen magnum in association with lambdoid synostosis. Cinalli et al reviewed 44 patients with Crouzon syndrome and 51 with Apert syndrome, and showed a 72.7 per cent incidence in Crouzon syndrome versus 1.9 per cent in the Apert group (Cinalli et al 1995). All the patients with Crouzon syndrome and progressive hydrocephalus had CTH, but of 32 individuals with Apert syndrome and CTH, only 15 had progressive hydrocephalus. This is consistent with the observation that intracranial hypertension is more common in Crouzon

syndrome (>15 mmHg in 63 per cent of cases) than in Apert syndrome, with an increased risk of visual loss, papilloedema, and optic atrophy.

The extracranial skeletal phenotype
Crouzon syndrome shares many of the extracranial features observed in Pfeiffer syndrome, which correlates with the crossover of their causative mutations. The most consistent difference in relation to Pfeiffer syndrome relates to the limb phenotypes. While Apert, Pfeiffer and Crouzon syndromes share the finding of progressive elbow anomalies and synostoses, elbow pathology is more common in the Apert (n=33, 67 per cent) and Pfeiffer (n=16, 68 per cent) phenotypes than in Crouzon syndrome (n=22, 36 per cent). The common findings are synostoses, subluxation of the radial head and humero – ulnar joint – and epiphyseal anomalies (Anderson et al 1998a). Such anomalies emphasise the role of FGFR signalling in both endochondral ossification – such as in the skull base and appendicular skeleton – and the membranous ossification of the calvarium.

Why the observed range of anomalies should be less severely manifest against the background of the Crouzon phenotype, compared to that of the Pfeiffer phenotype, remains unclear, but it is a consistent finding in the distal limb also. Pfeiffer syndrome is so defined by the broad and radially deviated thumb, and range of simple syndactyly. Crouzon syndrome, despite the similar genotype range, lacks a clinically morbid phenotype in the hands. However, radiographic examination of the Crouzon hand does reveal subclinical anomalies of the metacarpal and carpal bones, and clinodactyly and brachydactyly have also been reported (Proudman et al 1994, Anderson et al 1997a, Anderson and Evans 1998). Furthermore, the Crouzon phenotype has been reported to demonstrate subtle subclinical anomalies of the feet (n=18), as well as normal feet in cases sharing a 'Jackson–Weiss' mutation (Anderson et al 1997b). These data provide subtle evidence that the 'Crouzon–Pfeiffer' group of mutations generates syndromes that exhibit a linear range of severity in the limb phenotype, with crossover of phenotypic features between syndromes.

The range of severity in the craniofacial phenotype is less easy to define. While Apert syndrome and cleft palate co-segregate, the sutural fusion phenotype of the 'Crouzon–Pfeiffer' group might be considered to be 'worse' according to the pattern and number of sutures involved and the incidence of the 'cloverleaf' skull. Range of phenotypic severity amongst the related syndromes, however, is evident in the cervical spine, where progressive fusions and anomalies occurred in 44 (18 per cent) patients, commonly at the C2–3 level (Anderson et al 1997a), compared to the higher incidence in Pfeiffer and Apert syndromes.

Other phenotypic features of Crouzon syndrome
Kreiborg (1981) reported a number of further features, including hearing deficits in 55 per cent, and structural ear anomalies. Calcification of the stylohyhoid ligament was also reported in 88 per cent of patients (n=50), compared to 50 per cent of Proudman's series (Proudman et al 1994). Tracheal cartilage anomalies occur, in company with the Apert and Pfeiffer phenotypes. Visceral anomalies are less common than in the Pfeiffer

or Apert phenotypes, but may sporadically occur (7 per cent of Proudman's series, n=59).

The association of Crouzon syndrome with skin pathology has been variously reported, including a sporadic association with multiple congenital naevi (Gines et al 1996). A number of case reports relate the skin condition acanthosis nigricans to Crouzon syndrome (Reddy et al 1985, Suslak et al 1985, Breitbart et al 1989, Meyer et al 1995). The skin phenotype consists of rugated skin with thickening and hyperpigmentation, particularly affecting the flexure creases.

APERT SYNDROME

Apert syndrome is characterised by turribrachycephaly, midfacial retrusion with a variable degree of hypertelorism, and symmetrical complex complete syndactylies of the hands and feet. The first description of Apert syndrome is eponymously attributed to 1906 (Apert 1906), though previous postmortem cases had been described (Wheaton 1894). Apert reported a 15-month-old girl presenting in 1896 at the L'Hôpital Necker des Enfants-Malades in Paris with a high brachycephalic head, severe syndactyly of all four limbs and a cleft palate. Ten years later, he had collected eight more cases from the literature and coined the term acrocephalosyndactyly, to describe the appearance of a flattened occiput, tall forehead and the syndactyly deformity. A case series was reported in 1920 (Park and Powers 1920), and in 1960 a collection of 54 United Kingdom cases was reported and sub-classified (Blank 1960). Blank distinguished two clinical categories: 'typical' acrocephalosyndactyly, the group to which Apert's name now commonly applies; and other forms, comprising phenotypes now otherwise attributed, grouped as 'atypical' acrocephalosyndactyly. The 'true Apert' was distinguished by the mid-digital hand mass, or 'spatulate hand', with a single nail common to digits 2–4, found in Apert syndrome and lacking in the non-Apert group. Thirty-nine of the 54 in Blank's series were of the 'true Apert' type.

In Cohen's series, Apert syndrome is the second commonest craniofacial syndrome, after Crouzon syndrome, accounting for 4.5 per cent of all craniosynostosis cases (Cohen et al 1992). In our surgical series, Apert syndrome accounts for 7 per cent of cases, the same as Crouzon syndrome (Fig. 2.2). Estimates of the frequency of Apert syndrome vary. Pooled data from seven geographic areas (across North America, Denmark, Spain and Italy) give a birth prevalence of 15.5 per 1,000,000 births (Cohen et al 1992).

The craniofacial phenotype

Craniofacial features include a wide turribrachycephaly, which tapers down from the parietal to the supraorbital region. There is a steeply inclined, flattened forehead, and shortened, shallow posterior fossa with short, asymmetric cranial base. The anterior cranial fossa and tuberculum sellae, pituitary fossa, dorsum sellae and clivus are all shortened and widened. There is reduced orbital volume and significant proptosis, with hypertelorism, and an expanded, dysplastic ethmoidal labyrinth. The lesser wings of the sphenoid bone, forming the posterior wall of the orbit and upper border of the superior orbital fissure, are angled obliquely up and laterally, producing a characteristic radiographic sign. The summary effect is that of the skull base being foreshortened and angled, such that there is an increasing lateral angulation of the cranial fossae above.

The cranial sutures are affected in a broadly consistent fashion. There is a wide-open calvarial defect from the root of the nose to the posterior fontanelle in the mid-sagittal plane, encompassing the territory of the metopic and sagittal sutures and the anterior fontanelle. Progression to bony fusion in this mid-sagittal plane is by the formation of islands of bone in the presumptive mesenchymal connective tissue, which coalesce to bony fusion by 36 months without the sutures ever having been truly formed (Kreiborg and Cohen 1990). True frontal encephalocele probably does not occur but reflects protrusion of the frontal fossa anteriorly via the calvarial defect. The intracranial volume is consistently greater than that of controls (Cohen and Kreiborg 1994a, Gosain et al 1995), and the brain is large within the skull with an expanded head height, although the head circumference normalises at birth and slows thereafter. In contrast, true fusion of the coronal suture in most cases begins *in utero*, commencing at the cranial base and extending cephalad (Kreiborg and Cohen 1990). Cloverleaf skull has been reported in association with Apert syndrome (Gosain et al 1997), but occurs in a minority (4 per cent) of cases (Cohen and Kreiborg 1994b). Reports of open coronal sutures in Apert syndrome may reflect variance in age of onset (Cohen and Kreiborg 1994b, Lajeunie et al 1999), but are consistent with reports of persistently open synchondroses at the Apert skull base (Kreiborg et al 1993).

Patients with Apert syndrome demonstrate consistent and typical facial features (Fig. 2.8). There is severe midface retrusion and secondary ocular proptosis with lagophalmos. Ocular subluxation of the globe onto the cheek may occur, in conjunction with the retruded midface and marked protrusion of the greater wing of the sphenoid, with elevation of the lesser wing (Kreiborg et al 1999). Maxillary and nasal height is reduced; the nasal root is depressed, such that the nasal bridge is humped and beak-like. Deviated nasal septum is common. Hypertelorism, and down-slanting palpebral fissures, are common features (Cohen and Kreiborg 1996). A deeply wrinkled forehead skin is common. The retruded midfacial phenotype gives rise to a skeletal and dental class III malocclusion and relative pseudo-mandibular prognathia, though the mandible itself remains within control parameters (Kreiborg et al 1999). The upper dental arch is crowded and V-shaped, with an anterior open bite and posterior cross bite. Dental anomalies include severely delayed eruption, ectopic eruption, and shovel-shaped incisors. Malocclusion is severe, with a mandibular overjet, anterior and posterior crossbites, and severe crowding of teeth (Kreiborg and Cohen 1992).

The Apert craniofacial morphology (n=12) has been compared to that of Crouzon syndrome (n=19) in an age-banded series of cases studied with serial three-dimensional CT scans. While the operative history of some cases makes the interpretation of the upper calvaria data problematic, the study currently provides the best longitudinal analysis of the comparative cranial and skull base morphology of the two syndromic groups (Kreiborg et al 1993). See Table 2.2.

Ophthalmic manifestations include reported absence of the superior rectus muscle (Cuttone et al 1979, Morax and Pascal 1982) and intrinsic extraocular muscle dysplasia

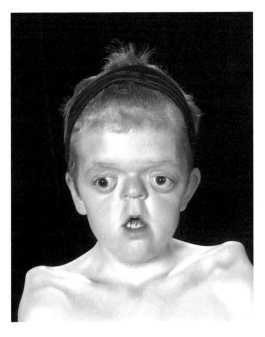

Fig. 2.8 Facial features of Apert syndrome.

(Margolis et al 1977b). Clinical sequelae of this include a consistent divergent upgaze and esotropic downgaze (Cohen and Kreiborg 1996). Ocular albinoid findings (Margolis et al 1977a), congenital glaucoma, keratoconus and ectopic lens are rare observations. Secondary ophthalmic concerns include corneal exposure keratitis and ocular subluxation. Visual loss and ocular atrophy are serious concerns and reflect untreated, sustained rises in intracranial pressure (Thompson et al 1995a, Taylor et al 2001).

Abnormalities of palatal morphology are common. Cleft palate is a consistent finding, and in the remaining population the palate is highly arched, with a deep median groove or 'pseudocleft' created by swelling in the upper arch mucosa (Peterson and Pruzansky 1974). Gorlin has postulated that the high-arched and laterally swollen palate results from compression of the upper dental arch during Apert craniofacial morphogenesis, and is secondary to the midfacial retrusion and hypertelorism (Gorlin et al 1990). However, similar palatal morphology in Crouzon syndrome, without the incidence of cleft palate (Peterson and Pruzansky 1974), suggests that the Apert mutations modulate a particularly sensitive role for FGFR2 in human palatogenesis. Furthermore, while the palates of both Apert and Crouzon patients are thicker and shorter than documented norms, no correlation between such parameters and palatal clefting can be demonstrated, thereby suggesting a molecular, rather than morphological, aetiology for Apert cleft palate.

Where it occurs, palatal clefting affects the secondary palate in variable severity, from complete clefts of the hard palate, to soft palatal clefts or simply bifid uvula. Reported frequencies of palatal clefting vary from 17 per cent to 43 per cent (Peterson and

TABLE 2.2
Cranial and skull base features of Apert and Crouzon syndromes (Kreiborg et al 1993)

	Apert	Crouzon
Calvaria Aged 0–1 year	Coronal synostosis Median sagittal diastema, including median plane fontanelles, with no midline sutures formed Open squamosal and lambdoid sutures Thin calvarial bone	Synostosis of coronal, sagittal, metopic, and squamosal sutures Fontanelles close early Lambdoid suture may remain unfused in early infancy Thin calvarial bone No median plane diastema Increased digital markings
Calvaria Aged 1–4 years	Delayed closure of fontanelles and median diastema by coalescing islands of bone formation No median plane sutures form Digital markings appear late	Pan-synostosis and progressive closure of fontanelles
Skull base	Open synchondroses in early infancy, which fuse late (>1 yr), with delayed closure of the spheno-occipital synchondrosis Enlarged sella turcica Widened ethmoid from birth with a depressed cribriform plate V-shaped anterior cranial fossa	Synchondroses close consistently early (<1 yr) in progressive manner Enlarged sella turcica with narrow floor Ethmoid not widened, and cribriform plate undisplaced Thin clivus and tendency for basilar kyphosis

Pruzansky 1974). The accuracy of reporting reflects the inclusion of milder phenotypes such as bifid uvula and occult cleft palate, where reported frequencies rise to 75 per cent (Kreiborg and Cohen 1992). The non-cleft hard palate is short, reflecting the reduced antero-posterior dimensions of the skull base. Nasopharyngeal height and depth are reduced (Peterson-Falzone et al 1981). There is no association with cleft lip, the Apert upper lip being characteristically intact in an open mouth, hood-like position at rest (Cohen and Kreiborg 1996), reflecting an anterior open bite beneath. The relationship of cleft palate to Eustachian tube malfunction may reflect the 71 per cent incidence of middle ear effusions in children with Apert syndrome (Park et al 1995). Conductive hearing loss occurs in 40 per cent of children with Apert syndrome and may reflect middle ear ossicular dysplasias revealed on computerised tomography of the middle temporal fossa.

Nasopharyngeal anomalies reflect the expected reduction in nasopharyngeal volume predicted by the cranioskeletal dysplasia. In a recent study of 13 Apert and 27 Crouzon patients, 40 per cent of patients with severe phenotypes demonstrated upper airway obstruction, caused by midface hypoplasia, tonsillar and adenoid hypertrophy, and choanal stenosis (Lo and Chen 1999). Choanal atresia/stenosis, which presents a surgical emergency, features in 23 per cent of Apert cases (Park et al 1995).

The extracranial phenotype

Perhaps the most distinguishing features of Apert syndrome, which set it apart from the rest of the syndromic craniosynostoses, are the hand and foot deformities (Fig. 2.9). The common features of the Apert hand are a short, radially deviated thumb; a complex, complete syndactyly and symbrachyphalangism which affects the 2-3-4 rays to form a mid-digital hand mass with single nail (synonychia); and a fifth-ray simple syndactyly. More severe forms completely incorporate the little finger (though only via soft tissue syndactyly) and thumb rays. The bony anomalies include a delta phalanx (longitudinally bracketed epiphysis) in the thumb ray; radial clinodactyly of the thumb, symphalangism (fused proximal and middle phalanges); 4–5 metaphyseal fusions of the metacarpals; and epiphyseal anomalies. Carpal fusions are common. The soft tissue anomalies include abnormal skin furrows and pilosebaceous activity, syndactyly, ectopic chondrification, and synonychia (Upton 1991, Cohen and Kreiborg 1995b, Holten et al 1997). Anomalous findings such as reduplications have also been reported (Anderson et al 1996b). Multiple anomalies of neurovascular and tendon anatomy are common (Upton 1991). More proximally, elbow fusions and elbow and shoulder joint anomalies have been commonly associated with the Apert limb phenotype (Upton 1991, Cohen and Kreiborg 1993a, Anderson et al 1998a). The classification of Upton remains the most common reference for the analysis of the Apert hand malformations (Table 2.3).

The Type 1 hand, the most common form (Upton 1991, Cohen and Kreiborg 1995b), has a thumb separated from the mid-digital hand mass by a shallow web. The mid-digital

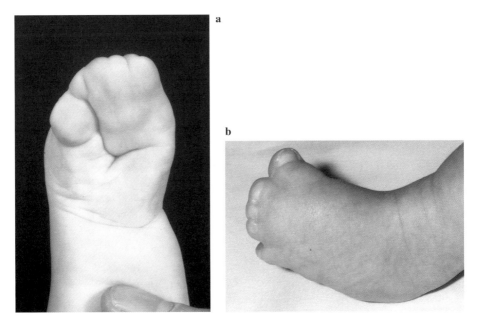

Fig. 2.9 (a) Apert hand. (b) Apert foot.

29

TABLE 2.3
Upton's classification of the Apert hand (Upton 1991)

Deformity	Type 1 (n=28)	Type 2 (n=24) 'Mitten hand'	Type 3 (n=16) 'Hoof hand'
Thumb radial clinodactyly	Present	Present	Present
Index radial clinodactyly	Absent	Present	Present
First web syndactyly	Simple (non-osseous)	Simple (non-osseous)	Complex (osseous)
Complex 2-3-4 syndactyly and symbrachyphalangism	Present	Present	Present
4-5 syndactyly	Simple, incomplete	Simple, incomplete	Simple, complete

hand mass, a 2-3-4 syndactyly, displays bone fusions of the distal phalanx at the metaphyseal and interphalangeal joint levels. There may be proximal osseous or cartilaginous fusion of the second and third rays. The fifth ray is joined by a variable soft tissue syndactyly only, and the hand position can present a flat palm.

The Type 2 hand has the thumb joined to the mid-digital hand mass by a simple soft tissue syndactyly, but the nail is separate and the distal phalangeal segment is radially deviated. The mid-digital hand mass features a severe fusion of the 2-3-4 distal phalanges, such that the proximal phalanges and metacarpals are splayed apart to create a 'mitten' or 'spoon' appearance with central concavity. The fifth ray is joined by a complete soft tissue syndactyly.

The Type 3 or 'hoof' hand is the most severe and least common variant. The 1-4 rays are joined by osseous or cartilaginous fusion, with a complex synonychia, such that the thumb and mid-digital hand mass are indistinguishable. The palm is deeply concave. The fifth ray is joined by a simple, complete syndactyly. Carpal and metacarpal coalitions are common.

The bony fusions of the Apert distal limb are progressive, beginning as cartilage ankyloses and ossifying with increasing maturity (Schauerte and St Aubin 1966).

Cohen and Kreiborg (1995b) studied 44 pairs of hands and 37 pairs of feet in Apert syndrome, using clinical and radiographic methods. In common with Upton (1991) they noted a more severe phenotype in the upper than the lower limb. Upton was unable to correlate upper and lower limb severity, but parallels were drawn by Cohen and Kreiborg (1995b), and the severity of upper and lower limb phenotypes has been significantly positively correlated more recently (Slaney et al 1996).

The foot deformity is also characteristic. Progressive synostosis occurs upon an unsegmented cartilaginous template. The first ray shortens with medial deviation of the great toe, secondary to growth abnormality and a delta phalanx (Mah et al 1991). The two phalanx digits characteristically go on to fusion, with maintenance of minimal motion at the metatarso-phalangeal joints. There is a 2-3-4 mid-digital mass analogous to that of the hand, with more severe forms incorporating progressively four, or all five, toes in the syndactyly (Cohen and Kreiborg 1995b, Slaney et al 1996). Progressive tarsal and metatarsal fusions occur and the midfoot and hindfoot fuse in a supinated position. There is prominence of the fifth metatarsal with callosities under the fifth and third metatarsal heads in all patients.

Cervical vertebral fusions are also common in Apert syndrome, occurring in up to 73 per cent of cases, and have also been shown to be progressive (Schauerte and St Aubin 1966, Thompson et al 1996). Kreiborg et al (1992) report fusion of cervical vertebrae in 68 per cent of patients with Apert syndrome: single fusions in 37 per cent and multiple fusions in 31 per cent. The C5–C6 level was most commonly involved. Similar figures have been observed independently (n=59 patients), and progressive fusion was noted in 10/17 patients in whom longitudinal radiographs were available (Thompson et al 1996). Complete bony fusion across the intervertebral disc space has been noted, and fusions most commonly involve the vertebral bodies and posterior elements in an apparent antero-posterior vector. The spinal canal is not compromised radiologically or clinically. In contrast, cervical fusion occurs in 18 to 25 per cent of patients with the Crouzon phenotype, which commonly involves C2–C3 (Kreiborg et al 1992, Anderson et al 1997a), the level also most commonly fused in the Pfeiffer phenotype (Anderson et al 1996a). Kreiborg et al (1992) concluded that when fusions are present, C5–C6 involvement in Apert syndrome and C2–C3 involvement in Crouzon syndrome separate the two conditions in most cases.

Intellectual performance and CNS anomalies
Patients with Apert syndrome generally have a decreased intellectual capability, though individuals with normal intelligence have been reported (Pantke et al 1975). In a review of 29 patients (aged 8–35 years) over a time period from 1952 to 1980, 14 (48 per cent) had a normal or borderline IQ, of which group 6/7 school leavers were in vocational training or full-time employment (Patton et al 1988). Nine patients had mild learning disability (IQ, 50–70), four were moderately compromised (IQ, 35–49), and two (7 per cent) were severely intellectually compromised (IQ less than 35). None had an IQ greater than 100. Early craniectomy, within the first year of life, did not appear to have improved intellectual outcome in this patient group, a conclusion supported by Cohen and Kreiborg (1990), who document a range of CNS anomalies, with malformations of the corpus callosum, the limbus, the hippocampus, the gyri, and pyramidal tracts. An absent or defective septum pellucidum was also noted. The authors observed that intracranial hypertension in the Apert group, given the tendency to increased intracranial volume (Kreiborg and Cohen 1990, Cohen and Kreiborg 1994b), would be unlikely to be a major contributor to the intellectual deficit. Early surgery for cranial vault decompression would therefore be unlikely to have a therapeutic effect upon poor intellectual capacity in the Apert group, which would most likely reflect neurodevelopmental abnormality. Evidence supporting a primarily neurodevelopmental cause for poor Apert intellectual performance is given by a series of 20 Apert children, assessed on psychometric scales, who displayed verbal skills that

31

were consistently lower than motor skills, despite the upper limb anomalies in the phenotype. Mean IQ was 73.6 (range 52–89), all children having undergone early cranial vault surgery (Lefebvre et al 1986).

Progressive hydrocephalus has been observed to be uncommon in the Apert group (Cohen and Kreiborg 1990), in comparison to the Crouzon phenotype, in which raised intracranial pressure, pansynostosis, and herniation of the cerebellar tonsils through the foramen magnum co-segregate (Cinalli et al 1995). Nevertheless, early craniectomy to improve intellectual outcome in Apert syndrome is advocated from a review of IQ in 70 children with Apert syndrome. An IQ greater than 70 was documented in 50 per cent of the children who had a skull decompression before 1 year of age, versus only 7.1 per cent in those operated on later in life (Renier et al 1996). Malformations of the corpus callosum (found in 12 per cent of cases in the series of Park et al 1995) and ventricular size did not correlate with the final IQ. Anomalies of the septum pellucidum had a significant negative effect, however, with the proportion of patients with an IQ over 70 increasing more than twofold in patients with a normal septum compared with patients with septal anomalies (p <0.04). In concert with findings from the general population, the third significant factor in intellectual achievement was the setting in which the children were brought up. Only 12.5 per cent of institutionalised children had a normal IQ, compared to 39.3 per cent of normal IQ cases living with their families.

Holten has reported CT data on 40 patients with Apert syndrome of mean age 4.1 years and median age of 12 months (Holten 1994). Ninety-eight per cent of patients had some form of ventriculomegaly, predominantly of the lateral (93 per cent) and third (68 per cent) ventricles, with mild to moderate dilatation. No particular pattern of dysmorphology could be established within or between ventricles. Despite ventriculomegaly being present in 39 of the 40 cases, only 8 of these 39 (20 per cent) had CT evidence of raised intracranial pressure and craniostenosis, with 11 cases demonstrating wide subarachnoid spaces and basal cisterns. Holten reports 13 anomalies of the septum pellucidum (32 per cent) in the Australian series of 40 cases, but was unable to demonstrate a particular effect of this anomaly upon the formal Wechsler IQ testing undertaken in only seven patients of the total group. Agenesis of the corpus callosum was noted in three cases. Other anomalies noted were: cerebellar hypoplasia, heterotopic grey matter, abnormal gyral patterns and schizogyria. The severity of the CNS phenotype may be related to the severity of the skeletal phenotype, but no objective correlating data are given.

The summary data therefore suggest that developmental impairment, in the form of a verbal skill deficit greater than the motor skill deficit, is a more common association than not in Apert syndrome (Shipster et al 2002). Intellectual deficit appears to correlate with primary neurodevelopmental malformation rather than raised intracranial pressure *per se*, and the incidence is in keeping with the role of FGF/FGFR signalling in neural differentiation (Chao 1992).

Visceral anomalies
Reports of visceral anomalies in Apert syndrome indicate a range of sporadic malformations affecting many systems. Blank reported that half of his autopsy group of 12 cases had

non-identical visceral anomalies (Blank 1960). Anal atresia in company with small bowel malrotation has also been reported (Park et al 1995). Cohen and Kreiborg, in a review of 136 patients of which 12 were postmortem autopsies, concluded a high rate of minor anomalies (Cohen and Kreiborg 1993b). The cardiovascular and genito-urinary systems were most commonly affected (10 per cent and 9.6 per cent respectively). A cardiovascular anomaly rate of 17 per cent has been independently reported, and urogenital abnormalities (hydronephrosis, nephrocalcinosis, hydrocele, cryptorchidism) in 19 per cent of cases of the same series (Park et al 1995).

In Holten's series of 48 Apert syndrome patients, 9 (19 per cent) had clinically detectable visceral anomalies (Holten 1994). The genito-urinary (14.6 per cent), cardiovascular (10.4 per cent) and gastro-intestinal (10.4 per cent) were the commonest systems affected. A respiratory system anomaly was diagnosed in one patient, which may have contributed to early death. Autopsy showed tracheal cartilage dysplasia with calcification of the whole trachea and bronchi and tracheal stenosis. This patient also demonstrated ectopic cartilage formation and calcification in the kidneys. Tracheal 'tube' cartilage in eight postmortem Apert cases has been reviewed (Cohen and Kreiborg 1992b), and this highly morbid anomaly has been reported in both Pfeiffer (Stone et al 1990) and Crouzon (Devine et al 1984, Sagehashi 1992) syndromes.

Dermatological changes
Cohen and Kreiborg commented on the cutaneous manifestations in a series of 136 cases of Apert syndrome (Cohen and Kreiborg 1995a). Hyperhydrosis is found in all patients, and a predilection for oily skin with cystic acne eruptions persists from adolescence to maturity. Apert skin biopsy data show expanded sebaceous gland tissue, and the acneiform lesions, which are very resistant to treatment (Henderson et al 1995), are particularly prevalent on the face, chest, back, and upper arms. The skin of the hand and forearm shows hyperhydrosis and excess pilosebaceous activity with a distribution of forearm acne that is characteristic of the syndrome.

SAETHRE–CHOTZEN SYNDROME
The Saethre–Chotzen syndrome (SCS) was eponymously named following initial reports in the early 1930s. In the family described by Saethre, a mother and two daughters showed mild craniosynostosis, facial asymmetry, low frontal hairline, brachydactyly and partial soft tissue syndactyly of index and middle fingers and the third and fourth toes (Saethre 1931). Chotzen described similar malformations in a father and two sons who also had hypertelorism, short stature, deafness and intellectual compromise (Chotzen 1932). The variability in the phenotype has been emphasised in many reports (Pantke et al 1975, Marini et al 1991, Niemann-Seyde et al 1991, Reardon and Winter 1994).

Characterising features include: mild and asymmetrical craniosynostosis, low-set frontal hairline, parrot-beaked nose with deviated septum, ptosis of the eyelids, strabismus, refractive error, tear duct stenosis, dystopia canthorum, brachydactyly and abnormal dermatoglyphic patterns. Muenke has suggested that minimal diagnostic criteria should include tear duct abnormalities, palatal anomalies including cleft palate, parietal foramina, brachydactyly, 2-3 simple syndactyly of hands, and bifid hallux with a lateral deviation (Muenke et al 1997).

The craniosynostosis phenotype most commonly comprises a bicoronal synostosis, but this may be asymmetric, producing the craniofacial scoliosis (Fig. 2.10). Metopic, lambdoid and sagittal suture involvement in variable patterns is also reported (Hunter et al 1976, Reardon and Winter 1994). Cranial defects include parietal foramina and late-closing fontanelles. Vertebral fusion is uncommon. Auricular malformations are common, including a long and prominent ear crus, reported as a consistent sign (Carter et al 1982). A small pinna, with short columella, mild simple syndactyly and craniosynostosis, has been described (Aase and Smith 1970, Kurczynski and Casperson 1988, Legius et al 1989), and other nasal anomalies, such as long thin nose, also occur. Extracranial skeletal mani-festations have been further catalogued by Anderson (Anderson et al 1996c, 1998a). Elbow synostosis, noted rarely by Reardon and Winter (1994), was not seen in this series, and only 3/15 cases had mild 2-3 syndactyly. The hand phenotype included radiographic evidence of anomalies of the thumbs, fingers, metacarpals, and the radius. Clinodactyly was a common finding. Epiphyseal anomalies of the distal phalanx of the thumb were noted in 7/15 patients. There was a variable delay of the bone age.

Saethre–Chotzen syndrome is predominantly familial, and of such great variability and subtlety of phenotype that figures of incidence are probably unreliable (Reardon and

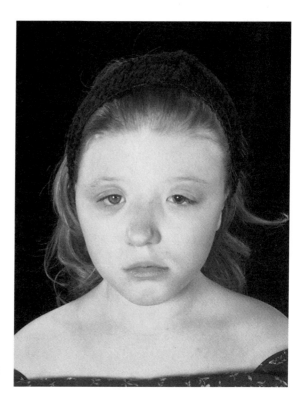

Fig. 2.10 Facial scoliosis and ptosis in Saethre–Chotzen syndrome.

Winter 1994), although 1 in 25,000 to 1 in 50,000 has been suggested (Howard et al 1997). The heterogeneity of the phenotype, with variable anomalies of both osseous and epithelial development, suggests that the causative gene is multifunctional in the control of the development of head mesenchyme, and that its effect is dose-dependent or modified by variable control mechanisms.

PFEIFFER SYNDROME

Pfeiffer syndrome is an autosomal dominant craniosynostosis syndrome, featuring patterns of sutural fusion varying from a mild bicoronal synostosis to pan-synostosis and cloverleaf skull.

The syndrome was originally defined as an entity in 1964 by the association of the craniofacial dysostosis with characteristic limb anomalies (Pfeiffer 1964). In addition to the craniofacial features, consistent limb anomalies were noted to include broad, short thumbs and big toes, with the proximal phalanx of the thumb often triangulated to cause a midline deviation of the thumb. Fusions between thumb phalanges (symphalangism) were also noted, together with partial soft tissue syndactylies of thumb and fingers. The recognition of this constellation of limb anomalies in conjunction with the craniofacial phenotype remains the major criterion for the clinical diagnosis and eponymous label (Cohen 1993a).

The pattern of cranial sutural synostosis in Pfeiffer syndrome is variable, although the coronal and sagittal sutures are most commonly involved. Cranial suture fusions combine to cause turribrachycephaly (tower-shaped skull), the most common Pfeiffer craniofacial phenotype. In severe cases, the syndrome is associated with the 'cloverleaf skull' or *kleeblattschadel* deformity in which the cranium has a trefoil shape with severe biparietal protrusion of the skull, turribrachycephaly, and a shallow posterior fossa (Cohen 1993a).

The cranial base in Pfeiffer syndrome is short, in company with the retruded midface (Fig. 2.11). True hypertelorism (increased inter-orbital distance) is less common than in Apert syndrome, and there is a much milder down-slanting cant to the face, with laterally down-slanting palpebral fissures. The ears are typically low-set. The dysmorphogenesis of the cranial base is also manifest in the auditory mechanism. In a study of nine patients with Pfeiffer syndrome, CT findings consisted of stenosis and/or atresia of the external auditory canal, hypoplasia of the middle ear cavity, and an enlarged middle ear cavity (Vallino-Napoli 1996). The ossicles may be hypoplastic, and ossicular synostosis has also been reported (Cremers 1981). These anomalies are associated with moderate to severe conductive or mixed hearing loss in most patients, despite the observation that inner ear anatomy is predominantly normal (Vallino-Napoli 1996).

The midfacial retrusion of Pfeiffer syndrome is accompanied by ocular proptosis and lagophthalmos (failure of corneal cover by the upper eyelid), which may progress to cause exposure keratitis and may result in recurrent subluxation of the entire globe onto the cheek. Ocular strabismus has been reported (Van Dyke et al 1983), which may reflect the dysmorphogenesis of the bony orbit and secondary mal-insertions of the extraocular musculature. The midfacial retrusion results in a relative mandibular prognathism, beaked

35

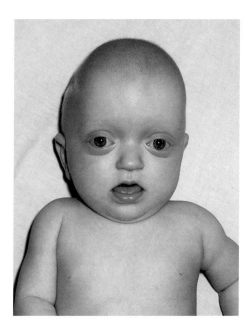

Fig. 2.11 Facial features of Pfeiffer syndrome.

nose, and class III skeletal and dental malocclusion, which is progressive through childhood
and adolescence to skeletal maturity. The maxillary dentition is crowded and malaligned,
and there is delayed eruption of the secondary dentition. The palate is high-arched, in
common with Apert syndrome, but cleft palate does not occur. The nasopharynx is of
restricted volume, and choanal stenosis, or less commonly choanal atresia, may occur.
Clinical problems of the upper airway are therefore common, and lower airway compromise
may also be noted. Primary tracheal anomalies have been reported in both Pfeiffer and
Crouzon syndromes (Devine et al 1984), including replacement of the cartilaginous rings
by a solid cartilaginous plate extending the full length of the trachea and beyond the carina
(Stone et al 1990).

The limb phenotype commonly consists of brachydactyly (short, broad digits),
primarily but not exclusively affecting the thumb or great toe (Cohen 1993a, Anderson
et al 1998b). Broad thumbs are the obligate diagnostic clue, and preaxial deviation of the
first digit, caused by a triangulated or trapezoidal first phalanx of thumb or toe is common.
A 'longitudinally bracketed epiphysis' or delta phalanx may occur. Subclinical tarsal
and metacarpal fusions and dysplasias of the feet are also common, particularly affecting
the first ray, and may be progressive. The feet may range from normal to those resembling
Apert syndrome with preaxial deviation of the first ray and multidigit syndactyly (Anderson
et al 1998b). Symmetrical ankyloses, radiographic and clinical anomalies of the elbow
(Anderson et al 1998a) and knee have been reported, and bear some correlation with the
global severity of the phenotype (Cohen 1993a, Anderson et al 1997b).

Developmental intelligence in Pfeiffer children is usually within normal limits,
though some cases are mildly intellectually impaired. Poor intellectual performance

co-segregates with the cloverleaf variant (Cohen 1993a), though a favourable prognosis in some of these cases is the author's experience and has been reported in response to aggressive mutidisciplinary clinical management (Moore et al 1995, Robin et al 1998). Intracranial abnormalities, including hydrocephalus, ventriculomegaly, tonsillar herniation, and intracranial venous sinus anomaly, are well recognised (Cohen 1993a, Taylor et al 2001). Untreated raised intracranial pressure may result in visual impairment by retinal damage, and intellectual compromise (Gosain et al 1996a).

Visceral anomaly in Pfeiffer syndrome is sporadic, and includes anal stenosis and cryptorchidism (Cohen 1993a).

The features of Pfeiffer syndrome detailed above exhibit a range of severity, and Cohen describes three subgroups of Pfeiffer syndrome, Types 1–3 (Cohen 1993a). The features of each are summarised in Table 2.4.

Various reports attest to the clinical variability of the Pfeiffer phenotype, which may range within families from a mild expression in the hallux and partial syndactyly in several generations, to the full craniofacial and limb presentation. The range of intra-familial variability includes the presentation of cloverleaf skull in the affected child of a mildly affected mother (Soekarman et al 1992). In a 1993 review, Cohen analysed seven previously published Pfeiffer syndrome pedigrees (three three-generation and four two-generation) and a number of sporadic cases. The variability of the clinical presentation of both the limb and craniofacial phenotypes in each generation of each family describes an autosomal

TABLE 2.4
Classification of Pfeiffer syndrome (Cohen 1993a)

Major characteristics	Associated anomaly	Functional outcome	Inheritance
Type 1 Turribrachycephaly, midface retrusion, broad thumbs and great toe, brachydactyly, variable syndactyly	Low frequency anomalies of viscera, cervical spine fusions	Survive to adulthood	Sporadic Autosomal dominant
Type 2 Cloverleaf skull, ocular proptosis, and severe midface retrusion Digital anomaly as Type 1	More severe limb and spinal phenotypes Elbow synostoses Intellectual compromise Intracranial and neurodevelopmental anomaly	Poor prognosis	Usually sporadic
Type 3 Severe midface retrusion without cloverleaf skull Ocular proptosis Class III malocclusion Distal limb features as Type 1	Elbow and knee synostoses Visceral anomaly Intellectual compromise Intracranial and neurodevelopmental anomaly	Poor prognosis	Usually sporadic

dominant syndrome with complete penetrance but very variable expressivity, particularly with reference to the limb phenotype. The presence of digital syndactyly, in particular, was highly variable, but was reported to most commonly involve the 2-3 web.

CLOVERLEAF SKULL – KLEEBLATTSCHADEL DEFORMITY

The *Kleeblattschadel* anomaly, or cloverleaf skull, is an uncommon and severe craniofacial phenotype resulting from multisutural fusion involving both coronal sutures and a combination of the metopic, lambdoid and sagittal sutures. The result is a broad bi-temporal and bi-parietal diameter, with a turricephalic vertex and steep forehead. The head has a flattened, trilobular configuration, caused by hydrocephalus in combination with extensive craniosynostosis. The midface is retruded, with the secondary ocular and dentoalveolar problems elsewhere described. There is a shallow posterior fossa, and herniation of the cerebellar tonsils via the foramen magnum is a common accompaniment (Thompson et al 1995b). The clinical prognosis is often poor, but improved by aggressive surgical management.

Cloverleaf skull has been reported in conjunction with a number of FGFR-related phenotypes, including 'Crouzonoid' non-specific craniosynostosis (Pulleyn et al 1996), Pfeiffer syndrome (Soekarman et al 1992, Meyers et al 1996), Crouzon syndrome (Hall et al 1972, Cohen 1975), Apert syndrome (Cohen and Kreiborg 1994b, Gosain et al 1997), Beare–Stevenson cutis gyrata syndrome (Hall et al 1992, Przylepa et al 1996) and thanatophoric dysplasia (Langer et al 1987, Machin 1992).

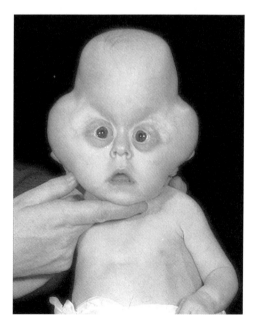

Fig. 2.12 Cloverleaf skull (*Kleeblattschadel*).

CARPENTER SYNDROME

This is a much less common syndrome than those described thus far, and the inheritance pattern is autosomal recessive. The condition is also known as acrocephalopolysyndactyly as preaxial polydactyly of the feet is a characteristic feature. The cranial deformity is often severe and asymmetric; it is the sagittal and lambdoid sutures that are primarily involved. Individuals are short and often obese and neurodevelopmental impairment is common.

ANTLEY–BIXLER SYNDROME

Craniosynostosis involves the coronal and often lambdoid sutures, resulting in a brachy-cephalic head shape; the ears are dysplastic and there are extensive extracranial skeletal abnormalities including joint contractures, radiohumeral synostosis, bowing of the femora and long tapering fingers. Upper airway obstruction has been responsible for a high mortality in this condition.

JACKSON–WEISS SYNDROME

This craniosynostosis syndrome was reported relatively recently in an Amish population (Jackson et al. 1976). This rare syndrome comprises craniosynostosis, midfacial hypoplasia and foot abnormalities comprising variable forms of syndactyly and bony aberrations of the tarsus and metatarsus.

MUENKE SYNDROME

This condition is of particular interest in that the syndrome was defined on the basis of the underlying molecular abnormality (Muenke et al 1997). In common with the other syndromes, involvement of the coronal sutures is seen in this condition. The coronal synostosis, however, is often unilateral; indeed many patients diagnosed with non-syndromic unicoronal craniosynostosis have been found to harbour the FGFR3 mutation.

There is now a vast array of clinical syndromes in which craniosynostosis is a recognised feature, and only the more commonly encountered syndromes have been addressed here. Many of the other syndromes are exceedingly rare and in some cases the craniosynostosis is of relatively minor clinical significance. More detailed accounts of these can be found in dysmorphology texts (Gorlin et al 2001).

REFERENCES

Aase JM, Smith DW (1970) Facial asymmetry and abnormalities of palms and ears: a dominantly inherited developmental syndrome. *J Pediatr* 76: 928–930.

Anderson PJ, Evans RD (1998) Re: Metacarpophalangeal analysis in Crouzon syndrome. *Am J Med Genet* 80: 439.

Anderson PJ, Hall CM, Evans RD, Jones BM, Harkness W, Hayward RD (1996a) Cervical spine in Pfeiffer's syndrome. *J Craniofac Surg* 7: 275–279.

Anderson PJ, Hall R, Smith PJ (1996b) Finger duplication in Apert's syndrome. *J Hand Surg (Br)* 21: 649–651.

Anderson PJ, Hall CM, Evans RD, Hayward RD, Jones BM (1996c) The hands in Saethre-Chotzen syndrome. *J Craniofac Genet Dev Biol* 16: 228–233.

Anderson PJ, Hall C, Evans RD, Harkness WJ, Hayward RD, Jones BM (1997a) The cervical spine in Crouzon syndrome. *Spine* 22: 402–405.

Anderson PJ, Hall CM, Evans RD, Jones BM, Hayward RD (1997b) The feet in Crouzon syndrome. *J Craniofac Genet Dev Biol* 17: 43–47.

Anderson PJ, Hall CM, Evans RD, Jones BM, Hayward RD (1997c) Hand anomalies in Crouzon syndrome. *Skeletal Radiol* 26: 113–115.

Anderson PJ, Hall CM, Evans RD, Hayward RD, Jones BM (1997d) Knee radiographs in Pfeiffer and Crouzon syndromes. *Plast Reconstr Surg* 100: 550.

Anderson PJ, Hall CM, Evans RD, Hayward RD, Jones BM (1998a) The elbow in syndromic craniosynostosis. *J Craniofac Surg* 9: 201–206.

Anderson PJ, Hall CM, Evans RD, Jones BM, Hayward RD (1998b) The feet in Pfeiffer's syndrome. *J Craniofac Surg* 9: 83–87.

Apert E (1906) De l'acrocephalosyndactylie. *Bull Soc Med Hop (Paris)* 23: 1310–1330.

Baum DJ, Searls D (1971) Head shape and size of pre-term low-birthweight infants. *Dev Med Child Neurol* 13: 576–581.

Blank CE (1960) Apert's syndrome (a type of acrocephalosyndactyly) – observations on a British series of thirty-nine cases. *Ann Hum Genet* 24: 151–164.

Boop FA, Chadduck WM, Shewmake K, Teo C (1996) Outcome analysis of 85 patients undergoing the pi procedure for correction of sagittal synostosis. *J Neurosurg* 85: 50–55.

Breitbart AS, Eaton C, McCarthy JG (1989) Crouzon's syndrome associated with acanthosis nigricans: ramifications for the craniofacial surgeon. *Ann Plast Surg* 22: 310–315.

Carter CO, Till K, Fraser V, Coffey R (1982) A family study of craniosynostosis, with probable recognition of a distinct syndrome. *J Med Genet* 19: 280–285.

Chadduck WM, Chadduck JB, Boop FA (1992) The subarachnoid spaces in craniosynostosis. *Neurosurgery* 30: 867–871.

Chao MV (1992) Growth factor signaling: where is the specificity? *Cell* 68: 995–997.

Chotzen F (1932) Eine eigenartige familiaere Entwicklungsstoerung (Akrocephalosyndaktylie, dysostosis craniofacialis und Hypertelorismus). *Monatschir Kinderheilkd* 55: 97–122.

Chumas PD, Cinalli G, Arnaud E, Marchac D, Renier D (1997) Classification of previously unclassified cases of craniosynostosis. *J Neurosurg* 86: 177–181.

Cinalli G, Renier D, Sebag G, Sainte-Rose C, Arnaud E, Pierre-Kahn A (1995) Chronic tonsillar herniation in Crouzon's and Apert's syndromes: the role of premature synostosis of the lambdoid suture. *J Neurosurg* 83: 575–582.

Cohen MM Jr (1975) An etiologic and nosologic overview of craniosynostosis syndromes. *Birth Defects Orig Artic Ser* 11: 137–189.

Cohen MM Jr (1993a) Pfeiffer syndrome update, clinical subtypes, and guidelines for differential diagnosis. *Am J Med Genet* 45: 300–307.

Cohen MM Jr (1993b) Sutural biology and the correlates of craniosynostosis. *Am J Med Genet* 47: 581–616.

Cohen MM Jr, Kreiborg S (1990) The central nervous system in the Apert syndrome. *Am J Med Genet* 35: 36–45.

Cohen MM Jr, Kreiborg S (1992a) Birth prevalence studies of the Crouzon syndrome: comparison of direct and indirect methods. *Clin Genet* 41: 12–15.

Cohen MM Jr, Kreiborg S (1992b) Upper and lower airway compromise in the Apert syndrome. *Am J Med Genet* 44: 90–93.

Cohen MM Jr, Kreiborg S (1993a) Skeletal abnormalities in the Apert syndrome. *Am J Med Genet* 47: 624–632.

Cohen MM Jr, Kreiborg S (1993b) Visceral anomalies in the Apert syndrome. *Am J Med Genet* 45: 758–760.

Cohen MM Jr, Kreiborg S (1994a) Cranial size and configuration in the Apert syndrome. *J Craniofac Genet Dev Biol* 14: 153–162.

Cohen MM Jr, Kreiborg S (1994b) Unusual cranial aspects of the Apert syndrome. *J Craniofac Genet Dev Biol* 14: 48–56.

Cohen MM Jr, Kreiborg S (1995a) Cutaneous manifestations of Apert syndrome. *Am J Med Genet* 58: 94–96.

Cohen MM Jr, Kreiborg S (1995b) Hands and feet in the Apert syndrome. *Am J Med Genet* 57: 82–96.

Cohen MM Jr, Kreiborg S (1996) A clinical study of the craniofacial features in Apert syndrome. *Int J Oral Maxillofac Surg* 25: 45–53.

Cohen MM Jr, Kreiborg S, Lammer EJ, Cordero JF, Mastroiacovo P, Erickson JD, Roeper P, Martinez-Frias ML (1992) Birth prevalence study of the Apert syndrome. *Am J Med Genet* 42: 655–659.

Cohen SR, Dauser RC, Gorski JL (1993) Insidious onset of familial craniosynostosis. *Cleft Palate Craniofac J* 30: 401–405.

Cremers CW (1981) Hearing loss in Pfeiffer's syndrome. *Int J Pediatr Otorhinolaryngol* 3: 343–353.

Crouzon O (1912) Dysostose cranio-faciale hereditaire. *Bull Soc Med Hop (Paris)* 33: 545–555.

Cuttone JM, Brazis PT, Miller MT, Folk ER (1979) Absence of the superior rectus muscle in Apert's syndrome. *J Pediatr Ophthalmol Strabismus* 16: 349–354.

Devine P, Bhan I, Feingold M, Leonidas JC, Wolpert SM (1984) Completely cartilaginous trachea in a child with Crouzon syndrome. *Am J Dis Child* 138: 40–43.

Di Rocco C, Velardi F (1988) Nosographic identification and classification of plagiocephaly. *Childs Nerv Syst* 4: 9–15.

Frydman M, Kauschansky A, Elian E (1984) Trigonocephaly: a new familial syndrome. *Am J Med Genet* 18: 55–59.

Gines E, Rodriguez-Pichardo A, Jorquera E, Moreno JC, Camacho F (1996) Crouzon disease with acanthosis nigricans and melanocytic nevi. *Pediatr Dermatol* 13: 18–21.

Glaser RL, Jiang W, Boyadjiev SA, Tran AK, Zachary AA, Van Maldergem L, Johnson D, Walsh S, Oldridge M, Wall SA, Wilkie AO, Jabs EW (2000) Paternal origin of FGFR2 mutations in sporadic cases of Crouzon syndrome and Pfeiffer syndrome. *Am J Hum Genet* 66: 768–777.

Golabi M, Edwards MS, Ousterhout DK (1987) Craniosynostosis and hydrocephalus. *Neurosurgery* 21: 63–67.

Gorlin RJ, Cohen MM Jr, Levin LS (1990) *Syndromes of the Head and Neck.* Oxford: Oxford University Press.

Gorlin RJ, Cohen MM Jr, Hennekam RC (2001) *Syndromes of the Head and Neck,* 2nd edn. Oxford: Oxford University Press.

Gosain AK, McCarthy JG, Glatt P, Staffenberg D, Hoffmann RG (1995) A study of intracranial volume in Apert syndrome. *Plast Reconstr Surg* 95: 284–295.

Gosain AK, McCarthy JG, Wisoff JH (1996a) Morbidity associated with increased intracranial pressure in Apert and Pfeiffer syndromes: the need for long-term evaluation. *Plast Reconstr Surg* 97: 292–301.

Gosain AK, Steele MA, McCarthy JG, Thorne CH (1996b) A prospective study of the relationship between strabismus and head posture in patients with frontal plagiocephaly. *Plast Reconstr Surg* 97: 881–891.

Gosain AK, Moore FO, Hemmy DC (1997) The kleeblattschadel anomaly in Apert syndrome: intracranial anatomy, surgical correction, and subsequent cranial vault development. *Plast Reconstr Surg* 100: 1796–1802.

Hall BD, Smith DW, Shiller JG (1972) Kleeblattschadel (cloverleaf) syndrome: severe form of Crouzon's disease? *J Pediatr* 80: 526–528.

Hall BD, Cadle RG, Golabi M, Morris CA, Cohen MM Jr (1992) Beare-Stevenson cutis gyrata syndrome. *Am J Med Genet* 44: 82–89.

Henderson CA, Knaggs H, Clark A, Highet AS, Cunliffe WJ (1995) Apert's syndrome and androgen receptor staining of the basal cells of sebaceous glands. *Br J Dermatol* 132: 139–143.

Holten IW (1994) Apert syndrome. Master of Surgery thesis, University of Adelaide, Adelaide, South Australia.

Holten IW, Smith AW, Bourne AJ, David DJ (1997) The Apert syndrome hand: pathologic anatomy and clinical manifestations. *Plast Reconstr Surg* 99: 1681–1687.

Howard TD, Paznekas WA, Green ED, Chiang LC, Ma N, Ortiz de Luna RI, Garcia DC, Gonzalez-Ramos M, Kline AD, Jabs EW (1997) Mutations in TWIST, a basic helix-loop-helix transcription factor, in Saethre-Chotzen syndrome. *Nat Genet* 15: 36–41.

Huang MH, Mouradian WE, Cohen SR, Gruss JS (1998) The differential diagnosis of abnormal head shapes: separating craniosynostosis from positional deformities and normal variants. *Cleft Palate Craniofac J* 35: 204–211.

Hunter AG, Rudd NL, Hoffmann HJ (1976) Trigonocephaly and associated minor anomalies in mother and son. *J Med Genet* 13: 77–79.

Jackson CE, Weiss L, Reynolds WA, Forman TF, Peterson JA (1976) Craniosynostosis, midfacial hypoplasia and foot abnormalities: an autosomal dominant phenotype in a large Amish kindred. *J Pediatr* 88: 963–968.

Kane AA, Mitchell LE, Craven KP, Marsh JL (1996) Observations on a recent increase in plagiocephaly without synostosis. *Pediatrics* 97: 877–885.

Kreiborg S (1981) Crouzon syndrome. A clinical and roentgencephalometric study. *Scand J Plast Reconstr Surg Suppl* 18: 1–198.

Kreiborg S, Cohen MM Jr (1990) Characteristics of the infant Apert skull and its subsequent development. *J Craniofac Genet Dev Biol* 10: 399–410.

41

Kreiborg S, Cohen MM Jr (1992) The oral manifestations of Apert syndrome. *J Craniofac Genet Dev Biol* 12: 41–48.

Kreiborg S, Barr M Jr, Cohen MM Jr (1992) Cervical spine in the Apert syndrome. *Am J Med Genet* 43: 704–708.

Kreiborg S, Marsh JL, Cohen MM Jr, Liversage M, Pedersen H, Skovby F, Borgesen SE, Vannier MW (1993) Comparative three-dimensional analysis of CT-scans of the calvaria and cranial base in Apert and Crouzon syndromes. *J Craniomaxillofac Surg* 21: 181–188.

Kreiborg S, Aduss H, Cohen MM Jr (1999) Cephalometric study of the Apert syndrome in adolescence and adulthood. *J Craniofac Genet Dev Biol* 19: 1–11.

Kurczynski TW, Casperson SM (1988) Auralcephalosyndactyly: a new hereditary craniosynostosis syndrome. *J Med Genet* 25: 491–493.

Lajeunie E, Le Merrer M, Bonaiti-Pellie C, Marchac D, Renier D (1995) Genetic study of nonsyndromic coronal craniosynostosis. *Am J Med Genet* 55: 500–504.

Lajeunie E, Le Merrer M, Bonaiti-Pellie C, Marchac D, Renier D (1996) Genetic study of scaphocephaly. *Am J Med Genet* 62: 282–285.

Lajeunie E, Le Merrer M, Marchac D, Renier D (1998) Syndromal and nonsyndromal primary trigonocephaly: analysis of a series of 237 patients. *Am J Med Genet* 75: 211–215.

Lajeunie E, Cameron R, El Ghouzzi V, de Parseval N, Journeau P, Gonzales M, Delezoide AL, Bonaventure J, Le Merrer M, Renier D (1999) Clinical variability in patients with Apert's syndrome. *J Neurosurg* 90: 443–447.

Lajeunie E, Barcik U, Thorne JA, Ghouzzi VE, Bourgeois M, Renier D (2001) Craniosynostosis and fetal exposure to sodium valproate. *J Neurosurg* 95: 778–782.

Langer LO Jr, Yang SS, Hall JG, Sommer A, Kottamasu SR, Golabi M, Krassikoff N (1987) Thanatophoric dysplasia and cloverleaf skull. *Am J Med Genet Suppl* 3: 167–179.

Lefebvre A, Travis F, Arndt EM, Munro IR (1986) A psychiatric profile before and after reconstructive surgery in children with Apert's syndrome. *Br J Plast Surg* 39: 510–513.

Legius E, Fryns JP, Van Den BH (1989) Auralcephalosyndactyly: a new craniosynostosis syndrome or a variant of the Saethre-Chotzen syndrome? *J Med Genet* 26: 522–524.

Littlefield TR, Beals SP, Manwaring KH, Pomatto JK, Joganic EF, Golden KA, Ripley CE (1998) Treatment of craniofacial asymmetry with dynamic orthotic cranioplasty. *J Craniofac Surg* 9: 11–17.

Lo LJ, Chen YR (1999) Airway obstruction in severe syndromic craniosynostosis. *Ann Plast Surg* 43: 258–264.

McCarthy JG, Glasberg SB, Cutting CB, Epstein FJ, Grayson BH, Ruff G, Thorne CH, Wisoff J, Zide BM (1995) Twenty-year experience with early surgery for craniosynostosis: I. Isolated craniofacial synostosis – results and unsolved problems. *Plast Reconstr Surg* 96: 272–283.

Machin GA (1992) Thanatophoric dysplasia in monozygotic twins discordant for cloverleaf skull: prenatal diagnosis, clinical and pathological findings. *Am J Med Genet* 44: 842–843.

Magge SN, Westerveld M, Pruzinsky T, Persing JA (2002) Long-term neuropsychological effects of sagittal craniosynostosis on child development. *J Craniofac Surg* 13: 99–104.

Mah J, Kasser J, Upton J (1991) The foot in Apert syndrome. *Clin Plast Surg* 18: 391–397.

Margolis S, Siegel IM, Choy A, Breinin GM (1977a) Oculocutaneous albinism associated with Apert's syndrome. *Am J Ophthalmol* 84: 830–839.

Margolis S, Pachter BR, Breinin GM (1977b) Structural alterations of extraocular muscle associated with Apert's syndrome. *Br J Ophthalmol* 61: 683–689.

Marini R, Temple K, Chitty L, Genet S, Baraitser M (1991) Pitfalls in counselling: the craniosynostoses. *J Med Genet* 28: 117–121.

Meyers GA, Orlow SJ, Munro IR, Przylepa KA, Jabs EW (1995) Fibroblast growth factor receptor 3 (FGFR3) transmembrane mutation in Crouzon syndrome with acanthosis nigricans. *Nat Genet* 11: 462–464.

Meyers GA, Day D, Goldberg R, Daentl DL, Przylepa KA, Abrams LJ, Graham JM Jr, Feingold M, Moeschler JB, Rawnsley E, Scott AF, Jabs EW (1996) FGFR2 exon IIIa and IIIc mutations in Crouzon, Jackson-Weiss, and Pfeiffer syndromes: evidence for missense changes, insertions, and a deletion due to alternative RNA splicing. *Am J Hum Genet* 58: 491–498.

Moore MH, Cantrell SB, Trott JA, David DJ (1995) Pfeiffer syndrome: a clinical review. *Cleft Palate Craniofac J* 32: 62–70.

Morax S, Pascal D (1982) [Absence of the right superior rectus muscle in Apert's syndrome (author's translation)]. *J Fr Ophtalmol* 5: 323–326.

42

Muenke M, Gripp KW, McDonald-McGinn DM, Gaudenz K, Whitaker LA, Bartlett SP, Markowitz RI, Robin NH, Nwokoro N, Mulvihill JJ, Losken HW, Mulliken JB, Guttmacher AE, Wilroy RS, Clarke LA, Hollway G, Ades LC, Haan EA, Mulley JC, Cohen MM Jr, Bellus GA, Francomano CA, Moloney DM, Wall SA, Wilkie AO (1997) A unique point mutation in the fibroblast growth factor receptor 3 gene (FGFR3) defines a new craniosynostosis syndrome. *Am J Hum Genet* 60: 555–564.

Niemann-Seyde SC, Eber SW, Zoll B (1991) Saethre-Chotzen syndrome (ACS III) in four generations. *Clin Genet* 40: 271–276.

Okajima K, Robinson LK, Hart MA, Abuelo DN, Cowan LS, Hasegawa T, Maumenee IH, Wang JE (1999) Ocular anterior chamber dysgenesis in craniosynostosis syndromes with a fibroblast growth factor receptor 2 mutation. *Am J Med Genet* 85: 160–170.

Opitz JM (1969) The C syndrome of multiple congenital anomalies. *Birth Defects* 5: 161–166.

Pantke OA, Cohen MM Jr, Witkop CJ Jr, Feingold M, Schaumann B, Pantke HC, Gorlin RJ (1975) The Saethre-Chotzen syndrome. *Birth Defects Orig Artic Ser* 11: 190–225.

Park EA, Powers GA (1920) Acrocephaly and scaphocephaly with symmetrically distributed malformations of the extremities. *Am J Dis Child* 20: 235–315.

Park WJ, Theda C, Maestri NE, Meyers GA, Fryburg JS, Dufresne C, Cohen MM Jr, Jabs EW (1995) Analysis of phenotypic features and FGFR2 mutations in Apert syndrome. *Am J Hum Genet* 57: 321–328.

Patton MA, Goodship J, Hayward R, Lansdown R (1988) Intellectual development in Apert's syndrome: a long term follow up of 29 patients. *J Med Genet* 25: 164–167.

Peterson-Falzone SJ, Pruzansky S, Parris PJ, Laffer JL (1981) Nasopharyngeal dysmorphology in the syndromes of Apert and Crouzon. *Cleft Palate J* 18: 237–250.

Peterson SJ, Pruzansky S (1974) Palatal anomalies in the syndromes of Apert and Crouzon. *Cleft Palate J* 11: 394–403.

Pfeiffer RA (1964) Dominant erbliche Akrocephalosyndaktylie. *Z Kinderheilkd* 90: 301–320.

Proudman TW, Moore MH, Abbott AH, David DJ (1994) Noncraniofacial manifestations of Crouzon's disease. *J Craniofac Surg* 5: 218–222.

Przylepa KA, Paznekas W, Zhang M, Golabi M, Bias W, Bamshad MJ, Carey JC, Hall BD, Stevenson R, Orlow S, Cohen MM Jr, Jabs EW (1996) Fibroblast growth factor receptor 2 mutations in Beare-Stevenson cutis gyrata syndrome. *Nat Genet* 13: 492–494.

Pulleyn LJ, Reardon W, Wilkes D, Rutland P, Jones BM, Hayward R, Hall CM, Brueton L, Chun N, Lammer E, Malcolm S, Winter RM (1996) Spectrum of craniosynostosis phenotypes associated with novel mutations at the fibroblast growth factor receptor 2 locus. *Eur J Hum Genet* 4: 283–291.

Reardon W, Winter RM (1994) Saethre-Chotzen syndrome. *J Med Genet* 31: 393–396.

Reddy BS, Garg BR, Padiyar NV, Krishnaram AS (1985) An unusual association of acanthosis nigricans and Crouzon's disease – a case report. *J Dermatol* 12: 85–90.

Reddy K, Hoffman H, Armstrong D (1990) Delayed and progressive multiple suture craniosynostosis. *Neurosurgery* 26: 442–448.

Renier D, Sainte-Rose C, Marchac D, Hirsch JF (1982) Intracranial pressure in craniostenosis. *J Neurosurg* 57: 370–377.

Renier D, Arnaud E, Cinalli G, Sebag G, Zerah M, Marchac D (1996) Prognosis for mental function in Apert's syndrome. *J Neurosurg* 85: 66–72.

Robin NH, Scott JA, Arnold JE, Goldstein JA, Shilling BB, Marion RW, Cohen MM Jr (1998) Favorable prognosis for children with Pfeiffer syndrome types 2 and 3: implications for classification. *Am J Med Genet* 75: 240–244.

Saethre H (1931) Beitrag zum Turmschaedelproblem (Pathogenese, Erblichkeit und Symptomatologie). *Dtsch Z Nervenheilkd* 119: 533–555.

Sagehashi N (1992) An infant with Crouzon's syndrome with a cartilaginous trachea and a human tail. *J Craniomaxillofac Surg* 20: 21–23.

Say B, Meyer J (1981) Familial trigonocephaly associated with short stature and developmental delay. *Am J Dis Child* 135: 711–712.

Schauerte EW, St Aubin PM (1966) Progressive synosteosis in Apert's syndrome (acrocephalosyndactyly), with a description of roentgenographic changes in the feet. *Am J Roentgenol Radium Ther Nucl Med* 97: 67–73.

Shillito J Jr, Matson DD (1968) Craniosynostosis: a review of 519 surgical patients. *Pediatrics* 41: 829–853.

Shipster C, Hearst D, Dockrell JE, Kilby E, Hayward R (2002) Speech and language skills and cognitive functioning in children with Apert syndrome: a pilot study. *Int J Lang Commun Disord* 37: 325–343.

43

Sidoti EJ Jr, Marsh JL, Marty-Grames L, Noetzel MJ (1996) Long-term studies of metopic synostosis: frequency of cognitive impairment and behavioral disturbances. *Plast Reconstr Surg* 97: 276–281.

Slaney SF, Oldridge M, Hurst JA, Moriss-Kay GM, Hall CM, Poole MD, Wilkie AO (1996) Differential effects of FGFR2 mutations on syndactyly and cleft palate in Apert syndrome. *Am J Hum Genet* 58: 923–932.

Soekarman D, Fryns JP, Van Den BH (1992) Pfeiffer acrocephalosyndactyly syndrome in mother and son with cloverleaf skull anomaly in the child. *Genet Couns* 3: 217–220.

Stone P, Trevenen CL, Mitchell I, Rudd N (1990) Congenital tracheal stenosis in Pfeiffer syndrome. *Clin Genet* 38: 145–148.

Suslak L, Glista B, Gertzman GB, Lieberman L, Schwartz RA, Desposito F (1985) Crouzon syndrome with periapical cemental dysplasia and acanthosis nigricans: the pleiotropic effect of a single gene? *Birth Defects Orig Artic Ser* 21: 127–134.

Taylor WJ, Hayward RD, Lasjaunias P, Britto JA, Thompson DN, Jones BM, Evans RD (2001) Enigma of raised intracranial pressure in patients with complex craniosynostosis: the role of abnormal intracranial venous drainage. *J Neurosurg* 94: 377–385.

Thompson DN, Harkness W, Jones B, Gonsalez S, Andar U, Hayward R (1995a) Subdural intracranial pressure monitoring in craniosynostosis: its role in surgical management. *Childs Nerv Syst* 11: 269–275.

Thompson DN, Hayward RD, Harkness WJ, Bingham RM, Jones BM (1995b) Lessons from a case of kleeblattschadel. Case report. *J Neurosurg* 82: 1071–1074.

Thompson DN, Malcolm GP, Jones BM, Harkness WJ, Hayward RD (1995c) Intracranial pressure in single-suture craniosynostosis. *Pediatr Neurosurg* 22: 235–240.

Thompson DN, Slaney SF, Hall CM, Shaw D, Jones BM, Hayward RD (1996) Congenital cervical spinal fusion: a study in Apert syndrome. *Pediatr Neurosurg* 25: 20–27.

Thompson DN, Harkness W, Jones BM, Hayward RD (1997) Aetiology of herniation of the hindbrain in craniosynostosis. An investigation incorporating intracranial pressure monitoring and magnetic resonance imaging. *Pediatr Neurosurg* 26: 288–295.

Upton J (1991) Apert syndrome. Classification and pathologic anatomy of limb anomalies. *Clin Plast Surg* 18: 321–355.

Vallino-Napoli LD (1996) Audiologic and otologic characteristics of Pfeiffer syndrome. *Cleft Palate Craniofac J* 33: 524–529.

Van Dyke DC, Zackai EH, Diamond GR (1983) Clinical observation: ocular abnormalities in a patient with Pfeiffer syndrome (acrocephalosyndactyly, type V). *J Clin Dysmorphol* 1: 2–5.

Virtanen R, Korhonen T, Fagerholm J, Viljanto J (1999) Neurocognitive sequelae of scaphocephaly. *Pediatrics* 103: 791–795.

Wheaton S (1894) Two specimens of congenital cranial deformity in infants associated with fusion of fingers and toes. *Trans Path Soc London* 45: 238–241.

3
SYNDROMIC CRANIOFACIAL DYSOSTOSIS: MOLECULAR AND DEVELOPMENTAL ASPECTS

Jonathan Britto and Willie Reardon

Introduction: FGFR mutations cause certain human skeletal dysplasias

The 'syndromic craniosynostoses' occur as a subset of a wider group of skeletal dysplasias, which, as the result of intensive research during the last decade, have been linked to a series of mutations in the FGFR (fibroblast growth factor receptor) genes 1–3. The clinical presentation of these conditions can be broadly classified into two groups:

1   The dwarfing chondrodysplasias, which primarily affect the appendicular skeleton and include hypochondroplasia (HCH), achondroplasia (ACH), and thanatophoric dysplasia (TD). These syndromes will be considered further only by way of example in this chapter.

2   The syndromic craniofacial dysostoses (including the 'acrocephalosyndactylies' such as Apert, Crouzon, and Pfeiffer syndromes), the clinical features of which have been described in Chapter 2.

All of the individual syndromes that are encoded by FGFR mutations are either inherited in an autosomal dominant manner or arise sporadically as a result of new dominant mutations. Several of the resulting conditions, because of reduced life expectancy, do not successfully reproduce, but do, nonetheless, represent dominant mutations. These mutations are thought to be the most frequent in the human genome. The chondrodysplasias are caused by a series of mutations in FGFR3, and, in displaying a dwarfing phenotype, implicate this gene in the regulation of the endochondral ossification of long bones. However, these phenotypes may also include craniofacial manifestations, such as a short skull base, macrocephaly, and craniosynostosis (including pan-synostosis causing 'cloverleaf' skull, as evidenced in cases of thanatophoric dysplasia). These clinical features thus implicate FGFR3 in the regulation of basicranial endochondral ossification, and also suggest that it plays a contributory role in the membranous ossification of the cranial vault and the regulation of cranial sutural development.

The syndromic craniofacial dysostoses of Apert, Pfeiffer, Crouzon, and Jackson–Weiss (a large and variable single kindred) are predominantly caused by mutations in the FGFR2 gene, and feature craniosynostosis as the common feature of a broad and overlapping range of phenotypes (see Chapter 2). Pfeiffer syndrome can also be caused by a mutation in FGFR1, and unicoronal and bicoronal synostoses (traditionally termed 'non-syndromic') by mutations in FGFR3. The extent of the clinical phenotypes suggests that the genes FGFR1–3 play a broad and functionally overlapping role in human development that extends beyond their role in skeletogenesis. In particular, however, in displaying similar ranges of cranial and limb dysplasia, the FGFR-syndromes demonstrate that common molecular control mechanisms regulate human skull and limb development.

A fundamental role for FGFR signalling in development is further indicated by the fact that members of the FGFR protein family display great sequence homology, and are highly conserved amongst a range of species including C. elegans, Drosophila, chicken, and higher mammalian vertebrates (Johnson and Williams 1993, Park et al 1995a). Human FGFR mutations have been demonstrated to affect a range of different sites throughout the receptor protein. Certain non-random, high-frequency mutations within the protein structure are common amongst the three FGFRs, however, and these mutations predict common functional effects upon receptor dimerisation and signal transduction. The 'gain of function', in turn, generates common phenotypic effects, which reflect patterns of isoform-specific FGFR expression during human development (Chan and Thorogood 1999, Britto et al 2001a, 2001b, 2001c, 2002). The variability of cranioskeletal presentation within and between these clinically related syndromes, and often between affected members of the same family (Jackson et al 1976, Baraitser et al 1980, Reardon and Winter 1994), suggests that there is great plasticity in the genotype–phenotype relationship. The clinical presentation probably reflects the functional effects of each specific FGFR mutation, the tissue-specific expression of the mutant genes throughout human development, the extent of co-regulation by modifier signalling pathways, and environmental influences.

Of the 'primary' syndromic forms of craniosynostosis, approximately 30 are considered to be single gene disorders. The FGFR genes were originally considered as candidate causative genes for human skeletal dysplasias following a number of corroborative observations (Table 3.1). Crouzon and Jackson–Weiss pedigrees had been mapped by genetic linkage studies to the chromosome regions 10q2, and 10q23–q26 respectively (Li et al 1994, Preston et al 1994, Ma et al 1995), having been excluded from a Saethre–Chotzen syndrome locus at chromosome 7p (Brueton et al 1992, Reardon et al 1994a, van Herwerden et al 1994). Human FGFR2 had been mapped to the same region 10q25–q26 (Johnson and Williams 1993), and initial studies in the mouse had defined expression domains for the bek/IgIIIc protein receptor isoform of murine fgfr2 in the frontal bones, maxilla and middle ear ossicles (Orr-Urtreger et al 1991, 1993).

Pfeiffer syndrome was linked to the peri-centromic region of chromosome 8 in 5/11 affected pedigrees in 1994 (Robin et al 1994), although genetic heterogeneity was implied by exclusion of linkage criteria in a further six families. Human FGFR1 maps to 8p11.2–p12 (Johnson and Williams 1993); and following observations in Crouzon syndrome, was thus considered a strong candidate gene. Mis-sense mutations in the linker sequence of the FGFR1 protein were subsequently reported in Pfeiffer syndrome in 1994 (Muenke et al 1994). Linkage of a further three Pfeiffer kindreds to chromosome 10q was reported in 1995, in whom a number of mutations in FGFR2 were identified (Schell et al 1995).

TABLE 3.1
FGFR mutations in craniosynostosis syndromes

	FGFR1	FGFR2	FGFR3
Pfeiffer	√	√	
Crouzon		√	√
Apert		√	
Muenke coronal synostosis			√
Jackson–Weiss		√	
Beare–Stevenson cutis gyrata		√	
Antley–Bixler		√	

The paucity of Apert kindreds (only 11 cases of vertical transmission had been recorded by 1995) had precluded classical genetic linkage studies in Apert syndrome. However, the similarity of aspects of the craniofacial and limb phenotypes to those of Crouzon and Pfeiffer syndromes resulted in FGFR1 and FGFR2 being strong potential candidates. FGFR2 mutations were found to be causal in 40 unrelated Apert cases in 1995 (Wilkie et al 1995).

Achondroplasia, a skeletal dwarfing condition inherited in an autosomal dominant fashion, was linked to chromosome 4p16 (Francomano et al 1994, Le Merrer et al 1994, Velinov et al 1994), the same position to which FGFR3 had been localised (Johnson and Williams 1993). *In situ* hybridisation studies in the mouse show that murine fgfr3 is strongly expressed throughout endochondral ossification (Peters et al 1993), and therefore presented FGFR3 as a candidate for achondroplasia. FGFR3 mutations causing achondroplasia were first reported in 1994 (Shiang et al 1994).

The following sections of this chapter review:

1   The relevant molecular biology of those members of the FGFR gene family that cause human skeletal dysplasias.
2   The effect that FGFR disease mutations have upon FGFR function.
3   The correlation of mutant FGFR function with clinical presentation in the affected individual.

FGFR signalling mechanisms: relevance to human craniofacial syndromes.
Human FGFR mutations follow non-random themes and result in mutant proteins that demonstrate 'gain of function' at the molecular level. Receptor functional gain results in the recognisable patterns of craniosynostosis affecting children presenting to craniofacial clinics, and studies to link these two ends of the pathogenetic pathway have been energetically pursued. A basic knowledge of FGFR biology is necessary to understand the link between genetic mutation and affected child.

THE GENERAL STRUCTURE OF FGFR
The FGFRs form a sub-family of the receptor tyrosine kinases. The FGF–FGFR interaction is facilitated by heparin and heparin sulphate proteoglycan, and there is evidence that the availability of HSPG is functionally limiting (Ornitz 2000). The human FGFR family

of genes encodes a group of structurally related protein receptors of the tyrosine kinase subclass IV which are predominantly membrane-bound and transduce ligand interaction to intracellular-signal cascades. Four FGFR gene loci are identified: FGFR1 on chromosome 8p; FGFR2 on chromosome 10q; FGFR3 on chromosome 4p; and FGFR4 on chromosome 5q (Johnson and Williams 1993).

The full-length mammalian receptors share basic structure consisting of an extracellular domain, a transmembrane (TM) domain, and an intracellular region, incorporating a juxtamembranous (JM) domain and a split tyrosine kinase (TK) domain (Givol and Yayon 1992, Johnson and Williams 1993). The extracellular domain incorporates a number of (usually three) immunoglobulin-like loops (IgI–III), named for their similarity in structure to immunoglobulins, which contain a similar distribution of intra-molecular Cys–Cys disulphide bonds (Fig. 3.1). The different human FGFR homologues show great sequence conservation, in particular within the IgII-loop, the IgII–III linker sequence, and the IgIIIc-loop isoforms of the extracellular domain. A table of human FGFR sequence homology is shown in Table 3.2.

Despite the high level of FGFR sequence homology, a high degree of receptor diversity results from mRNA splice events that generate protein receptors with variable sequence composition within the extracellular domain. Splice variance may generate extracellular domains variously lacking the IgI-loop, the acid box, and CAM homology domain (Johnson and Williams 1993). The 'short-form' receptors retain their ligand-binding ability, suggesting that the interaction between FGFR and ligand FGF is predominantly a function of the

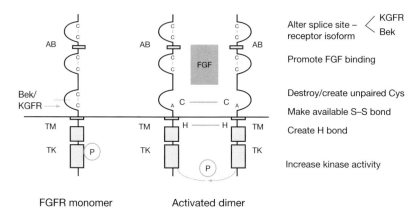

Fig. 3.1 Normal FGFR monomer structure is characterised by three, extracellular, immunoglobulin-like loops. These are maintained by disulphide links between the cysteine moieties (C). The 'bek' and 'kgfr' isoforms are characterised by different sequences in the 3rd Ig-like loop. The monomers form a dimer when activated by an FGF ligand, and the intracellular split tyrosine kinase moiety generates a phosphorylation, and thereby intracellular signal transduction. Mutated FGFRs generate gain-of-function by different mechanisms, including inter-monomer hydrogen bonds (H–H), inter-monomer disulphide bridges (C–C), facilitated FGF binding, increased kinase activity, and increased expression of alternative isoforms.

TABLE 3.2
The degree of amino acid identity between the IgIIIc isoforms
(3-Ig loop structure) of the receptor (Johnson and Williams 1993)

	FGFR2	FGFR3	FGFR4
FGFR1	72%	62%	55%
FGFR2		66%	57%
FGFR3			61%

IgII and IgIII loops and the intervening linker-region amino acid sequence (Hou et al 1992, Cheon et al 1994). In the membrane-bound FGFRs, the transmembrane domain anchors the protein to the hydophobic cell membrane and is accompanied by a relatively long juxtamembranous region (Johnson and Williams 1993). The intracellular split TK domain of the FGFR group contains a 13–14 sequence insert, which defines the receptor family amongst the receptor tyrosine kinases (Johnson and Williams 1993, Green et al 1996). It consists of a number of consensus tyrosine residues that may act as phosphate acceptors for autophosphorylation. The TK domain adjoins the intracellular COOH tail of the receptor, which contains tyrosine residues that may be phosphorylated upon receptor activation (Johnson and Williams 1993).

FGFR SPLICE VARIANCE AND LIGAND-RECEPTOR SPECIFICITY

FGFR variants are generated by alternative splicing of mRNA (Champion Arnaud et al 1991, Johnson et al 1991), to deliver an unprecedented degree of receptor diversity (Johnson and Williams 1993). The generic structure of the FGFR genes provides a basis for the number and types of splice variants observed. FGFR1 protein is encoded by 19 exons (Johnson et al 1991). The extracellular domain is encoded by nine exons, within which the IIIb isoform is encoded by exon 8, and the IIIc isoform is encoded by exon 9. Extended to FGFR2, which has a similar exon arrangement, the IgIIIa/c isoform (exons 7/9) is translated to the BEK (originally identified as bacterially expressed kinase) receptor, and the IgIIIa/b isoform (exons 7/8) forms the KGFR (keratinocyte growth factor receptor) protein in both humans and mice (Miki et al 1992, Werner et al 1992, Yayon et al 1992). Hence two functional receptor proteins are generated from a single gene, which differ within a confined internal amino acid sequence occupying a critical loop within the extracellular ligand-binding domain.

A hierarchy of mRNA splicing events determines a wide range of receptor protein variants (observed in FGFR1, 2 and 3) that differ in:

1   the number of Ig-like loops of the extracellular domain of the receptor;
2   the presence of the acid-box and the –COOH terminal sequence to generate variable 'short-form' receptors;
3   the presence of a TM domain, absence of which correlates with various secreted forms of FGFR. (It may be that the secreted and cytosolic forms act as a regulatory mechanism in the tissue matrix for the availability of FGF ligand.)

4   the presence and structural integrity of the the TK domain. (The truncated kinase form lacks the potential for self-phosphorylation. Such a receptor could theoretically play a modulatory functional role in the membrane by acting as a dominant-negative receptor in heterodimers with active receptors.)

The IgIIIb and IgIIIc isoforms of FGFR2 differ by a sequence of approximately 50 residues (Johnson and Williams 1993). Laboratory constructs of receptor 'chimeras' indicate that ligand-receptor specificity is dictated by the linker-region amino acid sequence and a few residues into each neighbouring (IgII and IgIII) loop (Wang et al 1995). Replacement of the BEK/IgIIIc sequence of FGFR2 with that of KGFR/IgIIIb donates the chimeric construct the high affinity binding for FGF7 of the KGFR-wild-type, and abrogates its affinity for FGF2 (Yayon et al 1992). FGFR1 and FGFR3 also demonstrate splice variance of the IgIII-loop, with IIIb and IIIc isoforms that differ in their ligand affinity.

The gene structure of FGFR is therefore demonstrated to allow for several forms of the receptor, generated by alternative splicing, splice-site skipping, and polyadenylation – which allows transcription of intronic sites (Givol and Yayon 1992). This receptor heterogeneity may account for some of the plasticity of the genotype–phenotype relationship.

The frequency of splice variation in the transcription of the FGFR genes is reflected by the variability of the clinical FGFR mutant forms in human skeletal dysplasias. Splice-site mutations affecting exon 7 of FGFR2 are established in a subgroup of mutant human FGFR2-phenotypes, recognised as Pfeiffer, Crouzon and Jackson–Weiss syndromes (Lajeunie et al 1995, Li et al 1995, Schell et al 1995). These mutations cause abnormal splice events in FGFR2 which yield stable transcript RNA and stable altered IgIIIc receptor. The upregulation of abnormal splice variants in human craniofacial (Britto et al 2001a, 2001c) and digital (Oldridge et al 1999, Britto et al 2001b) development, possibly facilitating

TABLE 3.3
Ligand affinity of FGFR isoforms

	FGF1	FGF2	FGF3	FGF4	FGF5	FGF6	FGF7	FGF8	FGF9
FGFR1 -IIIc	100	100	-	100	60	55	-	-	20
FGFR1 -IIIb	100	60	35	15	-	-	-	-	-
FGFR2 -IIIc	100	65	-	100	25	60	-	16	90
FGFR2 -IIIb	100	-	45	15	-	-	80	-	-
FGFR3 -IIIc	100	107	-	70	12	-	-	40	95
FGFR3 -IIIb	100	-	-	-	-	-	-	-	41
FGFR4	100	110	-	110	-	80	-	75	75

Note: Values represent % incorporation of (3H)-thymidine in standardised assay compared to response to FGF1 (De Moerlooze et al 2000, Kannan and Givol 2000).

the recruitment of a different ligand range, may be a contributary factor in the pathogenesis of the syndromic phenotypes.

FGFR ACTIVATION: THE ROLE OF LIGAND AND MATRIX CO-FACTORS

An increasing number of activating FGF ligands are identified, which act in a very wide range of developmental and physiological roles, including many facets of embryo-foetal development, neovascularisation and responses to wound healing (Johnson and Williams 1993, Mason, 1994, Green et al 1996). The FGFs are structurally related and highly conserved in vertebrate evolution. Human FGFs show a high level of sequence conservation (Givol and Yayon 1992), suggesting that this three-dimensional structure is likely to be a common theme within the group (FGF4 and FGF2 have ~40 per cent sequence homology, FGF5 and FGF2 have ~50 per cent homology, but FGF7 has only ~30 per cent homology with FGF2). This homogeneity of structure might indicate a high degree of functional redundancy within the group, and commonality of control mechanisms for ligand bio-availability and receptor signalling. FGF diversity is generated by alternative splicing, alternative translation events, and post-translational modifications, including glycosylation, methylation, phosphorylation and nucleotidylation (Mason 1994). FGFs are expressed throughout mammalian development and maturity (Johnson and Williams 1993) in an often overlapping but tissue-specific manner. FGF2, FGF4 and FGF7 are differentially expressed with their receptors in human craniofacial development (Britto et al 2001a, 2001c), and the availability of ligand is likely to be significant to the relationship between genotype and phenotype in development.

A number of studies correlate FGF/FGFR interaction with a limiting requirement for heparin or heparin sulphate proteoglycan. Heparin sulphate proteoglycans (HSPG) are a core constituent of many tissue matrices. Studies in Drosophila provide direct evidence of a physiological role for HSPGs in FGF/FGFR signalling (Ornitz 2000). This evidence of a limiting functional role for HSPG components in FGF/FGFR signalling, which is generally highly conserved, correlates with the diversity of human FGFR-phenotypes. It is probable that activating human FGFR mutations, set against a variable background of matrix composition, will generate variable phenotypic effects.

How do FGFR mutations cause disease phenotypes?

A CLASSIFICATION OF FGFR MUTATIONS: CORRELATING RECEPTOR
'GAIN-OF-FUNCTION' WITH CLINICAL PHENOTYPE

In general, the syndromic craniofacial dysostoses are primarily characterised by the presence of craniosynostosis and are caused by mutations of the extracellular domain of FGFR2. Exceptions include the predilection for proline to arginine substitutions in the IgII–IgIII linker, which occur in FGFR1 (Pro252Arg causing Pfeiffer syndrome), FGFR2 (Pro253Arg causing Apert syndrome) and FGFR3 (Pro250Arg defining a non-specific coronal synostosis syndrome). Furthermore, transmembrane mutations cause non-specific craniosynostosis (Pulleyn et al 1996), Beare–Stevenson cutis gyrata (Przylepa et al 1996), and Crouzon syndrome (Passos-Bueno et al 1999) in FGFR2; and Crouzon-acanthosis nigricans in

FGFR3 (Meyers et al 1995, Wilkes et al 1996). The phenotypes generated by these mutations implicate FGFR1, 2 and 3 proteins in both membranous (craniosynostosis, midface retrusion), and endochondral (skull base, tracheal anomalies, digital anomalies) ossification, as well as the developmental mechanisms of epithelio-mesenchymal signalling.

Most of the FGFR mutations causing human skeletal dysplasias are mis-sense, with a smaller number of splicing mutations, small insertions, and deletions. The mutations remain in-frame, and there are no non-sense or frame-shift mutations which might associate with loss-of-function (Wilkie 1997). In contrast, mutations of the TWIST gene causing Saethre–Chotzen syndrome are predominantly non-sense and 21 bp duplications, and are predicted, by analogy with experimental evidence in the analogous E47 transcription factor (Voronova and Baltimore 1990), to cause funtional loss. A strong clinical resemblance exists between some patients with the FGFR3-P250R mutation and the Saethre–Chotzen phenotype, which implies that TWIST and FGFR occupy the same signalling pathway.

There is considerable evidence that FGFR mutations will convey functional gain upon the receptor, while TWIST mutations result in haplo-insufficiency. All the FGFR mutations described thus far are dominantly acting. The mutant protein acts in a cellular environment containing the wild-type allele and all the various endogenous mechanisms for in-built functional redundancy. Whereas the TWIST null-heterozygote mouse has a craniofacial and limb phenotype that is reminiscent of the human heterozygote (El Ghouzzi et al 1997, Bourgeois et al 1998), models of FGFR loss of function do not model human skeletal dysplasia. Studies in Xenopus, chick and mouse, using dominant-negative receptor constructs expressed with tissue-specific promoters, imply non-redundant roles for FGFR in a variety of fundamental processes (Amaya et al 1991, 1993, Deng et al 1994, Peters et al 1994, Yamaguchi et al 1994, Deng et al 1997, Xu et al 1998). Theoretically, therefore, a dominant-negative mechanism for FGFR mutants in human disease, which donate absolute loss of function, would suggest *in utero* lethality. Various 'knock-out' models support this contention while demonstrating the fundamental role of fgfr-signalling which appears highly conserved throughout development. In this context it is interesting to note new evidence that Apert mutations, which can cause loss of FGFR-FGF binding specificity (Yu et al 2000), may act in a competitive, partially dominant-negative, exquisite loss of function manner to cause Apert cleft palate (Britto et al 2002).

PATHOLOGICAL FGFR MUTATIONS FOLLOW NON-RANDOM 'THEMES'
The extensive crossover between FGFR gene mutation and syndromic craniofacial dysostosis phenotype is well established. Many mutations in FGFR1 and FGFR2 generate phenotypic heterogeneity. Specific FGFR3 mutations generate craniofacial dysostoses without the dwarfism that characterises so many FGFR3 mutations (Moloney et al 1997, Muenke et al 1997). Despite the various complexities, human FGFR mutations follow non-random 'themes', and may be usefully divided into various groups according to their position within the highly conserved receptor structure, and/or the effect which they impose upon receptor function *in vivo*. In the subsequent sections, therefore, these mutations are grouped according to certain common features, by which some mutations may unavoidably fall into more than one class.

MUTATIONS THAT CHARACTERISE COMPARABLE POSITIONS IN
FGFR1, FGFR2 AND FGFR3 BUT ENCODE DIFFERENT PHENOTYPES

1 Proline-arginine substitutions in the IgII–IgIII linker
The substitution of the highly conserved proline residue by arginine in the extracellular
IgII–IgIII linker sequence (Pro-252 in FGFR1) is common to the three FGFRs associated
with human skeletal dysplasia (Bellus et al 1996). The substitution of arginine introduces
a bulky side-chain amino acid and creates a change of orientation in the linker. The P-R
is predicted to create aberrant interactions between ligand FGF and FGFR. A study of
the affinity of the Apert linker region for ligand indicates that both the Pro253Arg and the
Ser252Trp linker-region mutations display selectively altered binding affinity (Anderson
et al 1998a). The affinity of FGF2 for Ser252Trp is greater than that for Pro253Arg, which
is greater than that for wild-type. The effect is quantitatively less for FGF1, and no different
from wild-type with FGF4, thus providing functional evidence that the hydrogen-bonds
formed by the FGFR linker sequence and ligand sequences are exquisitely sensitive
(Plotnikov et al 2000). Recent evidence suggests that the Apert Ser252Trp and Pro253Arg
mutations in FGFR2 cause loss of ligand specificity of the IgIIIc/BEK and IgIIIb/KGFR
isoforms for FGF2, and FGF7 or FGF10, respectively (Yu et al 2000), further illustrating
the functional sensitivity of the linker sequence. The substitution of specific residues in the
linker has specific phenotypic consequences (Slaney et al 1996, Britto et al 2002), which
are thus likely to reflect specific ligand-receptor kinetics. Given the sequence conservation,
it seems likely that the P-R mutations of FGFR1 and FGFR3 will have similar functional
effect upon ligand kinetics, which will be conducted via both IgIIIb and IgIIIc forms of the
receptor protein.

The functional effect of the Pro252Arg mutation in FGFR1 (Pfeiffer syndrome) has been
modelled in Xenopus (Neilson and Friesel 1996). As might be predicted from the studies of
Anderson et al (1998), the Xenopus xfgfr1-P160R mutation consistently binds more radio-
labelled FGF1 and FGF2 than the wild-type receptor. However, the xfgfr1-P160R mutant,
in comparison to wild-type receptor, failed to show increases in tyrosine phosphorylation or
elongation of animal pole ectoderm, despite such increases displayed by Xenopus models
of other classes of activating FGFR mutation (Neilson and Friesel 1996). This raises the
possibility that the ligand-dependent mutations of the linker region of the extracellular domain
of the FGFRs may be quantitatively less activating than certain cysteine altering mutations
or transmembrane mutations examined in the same system. The different human clinical
phenotypes of the linker-region P-R mutations in each of FGFR1, 2 and 3 (Pfeiffer, Apert,
'non-syndromic' craniosynostosis, respectively) will, therefore, reflect the specifics of ligand-
receptor activation as well as their relative bioavailability in human skeletal development.

2 Comparable transmembrane region mutations in FGFR2 and FGFR3

2.1 Glycine-arginine mis-sense mutations. Glycine-to-arginine mutations in the transmembrane regions of FGFR2 and FGFR3 cause very different syndromes. Glycine is
substituted by arginine at Gly384 in FGFR2 to cause an unclassified craniosynostosis

(Gly384Arg), featuring coronal and sagittal synostosis and choanal stenosis (Pulleyn et al 1996). By contrast, the corresponding mutation in FGFR3, Gly380Arg, causes the relatively invariable achondroplasia phenotype with one of the highest mutation rates in the human genome. The neutral glycine residue is replaced by a basic, bulky, arginine in each case and, given the sequence homology between the receptors, could be expected to effect the same functional change.

Receptor chimeras of the Neu receptor with the transmembrane domain of wild-type or achondroplasia mutant FGFR3 are observed to generate different tyrosine kinase activity via the Neu-TK domain in NIH3T3-fibroblast cell lines (Webster and Donoghue 1996). The Gly380Arg construct showed a ligand-independent increase in kinase activity over the wild-type, and successfully transformed the NIH3T3 cells, an effect which was corroborated in full-length FGFR3. The Gly380Arg mutation significantly increased receptor tyrosine phosphorylation over control, with constitutive induction of mesodermal muscle-specific actin transcript, and the elongation of Xenopus cap mesoderm (Neilson and Friesel 1996). Receptor chimeras of the murine fgfr3-Gly380Arg receptor, with a substituted fgfr1-tyrosine-kinase domain, did not constitutively stimulate kinase activity, however, despite being moderately mitogenic in a BaF3 transfected cell line (Naski et al 1996).

The sequence homology of the TM region of FGFR2 and FGFR3 suggests that the Gly-Arg mis-sense substitution will have the same functional effect in the two receptors, which will be enacted through all the natural extracellular-domain isoforms of each. Both mutations generate relatively mild phenotypes within the range of clinical phenotypes to which each belongs: achondroplasia compared to severe thanatophoric dysplasia, and mild craniosynostosis compared to the Crouzon–Pfeiffer phenotypes. In each case the phenotype may reflect the relatively weak mutant receptor dimerisation, via putative hydrogen bonds created by the arginine substitution (Webster and Donoghue 1996). In comparison, the mutations causing thanatophoric dysplasia (Naski et al 1996, Webster et al 1996), and Crouzon-type phenotypes (Neilson and Friesel, 1995, 1996, Robertson et al 1998) are highly activating. Graded activation of the receptor by geographically distinct mutations may thus reflect severity of phenotype in both human mutant FGFR2 and FGFR3 syndromes. Furthermore, the difference between the craniofacial phenotypes of achondroplasia (FGFR3) and craniosynostosis (FGFR2) will reflect, in part, the differential expression of the receptors in human craniofacial development (Britto et al 2001c)

2.2 Cysteine substitutions in the juxtamembranous-transmembrane domain. Cysteine substitutions in the transmembrane regions of FGFR2 and FGFR3 also result in different skeletal dysplasia phenotypes. The Ser372Cys and Tyr375Cys mutations in FGFR2 result in Beare–Stevenson cutis gyrata, whereas the corresponding Tyr373Cys and Gly375Cys mutations in FGFR3 cause thanatophoric dysplasia type 1 and achondroplasia respectively. The introduction of cysteine residues to the transmembrane domain has been shown to be activating in independent systems (Thompson et al 1997). The Gly375Cys mutation in FGFR3, the less common of the two achondroplasia mutations, is activating in a chimera with the extracellular domain of the platelet derived growth factor receptor (PDGF) (Thompson et al 1997).

3 FGFR mutations which alter the functional availability of cysteine residues in the extracellular domain

The introduction or replacement of cysteine residues is a common and functionally defining theme of certain mutations in the extracellular domain of FGFR2 and FGFR3. The Cys278 and Cys342 in FGFR2 are very commonly mutated (Reardon et al 1994b, Park et al 1995b, Passos-Bueno et al 1999), and the non-specificity of the mis-sense replacement predicts that functional gain is delivered by the removal of the cysteine residue. Both these positions are crucial to the structure of the IgIII-loop of the protein. The cysteine residues form intra-molecular covalent disulphide bonds and are thus integral to the structural integrity of the protein. The removal of one of the cysteine residues would be predicted to unfurl the IgIII-loop and leave the partner residue free to form intra-molecular covalent bonds. Candidate molecules for such bonds include other mutant alleles within the membrane, and create the opportunity for mutant receptor dimerisation in the absence of ligand. The Cys278 and Cys342 residues are highly conserved between the members of the FGFR family, and mutations in the equivalent positions in FGFR1 have been shown to abolish ligand binding (Hou et al 1992). The loss of ligand binding by such mutants suggests that the structural integrity of the IgIII domain is functionally limiting in the interaction of FGFR and ligand FGF (Zhu et al 1997, Passos-Bueno et al 1999, Plotnikov et al 2000). These data provide the molecular basis for observations that certain FGFR2 IgIII-mutations in the Crouzon–Pfeiffer group of syndromes abrogate ligand binding and are constitutively activating (Neilson and Friesel 1995, 1996).

Constitutive activation of the receptor by mutations that directly or indirectly alter the functional availability of cysteine has been demonstrated in a number of systems. The Cys342Tyr mutation, modelled in Xenopus, induces ligand-independent FGFR-dimerisation, tyrosine kinase activity, expression of the mesodermal markers Xbra and muscle alpha actin, and the induction of mesodermal elongation (Neilson and Friesel 1995). The response is dose-dependent upon the amount of mutant receptor and provides a possible explanation for the range of phenotype severity in these syndromes, which may reflect the degree of activation established by each individual mutation. Further studies in the same system examine the Xenopus analogues of the common clinical mutation FGFR2 Cys-278; an xfgfr1-Cys249Tyr mutation which also results in an unpaired cysteine; and a double FGFR2 mutation that disrupts the IgIII-loop without the generation of an unpaired cysteine residue (xfgfr2-c268F/C332Y). Results suggest that it is the availability of cysteine that potentiates ligand-independent dimerisation and activation of the mutant receptor (Neilson and Friesel 1996, Robertson et al 1998).

The FGFR2-Cys342Tyr has been modelled in a chimera of the Neu-transmembrane and tyrosine kinase domains. The mutant extracellular domain of the FGFR2 was able to induce signal transduction via the Neu chimera and induce focus formation in the NIH3T3 fibroblast cell line. Similar results were obtained for the Cys342Arg and Cys342Ser mutations, as well as the Tyr340His and Ser254Cys mutations (Galvin et al 1996). All of the mutations induced tyrosine kinase activity and formed disulphide bonded dimers, thus raising the question whether non-cysteine mutations causing the Crouzon–Pfeiffer phenotypes can modulate similar effects to those directly creating free cysteine residues. The Trp290Gly and Thr341Pro mutations cause Crouzon (Park et al 1995b) and Pfeiffer (Rutland et al 1995) syndromes, respectively, and each is adjacent to a conserved IgIII-loop-dependent cysteine residue (Cys278 and Cys342) in the 3D structure (Plotnikov et al 2000). When expressed as FGFR2/Neu chimeras, both mutations cause transformation of NIH3T3 cells compared to the mis-sense substitutions Cys278Phe and Cys342Tyr acting as positive controls (Robertson et al 1998). Transforming activity was lost when these non-cysteine mutations were combined with double mutation constructs replacing the Cys278 and Cys342 with alanine, thereby suggesting that the non-cysteine mutations confer activation by virtue of their intact cysteine neighbour. These data suggest that mutations, which by their proximity to conserved cysteine residues disrupt the IgIII-loop Cys=Cys disulphide bond, activate the receptor when inter-molecular disulphide bonds are created by default (Plotnikov et al 2000). Such a mechanism might explain the observation that the FGFR2-Ser267Pro Crouzon-mutant receptors migrate as a dimer in polyacrylamide gel electrophoresis studies, despite abrogation of FGF2 ligand binding (Anderson et al 1998a).

4 Phenotypic diversity generated by cysteine-related and other mutations in FGFR2

Studies in Xenopus blastomeres indicate that FGFR2-Cys342Tyr mutant function is dose-dependent (Neilson and Friesel 1995). A range of phenotypes is described with this mutation, Crouzon and Pfeiffer syndromes in particular, and the observed range reflects the degree of functional gain, as well as epigenetic influences and the genetic environment of the individual. Epigenetic influences, such as the effect of the growing brain on the neurocranium, or influences *in utero*, may influence the range of phenotypes generated by specific mutations. Such phenomena might explain the variability of phenotype within the FGFR2-A334G Jackson–Weiss kindred (Winter and Reardon 1996), the phenotypes from the splicing mutation G1044A at codon 344 of FGFR2 (Steinberger et al 1996), and the FGFR3-P250R group of phenotypes.

5 Amino acid substitutions with sensitive effects upon the phenotype

5.1 Linker-region substitutions in FGFR2 and FGFR3.   The degree of conservation of the IgII–IgIII linker-region sequence, and the demonstration of the exquisite specificity and functional sensitivity of the region to disruption (Anderson et al 1998a, Plotnikov et al 2000), provide a basis for the observation that the phenotypes generated by mutations in the linker are highly specific. Ser252Trp and Ser252Phe result in Apert syndrome, whereas Ser252Leu generates both mild Crouzon and normal phenotypes in the same family (Oldridge et al 1997). The Ser252Leu mutation demonstrates normal FGF dissociation kinetics under experimental conditions compared to the selective increased ligand affinity displayed by Ser252Trp and Pro253Arg (Anderson et al 1998a). It may be that the Ser252Leu mutation facilitates the genetic background for epigenetic influences to propagate a mild craniofacial dysostosis phenotype. A similar theory has been advanced to explain unicoronal synostosis resulting from the FGFR2-Ala315Ser mutation and breech presentation (Johnson et al 2000a). Further evidence of the genotype-phenotype specificity

56

demonstrated by the linker-region mis-sense substitutions is given by the rare double mutation Ser252Phe and Pro253Ser, which generates a Pfeiffer phenotypic variant, with mild craniosynostosis, broad thumbs and toes, digital joint anomalies but minimal syndactyly. It may be that certain 'Apert' phenotypic features which demonstrate a range of expressivity, such as syndactyly or cleft palate (in only 70 per cent of Apert cases), become manifest under variable conditions of specific ligand-mutant receptor kinetics (Britto et al 2001b, 2002).

The sensitivity of the phenotype to specific linker-region mutations is demonstrated by the Arg248Cys mutation and the Pro250Arg neighbouring substitution in FGFR3, which cause the mutually exclusive phenotypes of thanatophoric dysplasia (TD) I and coronal synostosis, respectively. The FGFR3-Pro250Arg probably causes a selective increase in ligand affinity and is moderately activating by analogy with the Xenopus xfgfr1 mutant (Neilson and Friesel 1996). In contrast, the Arg248Cys mutation, modelled in the BaF3 transfected cell line, is highly activating, demonstrating maximal mitogenicity against positive and negative controls (Naski et al 1996). The introduction of the cysteine confers constitutive dimerisation and tyrosine phosphorylation, which can be further stimulated by ligand FGF1 to higher levels of kinase activity (Naski et al 1996). The substitution of the cysteine residue appears to be critical to the activating effect of the mutation. FGFR3-Arg248Cys is dimerising and comparatively highly activating as a Neu/FGFR3 chimera in NIH3T3 fibroblasts, which are driven to focus formation by the mutant constructs (D'Avis et al 1998) compared to control.

The differential activation conferred by the two mutations has a parallel in their phenotypes. TD1, the result of the consitutive Arg248Cys mutation, has a particularly severe skeletogenic phenotype, whereas the Pro250Arg, presumptively a ligand-dependent muta-tion, generates a variable phenotype without substantial effects upon stature. The different craniofacial phenotypes of the two mutations may reflect their differential activation and the expression of FGFR3 in human basicranial development (Britto et al 2001c).

6 FGFR mutations which create stable splice variants
Several mutations causing craniosynostosis phenotypes are proposed to cause aberrant splicing of FGFR2 (Reardon et al 1994b, Lajeunie et al 1995, Li et al 1995, Schell et al 1995, Meyers et al 1996, Steinberger et al 1996). These mutations are projected to yield various stable transcript RNAs and stable altered receptor proteins. An interesting set of splicing mutations may correlate with the pathogenesis of variable syndactyly in the limb phenotype of FGFR2-craniofacial dysostosis syndromes (Schell et al 1995, Passos-Bueno et al 1997, Anderson et al 1998b, Oldridge et al 1999, Britto et al 2001b).

Oldridge et al (1999) correlated the site of these mutations with the probability that they create stable splice variants of FGFR2 transcripts, and demonstrated in three patients an upregulation of the IgIIIb/KGFR mRNA in fibroblast cell lines derived from skin. The authors' attempt to quantify the relative upregulation of KGFR as a percentage of the expression of both IgIIIc/BEK and KGFR can be criticised, and the resulting conclusions cannot be applied unchallenged to the *in vivo* model. However, the selective expression of KGFR in the metaphyseal domain in human digital development, and its upregulation in human craniosynostosis, correlates with both the syndactyly and suture fusion human phenotypes (Britto et al 2001a, 2001b).

7 Variable pathways of FGFR activation may contribute to phenotype diversity
Activating FGFR mutations may result in accelerated membranous osseous differentiation but inhibition of chondrogenesis. This suggests that the mechanisms of activation of FGFR are multiple and may be cell-type specific. Several intracellular pathways may be activated by FGFRs, involving Ras and Raf proteins, mitogen activated protein kinase (MAPK), phosphatidyl-inositol 3 kinase (PI-3K), protein tyrosine phosphatases, and phospholipase C1 (Wilson 1994). Ras and MAPK are involved in a linear signalling pathway, which maintains the level of MAPK activation above a threshold level to enable phosphorylation of target molecules, including transcription factors, which may then modify gene expression. Dominant-negative Ras proteins and MAPK-inhibitors may be used to successfully inhibit FGFR activation in models of human mutations (Neilson and Friesel 1995, Naski et al 1996, Neilson and Friesel 1996). Similarly, dominantly active signalling by Ras can induce vertebrate neuronal differentiation in a manner similar to FGFR, which is reversed in a dominant-negative Ras model (Chao 1992). Linear activation of the Ras-MAPK pathway can be achieved by the alternate/combined use of intracellular cascades involving phospholipase C and protein kinase C; and increased complexity is generated by the utilisation of different molecular variants of individual proteins in these pathways (Wilson 1994).

The Ras-MAPK pathway is highly conserved, and its major steps are non-redundant (Wilson 1994). Genetic modelling in Drosophila raises the possibility that in certain systems the absolute level of MAPK activation is the major prerequisite for a phenotypic response, and that the specific activating ligand-receptor event is at least partially redundant. If this was the case in vertebrate skeletogenesis *in vivo*, one might expect gain-of-function human mutant FGFR signalling in cells of osteogenic lineage to be modified by parallel pathways reducing MAPK activation in a variable dominant-negative fashion. Phenotypic response may depend on the degree of MAPK activation, and might provide an alternative molecular mechanism for human phenotypic diversity amongst FGFR-syndromic patients. Further and independent activation pathways include the internalisation of FGF and its direct effect upon the nucleus (Mason 1994, Prudovsky et al 1996), which will elicit a phenotypic response independently of the Ras-MAPK system (Legeai-Mallet et al 1998).

How does FGFR gain of function cause human skeletal prematurity?
Receptor 'gain of function' causes human disease phenotypes, which are characterised by skeletal fusions (digits, elbows, vertebrae, cranial sutures), and osseous prematurity (midface retrusion, skull base stenosis). The link between receptor functional gain and affected child can be found in studies that investigate FGFR function in skeletogenesis. A number of studies demonstrate that a tissue-specific control of FGFR signalling is achieved by the differential expression of FGFR homologues in chicken (Patstone et al 1993, Wilke et al 1997), mouse (Orr-Urtreger et al 1991, Peters et al 1992, 1993) and human (Delezoide et al 1998, Chan and Thorogood, 1999). The expression patterns of the various genes in human development *in situ* further provide a means to correlate mutant gene

function with clinical phenotype (Britto et al 2001a, 2001b, 2001c, 2002). Many of the FGFR2 mutations causing human craniofacial dysostosis are predicted to affect both major functional splice variants of FGFR2 protein (BEK or FGFR2-IgIIIc; and KGFR or FGFR2-IgIIIb), and thus may allow genotype–phenotype correlation by means of their differential tissue expression.

Studies in human cranial suture fusion indicate that FGFR1 expression characterises a proliferative osteogenic precursor, whereas FGFR2-BEK expression characterises the differentiated osteoblast. The FGFR2-KGFR isoform is transiently upregulated in the sutural osteogenic front during human suture fusion (Britto et al 2001a). Thus FGFR2 expression is consistent with membranous osseous differentiation, whereas FGFR1 expression accompanies a pre-differentiated, proliferative phenotype, which is highly consistent with the clinical phenotypes. FGFR2 syndromes show patterns of advanced coronal sutural fusions and midface retrusion, whereas the FGFR1-Pfeiffer syndrome is considered to be a milder phenotype (Muenke and Schell 1995, Rutland et al 1995, Schell et al 1995). It should be noted that murine FGFR1 expression has been correlated with osseous differentiation and murine FGFR2 expression with proliferation (Iseki et al 1999, Johnson et al 2000b). This is consistent with a mouse Pfeiffer syndrome FGFR1-model (Zhou et al 2000), but not with the human clinical situation. It is probable, therefore, that subtle, species-specific differences in FGFR function exist. In these circumstances, the application of experimentation in mouse models to the development of human therapies must be suitably guarded.

In vitro studies in human osteoblasts further indicate that FGFR2 signalling promotes osteogenesis. FGFR2 mutations in Apert osteoblasts in culture demonstrate an increased calcified bone matrix, and an increased expression of molecular markers of osseous differentiation (alkaline phosphatase, osteocalcin, and type 1 collagen), compared to age-matched controls (Lomri et al 1998). Increases in matrix molecule production are observed in Apert fibroblasts (Bodo et al 1997) and osteoblasts (Locci et al 1999), and increased transforming growth factor ß1 production and secretion are also observed over control osteoblasts (Locci et al 1999). No differences are observed in Apert osteoblast growth or the cellular incorporation of tritiated thymidine, however, suggesting that the activating Apert (Ser252Trp) FGFR2 mutation causes accelerated differentiation, rather than a proliferative effect (Lomri et al 1998). Consistent with this, activated FGFR2 mutant osteoblasts from Apert (Pro253Arg) and Pfeiffer (Cys342Arg) patients exhibit lower proliferation rates than control osteoblasts (Fragale et al 1999), and the heterogeneous phenotypes for osseous differentiation that are observed reflect the maturity differences in the various calvariae examined.

Can FGFR expression in human craniofacial development explain phenotype diversity?

FGFR3 PHENOTYPES
FGFR3 is the least uniformly expressed FGFR homologue as protein in the human cranial suture, and throughout human cranial development. Consistently, FGFR3 protein is also

weakly expressed in the cranial mesenchyme and dura mater at 10 weeks of human cranial development (Britto et al 2001c). This suggests that FGFR3 has a limited, possibly redundant, role in human cranial morphogenesis and sutural molecular signalling pathways. Nevertheless, human craniosynostosis results from the activating FGFR3-Pro250Arg mutation (Moloney et al 1997, Muenke et al 1997, Reardon et al 1997), and pan-synostosis occurs in conjunction with activating mutations of the transmembrane and tyrosine kinase domains (Tavormina et al 1995, Wilcox et al 1998). Given the relative paucity of FGFR3 expression in the human suture, it is likely that these severe synostosis phenotypes are generated by mutant FGFR3-heterodimers, recruiting FGFR1/2 signalling pathways in the sutural osteogenic precursor. Experimental evidence and FGFR sequence conservation suggest that the P250R mutation may be ligand-dependent and less functionally activating than the transmembrane or tyrosine kinase mutations (Neilson and Friesel 1996, Mangasarian et al 1997, Anderson et al 1998a, Mansukhani et al 2000), and this is reflected in the variability of the P250R craniosynostosis phenotype. The pathogenesis of severe sutural synostosis in Crouzon-acanthosis nigricans and the thanatophoric dysplasias may thus reflect both the degree of mutant receptor activation and the ability of each mutant to form heterodimers in the induction of sutural osseous differentiation. FGFR-heterodimerisation occurs in the natural state in cells expressing FGFR homologues (Johnson and Williams 1993), and the use of dominant-negative constructs has demonstrated this phenomenon in several experimental models (Ueno et al 1992, Neilson and Friesel 1996). The great variability and cross-over of FGFR-associated craniosynostosis phenotype is, perhaps, the clinically evident reflection of the *in vivo* 'net' signal transduction in the sutural cell, influenced by the mutant FGFR (Nguyen et al 1997).

Despite some overlap (Bellus et al 1996), FGFR3 phenotypes tend to lack a midface retrusion phenotype compared to those of FGFR2 and FGFR1, but rather have a very variable craniosynostosis and limb involvement (Moloney et al 1997, Muenke et al 1997, Gripp et al 1998). It is, therefore, a notable correlate that while FGFR1 and FGFR2 isoforms are expressed in human midfacial osteogenesis, FGFR3 is very poorly expressed in the developing human midface (Britto et al 2001c). By contrast, highly specific FGFR3 regulation characterises human basicranial chondrogenic ossification (Britto et al 2001c). Various studies implicate FGFR3 in the negative regulation of endochondral ossification (Deng et al 1996, Chen et al 1999), and suggest that skull base ossification in FGFR3-mutants might progress upon a dysplastic cartilage template. This is consistent with observations of the cranial base in the mouse model of the activating achondroplasia FGFR3-Gly375Cys mutation. Premature ossification and closure of the basicranial synchondroses occurs, which results in an antero-posterior shortening of the skull base and secondary macrocephaly compared to age-matched wild-type (Chen et al 1999). The clinical correlate of this is the asymmetrical and dysplastic skull base observed in the chondrodysplasias, Crouzon-acanthosis nigricans, and the coronal synostoses.

Why do Apert and the Crouzon–Pfeiffer phenotypes differ, despite similarity of mutant genotype in FGFR2?

Apert syndrome (Apert 1906) features a narrow range of craniofacial dysmorphism including: pterional indrawing, a markedly foreshortened skull base, turribrachycephaly, severe midfacial retrusion with hypertelorism; and coronal sutural synostosis, with a widely unossified median sagittal diastema in place of metopic and sagittal sutures (Kreiborg and Cohen 1990, Kreiborg et al 1993, Cohen and Kreiborg 1994). The characteristic Apert cranial phenotype reflects a narrow mutational range within the FGFR2 gene. Two neighbouring 'linker-region' mutations in the IgIIIa extracellular subdomain of FGFR2 cause 98 per cent of Apert cases (Wilkie et al 1995) as a result of ligand-dependent 'gain of function' (Anderson et al 1998a).

By contrast, the related syndromes of Crouzon, Pfeiffer and Jackson–Weiss show a more variable and overlapping craniofacial dysmorphism. The basicranial sutures generally fuse earlier than in Apert syndrome, and the metopic and sagittal sutures form and fuse without the unossified median diastema (Kreiborg et al 1993, Cinalli et al 1995). Furthermore, facial retrusion may range from negligible to severe; and may variably affect the supraorbital or midfacial skeleton, with minimal pterional indrawing. The phenotypic variability within and between these syndromes reflects their mutational base. A wide range of mutations encompassing the extracellular and transmembrane domains of FGFR2 causes the 'Crouzon–Pfeiffer' group of syndromes, with greatest frequency in the IgIIIc subdomain of the FGFR2-IgIIIa/c (BEK) splice variant (Burke et al 1998). Many of these mutations result in the creation or removal of an unpaired cysteine residue, or affect a neighbouring site to cause conformational change and confer ligand-independent functional gain (Neilson and Friesel 1995, Galvin et al 1996, Neilson and Friesel 1996, Mangasarian et al 1997, Robertson et al 1998).

Studies in human tissues show that cases of Apert (FGFR2-P250R) and Pfeiffer (FGFR2-C278F) cranial morphogenesis cause negative autoregulation of FGFR2 expression in the *in situ* environment of human matrix co-factors and ligands (Britto et al 2001a). In concert with this process, the developing human basicranium is normally characterised by FGFR2 expression in concert with a more differentiated, mature stage of skeletogenesis, whereas the less skeletally mature mesenchyme towards the skull vertex is characterised by the expression of FGFR1. Apert mutant 'gain-of-function' (Anderson et al 1998a), phenotypically represented as premature ossification at the cellular level (Lomri et al 1998, Fragale et al 1999), is thus maximally demonstrated through a restricted and relatively mature domain of osteoblasts in the basicranial osteoid compared to the pre-osseous mesenchyme towards the cranial vertex. This correlates with the 'classic' clinical phenotype of the markedly foreshortened Apert basicranium and widely unossified vertical median diastema (Kreiborg and Cohen 1990). Apert frontal and parietal bone-fronts become widely splayed by the disproportionate basicranial ossification, such that initiation of Apert metopic and sagittal sutural morphogenesis (Johansen and Hall 1982) never occurs, and delayed ossification by coalescing islands of bone results by default (Kreiborg and Cohen 1990, Kreiborg et al 1993). Apert coronal synostosis, however, begins at the sphenoidal skull base. It is therefore suggested that Apert gain-of-function mutations, promoting mutant

FGFR2-homodimerisation (Anderson et al 1998a), 'drive' coronal sutural osteogenesis (Lemonnier et al 2000), despite normal dural influences to maintain sutural patency (Opperman et al 1995). The negative autoregulation of FGFR2-BEK, and differential FGFR expression relative to osteoblast maturity, also correlate with the marked infant Apert pterional stenosis phenotype. Apert pterional prematurity correlates with regulated FGFR2 expression in the 'pro-differentiated' membranous basicranium, whereas osteogenic precursor cells recruited into the early osteogenic pathway in domains towards the vertex will express FGFR1 predominantly.

Whereas 98 per cent of Apert cases are caused by ligand-dependent mutations in the extracellular 'linker region' (IgIIIa subdomain) of FGFR2 (Wilkie et al 1995, Oldridge et al 1999), Pfeiffer, Crouzon and related phenotypes show greater genetic heterogeneity. Although Pfeiffer syndrome may result from an FGFR1 mutation (Muenke et al 1994, Schell et al 1995), and a Crouzon variant arises from FGFR3 mutants (Meyers et al 1995), the majority of causative mutations are spread throughout the extracellular IgIIIc subdomain of the FGFR2-IgIIIa/c (BEK) isoform (Cornejo-Roldan et al 1999), mutations in which cause a variety of other craniosynostoses (Jabs et al 1994, Gorry et al 1995, Park et al 1995b, Przylepa et al 1996, Steinberger et al 1996, Tartaglia et al 1997, Reardon et al 2000). Many of these phenotypes are ascribed to different syndromes (Passos-Bueno et al 1999), which change longitudinally with time (Pulleyn et al 1996), giving rise to diagnostic confusion (Mulliken et al 1999). These variable 'Crouzon–Pfeiffer' phenotypes, lacking the Apert-type median diastema, markedly shortened skull base, and pterional indrawing, may be explained by the possible effect of ligand-independent FGFR heterodimerisation. Activated by mutations conferring ligand independence, these mutant FGFR2 proteins may form heterodimers (Ueno et al 1992, Johnson and Williams 1993) with FGFR1 and FGFR3, with which they are co-expressed in human membranous cranial ossification. Both homodimerisation and heterodimerisation by non-Apert FGFR2 mutants will occur in human tissues with a variable net intracellular signal as a result (Nguyen et al 1997). The variable osteoblast phenotype that results is in contrast to that of the pro-differentiated Apert osteoblast (Lomri et al 1998, Fragale et al 1999). Mutant FGFR2-heterodimerisation by constitutive mutations causing 'Crouzon–Pfeiffer' phenotypes would allow recruitment of the FGFR1 and FGFR3 expression domains. In this case, constitutive heterodimers would recruit the pre-osseous cranial mesenchyme by means of FGFR1 and FGFR3 signalling pathways, to promote cranial osteogenesis beyond the negatively-autoregulated mutant FGFR2 domain. The resultant 'Crouzon–Pfeiffer' phenotypes lack the distinctive pterional stenosis of Apert syndrome, by encompassing a wide domain of cranial mesenchyme in the pathogenic process via FGFR1 or FGFR3 heterodimers. Thus there is no median mesenchymal diastema, and a variable pattern of craniosynostosis that may involve all sutures results.

Epithelio-mesenchymal interactions account for a variety of normal processes in craniofacial development (Hall 1981, Wedden 1987, Richman and Tickle 1992, Matovinovic and Richman 1997, Francis-West et al 1998). The development of cranial mesenchyme is dependent upon epidermis (Tyler 1983), and osseoinduction by the dura mater can be driven by epithelium in heterotopic sites (Yu et al 1997). The KGFR isoform of FGFR2 is normally poorly expressed in both 14-week and 10-month human cranial ossification. KGFR is, however, strongly expressed in the osteoblasts of the para-sagittal osteogenic front of the 27-week C278F Pfeiffer fetus, and is also expressed in the mesenchymal domain (Britto et al 2001a). This preliminary evidence that KGFR is ectopically expressed in forms of cranial ossification correlates with the observation that splicing mutations in FGFR2 may upregulate KGFR and provide a novel pathogenetic mechanism for syndactyly (Oldridge et al 1999, Britto et al 2001b). The ectopic expression of KGFR in craniofacial dysostosis/ craniosynostosis would recruit a specific group of high-affinity FGF ligands, perhaps made available by the overlying dermis or subjacent dura mater/brain. The FGF4 and FGF7 genes are not co-expressed with KGFR, but other possible ligands include FGF10 (Igarashi et al 1998, Xu et al 1998) and FGF3, the over-expression of which causes craniosynostosis and a Crouzon-phenocopy in the murine model (Carlton et al 1998). The range of human FGFR2-associated craniofacial dysostosis phenotypes is very broad, and encompasses great variability in the observed pattern of craniosynostosis. The possibility that this may reflect the balance between negative regulation of the BEK isoform of FGFR2 and ectopic expression of KGFR has yet to be tested in model systems.

Why does Apert syndrome display a cleft palate despite a similar midface morphology to Crouzon–Pfeiffer syndromes?

Clinical observation suggests that mechanical obstruction will perturb human palatogenesis, for example by basal encephalocele (Shimizu et al 1999) or intraoral space-occupying lesions (Britto et al 2000). Under these circumstances, it might seem that the cleft palate phenotype in Apert syndrome occurs secondarily to the constriction effect of the Apert midface retrusion. However, the 'Crouzon–Pfeiffer' group of craniofacial dysostoses, in which severe midfacial retrusion may occur in combination with similar palatal (Peterson and Pruzansky 1974) and nasopharyngeal (Peterson-Falzone et al 1981) morphology to Apert syndrome, do not display cleft palate (Kreiborg and Cohen 1992) despite their association with activating FGFR2 mutations. Furthermore, Apert cleft palate significantly co-segregates with the Ser252Trp mutation (Slaney et al 1996). Consistent with this, both the KGFR and BEK isoforms of FGFR2 are co-expressed with FGFR1, FGFR3, and TGF beta isoforms in the fusing palatal epithelium during sequential stages of human palato-genesis (Britto et al 2002). Independent evidence shows that the FGFR2-IgIIIa/b (KGFR) homozygous null mouse has a cleft palate phenotype (De Moerlooze et al 2000), whereas the heterozygote is normal. This implies a dose-dependent functional role for KGFR signalling in normal murine palatogenesis.

In Apert syndrome, cleft palate occurs in 75 per cent of cases (Kreiborg and Cohen 1992), and the incomplete expressivity is consistent with a dose-dependent effect of Apert-FGFR2 mutations upon human palatal shelf fusion via the IgIIIb/KGFR isoform. To remain consistent with the cleft palate phenotype of the KGFR-null mouse, the Apert mutations might be predicted to confer a dominant-negative functional effect upon KGFR in human palatal epithelia, resulting in failure of normal palatal shelf fusion. It may be, therefore, that the Ser252Trp mutation confers a specific functional effect upon KGFR signalling, perhaps via changes in the normally high-affinity FGF4/KGFR binding association (Orr-Urtreger et al 1993), to result in a disruption of human palatal shelf fusion by dose-dependent dominant-negative means. Both the Ser252Trp and Pro253Arg mutations in Apert syndrome cause changes in ligand specificity for the IgIIIb/KGFR and IgIIIc/BEK receptor proteins (Yu et al 2000); and this might reduce the functional efficiency of IgIIIb/KGFR expressed in the human palatal epithelia. Further support for this theory comes from the observation of a cleft palate phenotype in E18.5 transgenic mice in which a soluble, dominant-negative, kinase-deficient kgfr protein is expressed as a chimera with mouse immunoglobulin (Celli et al 1998). Thus specific KGFR/FGFR2-IgIIIb loss of function co-segregates with murine cleft palate in a dose-dependent manner. The possible competitive, dominant-negative effect of KGFR signalling at work in Apert palatogenesis is at odds with the expected functional gain mechanism discussed above in Apert osteogenesis. The evidence is accumulating, however, and demonstrates the complexity of the molecular pathogenesis of the Apert syndrome.

Conclusions

The phenotypic diversity and molecular complexity of the craniofacial dysostoses provide a wonderful system in which to study human genetics and developmental pathology. Much remains to be learned. The mechanisms that generate the phenotype diversity are particularly intriguing and also, in this context, the role of epigenetic, environmental factors in the generation of craniofacial phenotypes. *In utero* constraint appears to be an important mechanism allied to FGFR genotype in some cases (Johnson et al 2000a). Constraint may be more important than genotype in the sagittal and metopic synostoses; whereas the coronal synostoses (including the eponymous syndromes) clearly reflect powerful molecular developmental mechanisms.

Other aspects of the phenotypes, such as intracranial hypertension, limb pathologies, and ocular pathologies will come under increasing scrutiny against the background of molecular pathology. Already it is possible to advise expectant parents who have undergone molecular analysis of a pregnancy about what to expect from the severity of their child's condition, and the protocols of the craniofacial team. Molecular correlations with phenotype severity have been useful in this regard (Taylor et al 2001). Will these studies yield a surgical, clinical benefit? The jury is out; however, increasing surgical awareness of the influence of molecular mechanisms will serve to stimulate the analysis of surgical results and the presentation of patients in a 'molecular light'. Surgical therapies, such as distraction osteogenesis, may have an outcome that reflects the molecular background of the patient. This in turn will influence the surgical protocols, and truly justify, in clinical terms, the resources invested in the investigation of the molecular pathology of the syndromic craniosynostoses.

REFERENCES

Amaya E, Musci TJ, Kirschner MW (1991) Expression of a dominant negative mutant of the FGF receptor disrupts mesoderm formation in Xenopus embryos. *Cell* 66: 257–270.
Amaya E, Stein PA, Musci TJ, Kirschner MW (1993) FGF signalling in the early specification of mesoderm in Xenopus. *Development* 118: 477–487.

Anderson J, Burns HD, Enriquez-Harris P, Wilkie AM, Heath JK (1998a) Apert syndrome mutations in fibroblast growth factor receptor 2 exhibit increased affinity for FGF ligand. *Hum Mol Genet* 7: 1475–1483.

Anderson PJ, Hall CM, Evans RD, Jones BM, Hayward RD (1998b) The feet in Pfeiffer's syndrome. *J Craniofac Surg* 9: 83–87.

Apert E (1906) De l'acrocephalosyndactylie. *Bull Soc Med Hop* (Paris) 23: 1310–1330.

Baraitser M, Bowen-Bravery M, Saldana-Garcia P (1980) Pitfalls of genetic counselling in Pfeiffer's syndrome. *J Med Genet* 17: 250–256.

Bellus GA, Gaudenz K, Zackai EH, Clarke LA, Szabo J, Francomano CA, Muenke M (1996) Identical mutations in three different fibroblast growth factor receptor genes in autosomal dominant craniosynostosis syndromes. *Nat Genet* 14: 174–176.

Bodo M, Carinci F, Baroni T, Giammarioli M, Bellucci C, Bosi G, Pezzetti F, Becchetti E, Evangelisti R, Carinci P (1997) Apert's syndrome: differential in vitro production of matrix macromolecules and its regulation by interleukins. *Eur J Clin Invest* 27: 36–42.

Bourgeois P, Bolcato-Bellemin AL, Danse JM, Bloch-Zupan A, Yoshiba K, Stoetzel C, Perrin-Schmitt F (1998) The variable expressivity and incomplete penetrance of the twist-null heterozygous mouse phenotype resemble those of human Saethre–Chotzen syndrome. *Hum Mol Genet* 7: 945–957.

Britto JA, Ragoowansi RH, Sommerlad BC (2000) Double tongue, intraoral anomalies, and cleft palate – case reports and a discussion of developmental pathology. *Cleft Palate Craniofac J* 37: 410–415.

Britto JA, Moore RL, Evans RD, Hayward RD, Jones BM (2001a) Negative auto-regulation of fibroblast growth factor 2 expression characterising cranial development in cases of Apert (P253R mutation) and Pfeiffer (C278F mutation) syndromes and suggesting a basis for differences in their cranial phenotypes. *J Neurosurg* 95: 660–673.

Britto JA, Chan C-TJ, Evans RD, Hayward RD, Jones BM (2001b) Differential expression of FGFRs in human digital development suggests common pathogenesis in complex acrosyndactyly and craniosynostosis. *Plast Reconstr Surg* 107: 1331–1338.

Britto JA, Evans RD, Hayward RD, Jones BM (2001c) From genotype to phenotype: the differential expression of FGF, FGFR, and TGF genes characterises human cranioskeletal development, and reflects clinical presentation in FGFR-syndromes. *Plast Reconstr Surg* 108: 2026–2039.

Britto JA, Hayward RD, Evans RD, Jones BM. *FGF* and *FGFR* expression co-regulates with human calvarial osteoblast maturity and human craniosynostosis *in situ*. (Submitted manuscript.)

Britto JA, Evans RD, Hayward RD, Jones BM (2002) Towards pathogenesis of Apert cleft palate – FGF, FGFR, and TGF beta genes are differentially expressed in sequential stages of human palatal shelf fusion. *Cleft Palate Craniofac J* 39: 332–340.

Brueton LA, van Herwerden L, Chotai KA, Winter RM (1992) The mapping of a gene for craniosynostosis: evidence for linkage of the Saethre–Chotzen syndrome to distal chromosome 7p. *J Med Genet* 29: 681–685.

Burke D, Wilkes D, Blundell TL, Malcolm S (1998) Fibroblast growth factor receptors: lessons from the genes. *Trends Biochem Sci* 23: 59–62.

Carlton MB, Colledge WH, Evans MJ (1998) Crouzon-like craniofacial dysmorphology in the mouse is caused by an insertional mutation at the Fgf3/Fgf4 locus. *Dev Dyn* 212: 242–249.

Celli G, LaRochelle WJ, Mackem S, Sharp R, Merlino G (1998) Soluble dominant-negative receptor uncovers essential roles for fibroblast growth factors in multi-organ induction and patterning. *EMBO J* 17: 1642–1655.

Champion Arnaud P, Ronsin C, Gilbert E, Gesnel MC, Houssaint E, Breathnach R (1991) Multiple mRNAs code for proteins related to the BEK fibroblast growth factor receptor. *Oncogene* 6: 979–987.

Chan C-TJ, Thorogood P (1999) Pleiotropic features of syndromic craniosynostoses correlate with differential expression of fibroblast growth factor receptors 1 and 2 during human craniofacial development. *Pediatr Res* 45: 1–8.

Chao MV (1992) Growth factor signaling: where is the specificity? *Cell* 68: 995–997.

Chen L, Adar R, Yang X, Monsonego EO, Li C, Hauschka PV, Yayon A, Deng CX (1999) Gly369Cys mutation in mouse FGFR3 causes achondroplasia by affecting both chondrogenesis and osteogenesis. *J Clin Invest* 104: 1517–1525.

Cheon HG, LaRochelle WJ, Bottaro DP, Burgess WH, Aaronson SA (1994) High-affinity binding sites for related fibroblast growth factor ligands reside within different receptor immunoglobulin-like domains. *Proc Natl Acad Sci USA* 91: 989–993.

Cinalli G, Renier D, Sebag G, Sainte-Rose C, Arnaud E, Pierre-Kahn A (1995) Chronic tonsillar herniation in Crouzon's and Apert's syndromes: the role of premature synostosis of the lambdoid suture. *J Neurosurg* 83: 575–582.

Cohen MMJ, Kreiborg S (1994) Cranial size and configuration in the Apert syndrome. *J Craniofac Genet Dev Biol* 14: 153–162.

Cornejo-Roldan LR, Roessler E, Muenke M (1999) Analysis of the mutational spectrum of the FGFR2 gene in Pfeiffer syndrome. *Hum Genet* 104: 425–431.

D'Avis PY, Robertson SC, Meyer AN, Bardwell WM, Webster MK, Donoghue DJ (1998) Constitutive activation of fibroblast growth factor receptor 3 by mutations responsible for the lethal skeletal dysplasia thanatophoric dysplasia type I. *Cell Growth Differ* 9: 71–78.

Delezoide AL, Benoist-Lasselin C, Legeai-Mallet L, Le Merrer M, Munnich A, Vekemans M, Bonaventure J (1998) Spatio-temporal expression of FGFR 1, 2 and 3 genes during human embryo-fetal ossification. *Mech Dev* 77: 19–30.

De Moerlooze L, Spencer-Dene B, Revest J, Hajihosseini M, Rosewell I, Dickson C (2000) An important role for the IIIb isoform of fibroblast growth factor receptor 2 (FGFR2) in mesenchymal-epithelial signalling during mouse organogenesis. *Development* 127: 483–492.

Deng CX, Wynshaw-Boris A, Shen MM, Daugherty C, Ornitz DM, Leder P (1994) Murine FGFR-1 is required for early postimplantation growth and axial organization. *Genes Dev* 8: 3045–3057.

Deng C, Wynshaw-Boris A, Zhou F, Kuo A, Leder P (1996) Fibroblast growth factor receptor 3 is a negative regulator of bone growth. *Cell* 84: 911–921.

Deng C, Bedford M, Li C, Xu X, Yang X, Dunmore J, Leder P (1997) Fibroblast growth factor receptor-1 (FGFR-1) is essential for normal neural tube and limb development. *Dev Biol* 185: 42–54.

El Ghouzzi V, Le Merrer M, Perrin-Schmitt F, Lajeunie E, Benit P, Renier D, Bourgeois P, Bolcato-Bellemin A-L, Munnich A, Bonaventure J (1997) Mutations of the TWIST gene in the Saethre–Chotzen syndrome. *Nat Genet* 15: 42–46.

Fragale A, Tartaglia M, Bernardini S, Di Stasi AM, Di Rocco C, Velardi F, Teti A, Battaglia PA, Migliaccio S (1999) Decreased proliferation and altered differentiation in osteoblasts from genetically and clinically distinct craniosynostotic disorders. *Am J Pathol* 154: 1465–1477.

Francis-West P, Graveson A, Barlow A, Ladher R (1998) Signalling interactions during facial development. *Mech Dev* 75: 3–28.

Francomano CA, Ortiz de Luna RI, Hefferon TW, Bellus GA, Turner CE, Taylor E, Meyers DA, Blanton SH, Murray JC, McIntosh I (1994) Localization of the achondroplasia gene to the distal 2.5 Mb of human chromosome 4p. *Hum Mol Genet* 3: 787–792.

Galvin BD, Hart KC, Meyer AN, Webster MK, Donoghue DJ (1996) Constitutive receptor activation by Crouzon syndrome mutations in fibroblast growth factor receptor (FGFR)2 and FGFR2/Neu chimeras. *Proc Natl Acad Sci USA* 93: 7894–7899.

Givol D, Yayon A (1992) Complexity of FGF receptors: genetic basis for structural diversity and functional specificity. *FASEB J* 6: 3362–3369.

Gorry MC, Preston RA, White GJ, Zhang Y, Singhal VK, Losken HW, Parker MG, Nwokoro NA, Post JC, Ehrlich GD (1995) Crouzon syndrome: mutations in two spliceoforms of FGFR2 and a common point mutation shared with Jackson–Weiss syndrome. *Hum Mol Genet* 4: 1387–1390.

Green PJ, Walsh FS, Doherty P (1996) Promiscuity of fibroblast growth factor receptors. *Bioessays* 18: 639–646.

Gripp KW, McDonald-McGinn DM, Gaudenz K, Whitaker LA, Bartlett SP, Glat PM, Cassileth LB, Mayro R, Zackai EH, Muenke M (1998) Identification of a genetic cause for isolated unilateral coronal synostosis: a unique mutation in the fibroblast growth factor receptor 3. *J Pediatr* 132: 714–716.

Hall BK (1981) The induction of neural crest-derived cartilage and bone by embryonic epithelia: an analysis of the mode of action of an epithelial-mesenchymal interaction. *J Embryol Exp Morphol* 64: 305–320.

Hou J, Kan M, Wang F, Xu JM, Nakahara M, McBride G, McKeehan K, McKeehan WL (1992) Substitution of putative half-cystine residues in heparin-binding fibroblast growth factor receptors. Loss of binding activity in both two and three loop isoforms. *J Biol Chem* 267: 17804–17808.

Igarashi M, Finch PW, Aaronson SA (1998) Characterization of recombinant human fibroblast growth factor (FGF)-10 reveals functional similarities with keratinocyte growth factor (FGF-7). *J Biol Chem* 273: 13230–13235.

Iseki S, Wilkie AO, Morriss-Kay GM (1999) Fgfr1 and Fgfr2 have distinct differentiation- and proliferation-related roles in the developing mouse skull vault. *Development* 126: 5611–5620.

Jabs EW, Li X, Scott AF, Meyers G, Chen W, Eccles M, Mao JI, Charnas LR, Jackson CE, Jaye M (1994) Jackson–Weiss and Crouzon syndromes are allelic with mutations in fibroblast growth factor receptor 2. *Nat Genet* 8: 275–279. (Published erratum appears in *Nat Genet* (1995) 9(4): 451.)

66

Jackson CE, Weiss L, Reynolds WA, Forman TF, Peterson JA (1976) Craniosynostosis, midfacial hypoplasia and foot abnormalities: an autosomal dominant phenotype in a large Amish kindred. *J Pediatr* 88: 963–968.

Johansen VA, Hall SH (1982) Morphogenesis of the mouse coronal suture. *Acta Anat* 114: 58–67.

Johnson DE, Williams LT (1993) Structural and functional diversity in the FGF receptor multigene family. *Adv Cancer Res* 60: 1–41.

Johnson DE, Lu J, Chen H, Werner S, Williams LT (1991) The human fibroblast growth factor receptor genes: a common structural arrangement underlies the mechanisms for generating receptor forms that differ in their third immunoglobulin domain. *Mol Cell Biol* 11: 4627–4634.

Johnson D, Wall SA, Mann S, Wilkie AO (2000a) A novel mutation, Ala315Ser, in FGFR2: a gene-environment interaction leading to craniosynostosis? *Eur J Hum Genet* 8: 571–577.

Johnson D, Iseki S, Wilkie AO, Morriss-Kay GM (2000b) Expression patterns of Twist and Fgfr1, -2 and -3 in the developing mouse coronal suture suggest a key role for twist in suture initiation and biogenesis. *Mech Dev* 91: 341–345.

Kannan K, Givol D (2000) FGF receptor mutations: dimerization syndromes, cell growth suppression, and animal models. *IUBMB Life* 49: 197–205.

Kreiborg S, Cohen MM Jr (1990) Characteristics of the infant Apert skull and its subsequent development. *J Craniofac Genet Dev Biol* 10: 399–410.

Kreiborg S, Cohen MM Jr (1992) The oral manifestations of Apert syndrome. *J Craniofac Genet Dev Biol* 12: 41–48.

Kreiborg S, Marsh JL, Cohen MMJ, Liversage M, Pedersen H, Skovby F, Borgesen SE, Vannier MW (1993) Comparative three-dimensional analysis of CT-scans of the calvaria and cranial base in Apert and Crouzon syndromes. *J Craniomaxillofac Surg* 21: 181–188.

Lajeunie E, Ma HW, Bonaventure J, Munnich A, Merrer ML, Renier D (1995) FGFR2 mutations in Pfeiffer syndrome. *Nat Genet* 9: 108.

Legeai-Mallet L, Benoist-Lasselin C, Delezoide AL, Munnich A, Bonaventure J (1998) Fibroblast growth factor receptor 3 mutations promote apoptosis but do not alter chondrocyte proliferation in thanatophoric dysplasia. *J Biol Chem* 273: 13007–13014.

Le Merrer M, Rousseau F, Legeai-Mallet L, Landais JC, Pelet A, Bonaventure J, Sanak M, Weissenbach J, Stoll C, Munnich A (1994) A gene for achondroplasia-hypochondroplasia maps to chromosome 4p. *Nat Genet* 6: 318–321.

Lemonnier J, Delannoy P, Hott M, Lomri A, Modrowski D, Marie PJ (2000) The Ser252Trp fibroblast growth factor receptor-2 (FGFR-2) mutation induces PKC-independent downregulation of FGFR-2 associated with premature calvaria osteoblast differentiation. *Exp Cell Res* 256: 158–167.

Li X, Lewanda AF, Eluma F, Jerald H, Choi H, Alozie I, Proukakis C, Talbot CCJ, Vander Kolk C, Bird LM (1994) Two craniosynostotic syndrome loci, Crouzon and Jackson–Weiss, map to chromosome 10q23–q26. *Genomics* 22: 418–424.

Li X, Park WJ, Pyeritz RE, Jabs EW (1995) Effect on splicing of a silent FGFR2 mutation in Crouzon syndrome. *Nat Genet* 9: 232–233.

Locci P, Baroni T, Pezzetti F, Lilli C, Marinucci L, Martinese D, Becchetti E, Calvitti M, Carinci F (1999) Differential in vitro phenotype pattern, transforming growth factor-beta(1) activity and mRNA expression of transforming growth factor-beta(1) in Apert osteoblasts. *Cell Tissue Res* 297: 475–483.

Lomri A, Lemonnier J, Hott M, de Parseval N, Lajeunie E, Munnich A, Renier D, Marie PJ (1998) Increased calvaria cell differentiation and bone matrix formation induced by fibroblast growth factor receptor 2 mutations in Apert syndrome. *J Clin Invest* 101: 1310–1317.

Ma HW, Lajeunie E, Le Merrer M, de Parseval N, Serville F, Weissenbach J, Munnich A, Renier D (1995) No evidence of genetic heterogeneity in Crouzon craniofacial dysostosis. *Hum Genet* 96: 731–735.

Mangasarian K, Li Y, Mansukhani A, Basilico C (1997) Mutation associated with Crouzon syndrome causes ligand-independent dimerization and activation of FGF receptor-2. *J Cell Physiol* 172: 117–125.

Mansukhani A, Bellosta P, Sahni M, Basilico C (2000) Signaling by fibroblast growth factors (FGF) and fibroblast growth factor receptor 2 (FGFR2)-activating mutations blocks mineralization and induces apoptosis in osteoblasts. *J Cell Biol* 149: 1297–1308.

Mason IJ (1994) The ins and outs of fibroblast growth factors. *Cell* 78: 547–552.

Matovinovic E, Richman JM (1997) Epithelium is required for maintaining FGFR-2 expression levels in facial mesenchyme of the developing chick embryo. *Dev Dyn* 210: 407–416.

Meyers GA, Orlow SJ, Munro IR, Przylepa KA, Jabs EW (1995) Fibroblast growth factor receptor 3 (FGFR3) transmembrane mutation in Crouzon syndrome with acanthosis nigricans. *Nat Genet* 11: 462–464.

Meyers GA, Day D, Goldberg R, Daentl DL, Przylepa KA, Abrams LJ, Graham JMJ, Feingold M, Moeschler JB, Rawnsley E, Scott AF, Jabs EW (1996) FGFR2 exon IIIa and IIIc mutations in Crouzon, Jackson–Weiss, and Pfeiffer syndromes: evidence for missense changes, insertions, and a deletion due to alternative RNA splicing. *Am J Hum Genet* 58: 491–498.

Miki T, Bottaro DP, Fleming TP, Smith CL, Burgess WH, Chan AM, Aaronson SA (1992) Determination of ligand binding specificity by alternative splicing: two distinct growth factor receptors encoded by a single gene. *Proc Natl Acad Sci* USA 89: 246–250.

Moloney DM, Wall SA, Ashworth GJ, Oldridge M, Glass IA, Francomano CA, Muenke M, Wilkie AO (1997) Prevalence of Pro250Arg mutation of fibroblast growth factor receptor 3 in coronal craniosynostosis. *Lancet* 349: 1059–1062.

Muenke M, Schell U (1995) Fibroblast-growth-factor receptor mutations in human skeletal disorders. *Trends Genet* 11: 308–313.

Muenke M, Schell U, Hehr A, Robin NH, Losken HW, Schinzel A, Pulleyn LJ, Rutland P, Reardon W, Malcolm S (1994) A common mutation in the fibroblast growth factor receptor 1 gene in Pfeiffer syndrome. *Nat Genet* 8: 269–274.

Muenke M, Gripp KW, McDonald-McGinn DM, Gaudenz K, Whitaker LA, Bartlett SP, Markowitz RI, Robin NH, Nwokoro N, Mulvihill JJ, Losken HW, Mulliken JB, Guttmacher AE, Wilroy RS, Clarke LA, Hollway G, Ades LC, Haan EA, Mulley JC, Cohen MMJ, Bellus GA, Francomano CA, Moloney DM, Wall SA, Wilkie AO (1997) A unique point mutation in the fibroblast growth factor receptor 3 gene (FGFR3) defines a new craniosynostosis syndrome. *Am J Hum Genet* 60: 555–564.

Mulliken JB, Steinberger D, Kunze S, Muller U (1999) Molecular diagnosis of bilateral coronal synostosis. *Plast Reconstr Surg* 104: 1603–1615.

Naski MC, Wang Q, Xu J, Ornitz DM (1996) Graded activation of fibroblast growth factor receptor 3 by mutations causing achondroplasia and thanatophoric dysplasia. *Nat Genet* 13: 233–237.

Neilson KM, Friesel RE (1995) Constitutive activation of fibroblast growth factor receptor-2 by a point mutation associated with Crouzon syndrome. *J Biol Chem* 270: 26037–26040.

Neilson KM, Friesel R (1996) Ligand-independent activation of fibroblast growth factor receptors by point mutations in the extracellular, transmembrane, and kinase domains. *J Biol Chem* 271: 25049–25057.

Nguyen HB, Estacion M, Gargus JJ (1997) Mutations causing achondroplasia and thanatophoric dysplasia alter bFGF-induced calcium signals in human diploid fibroblasts. *Hum Mol Genet* 6: 681–688.

Oldridge M, Lunt PW, Zackai EH, McDonald-McGinn DM, Muenke M, Moloney DM, Twigg SR, Heath JK, Howard TD, Hoganson G, Gagnon DM, Jabs EW, Wilkie AO (1997) Genotype–phenotype correlation for nucleotide substitutions in the IgII–IgIII linker of FGFR2. *Hum Mol Genet* 6: 137–143.

Oldridge M, Zackai EH, McDonald-McGinn DM, Iseki S, Morriss-Kay GM, Twigg SR, Johnson D, Wall SA, Jiang W, Theda C, Jabs EW, Wilkie AO (1999) De novo alu-element insertions in FGFR2 identify a distinct pathological basis for Apert syndrome. *Am J Hum Genet* 64: 446–461.

Opperman LA, Passarelli RW, Morgan EP, Reintjes M, Ogle RC (1995) Cranial sutures require tissue interactions with dura mater to resist osseous obliteration in vitro. *J Bone Miner Res* 10: 1978–1987.

Ornitz DM (2000) FGFs, heparan sulfate and FGFRs: complex interactions essential for development. *Bioessays* 22: 108–112.

Orr-Urtreger A, Givol D, Yayon A, Yarden Y, Lonai P (1991) Developmental expression of two murine fibroblast growth factor receptors, flg and bek. *Development* 113: 1419–1434.

Orr-Urtreger A, Bedford MT, Burakova T, Arman E, Zimmer Y, Yayon A, Givol D, Lonai P (1993) Developmental localization of the splicing alternatives of fibroblast growth factor receptor-2 (FGFR2). *Dev Biol* 158: 475–486.

Park WJ, Bellus GA, Jabs EW (1995a) Mutations in fibroblast growth factor receptors: phenotypic consequences during eukaryotic development. *Am J Hum Genet* 57: 748–754.

Park WJ, Meyers GA, Li X, Theda C, Day D, Orlow SJ, Jones MC, Jabs EW (1995b) Novel FGFR2 mutations in Crouzon and Jackson–Weiss syndromes show allelic heterogeneity and phenotypic variability. *Hum Mol Genet* 4: 1229–1233.

Passos-Bueno MR, Sertie AL, Zatz M, Richieri-Costa A (1997) Pfeiffer mutation in an Apert patient: how wide is the spectrum of variability due to mutations in the FGFR2 gene? *Am J Med Genet* 71: 243–245. (Letter.)

Passos-Bueno MR, Wilcox WR, Jabs EW, Sertie AL, Alonso LG, Kitoh H (1999) Clinical spectrum of fibroblast growth factor receptor mutations. *Hum Mutat* 14: 115–125.

Patstone G, Pasquale EB, Maher PA (1993) Different members of the fibroblast growth factor receptor family are specific to distinct cell types in the developing chicken embryo. *Dev Biol* 155: 107–123.

Peters KG, Werner S, Chen G, Williams LT (1992) Two FGF receptor genes are differentially expressed in epithelial and mesenchymal tissues during limb formation and organogenesis in the mouse. *Development* 114: 233–243.

Peters K, Ornitz D, Werner S, Williams L (1993) Unique expression pattern of the FGF receptor 3 gene during mouse organogenesis. *Dev Biol* 155: 423–430.

Peters K, Werner S, Liao X, Wert S, Whitsett J, Williams L (1994) Targeted expression of a dominant negative FGF receptor blocks branching morphogenesis and epithelial differentiation of the mouse lung. *EMBO J* 13: 3296–3301.

Peterson SJ, Pruzansky S (1974) Palatal anomalies in the syndromes of Apert and Crouzon. *Cleft Palate J* 11: 394–403.

Peterson-Falzone SJ, Pruzansky S, Parris PJ, Laffer JL (1981) Nasopharyngeal dysmorphology in the syndromes of Apert and Crouzon. *Cleft Palate J* 18: 237–250.

Plotnikov AN, Hubbard SR, Schlessinger J, Mohammadi M (2000) Crystal structures of two FGF-FGFR complexes reveal the determinants of ligand-receptor specificity. *Cell* 101: 413–424.

Preston RA, Post JC, Keats BJ, Aston CE, Ferrell RE, Priest J, Nouri N, Losken HW, Morris CA, Hurtt MR (1994) A gene for Crouzon craniofacial dysostosis maps to the long arm of chromosome 10. *Nat Genet* 7: 149–153.

Prudovsky IA, Savion N, LaVallee TM, Maciag T (1996) The nuclear trafficking of extracellular fibroblast growth factor (FGF)-1 correlates with the perinuclear association of the FGF receptor-1alpha isoforms but not the FGF receptor-1beta isoforms. *J Biol Chem* 271: 14198–14205.

Przylepa KA, Paznekas W, Zhang M, Golabi M, Bias W, Bamshad MJ, Carey JC, Hall BD, Stevenson R, Orlow S, Cohen MMJ, Jabs EW (1996) Fibroblast growth factor receptor 2 mutations in Beare–Stevenson cutis gyrata syndrome. *Nat Genet* 13: 492–494.

Pulleyn LJ, Reardon W, Wilkes D, Rutland P, Jones BM, Hayward R, Hall CM, Brueton L, Chun N, Lammer E, Malcolm S, Winter RM (1996) Spectrum of craniosynostosis phenotypes associated with novel mutations at the fibroblast growth factor receptor 2 locus. *Eur J Hum Genet* 4: 283–291.

Reardon W, Winter RM (1994) Saethre–Chotzen syndrome. *J Med Genet* 31: 393–396.

Reardon W, van Herwerden L, Rose C, Jones B, Malcolm S, Winter RM (1994a) Crouzon syndrome is not linked to craniosynostosis loci at 7p and 5qter. *J Med Genet* 31: 219–221.

Reardon W, Winter RM, Rutland P, Pulleyn LJ, Jones BM, Malcolm S (1994b) Mutations in the fibroblast growth factor receptor 2 gene cause Crouzon syndrome. *Nat Genet* 8: 98–103.

Reardon W, Wilkes D, Rutland P, Pulleyn LJ, Malcolm S, Dean JC, Evans RD, Jones BM, Hayward R, Hall CM, Nevin NC, Baraister M, Winter RM (1997) Craniosynostosis associated with FGFR3 pro250arg mutation results in a range of clinical presentations including unisutural sporadic craniosynostosis. *J Med Genet* 34: 632–636.

Reardon W, Smith A, Honour JW, Hindmarsh P, Das D, Rumsby G, Nelson I, Malcolm S, Ades L, Sillence D, Kumar D, DeLozier-Blanchet C, McKee S, Kelly T, McKeehan WL, Baraitser M, Winter RM (2000) Evidence for digenic inheritance in some cases of Antley–Bixler syndrome? *J Med Genet* 37: 26–32.

Richman JM, Tickle C (1992) Epithelial-mesenchymal interactions in the outgrowth of limb buds and facial primordia in chick embryos. *Dev Biol* 154: 299–308.

Robertson SC, Meyer AN, Hart KC, Galvin BD, Webster MK, Donoghue DJ (1998) Activating mutations in the extracellular domain of the fibroblast growth factor receptor 2 function by disruption of the disulfide bond in the third immunoglobulin-like domain. *Proc Natl Acad Sci USA* 95: 4567–4572.

Robin NH, Feldman GJ, Mitchell HF, Lorenz P, Wilroy RS, Zackai EH, Allanson JE, Reich EW, Pfeiffer RA, Clarke LA (1994) Linkage of Pfeiffer syndrome to chromosome 8 centromere and evidence for genetic heterogeneity. *Hum Mol Genet* 3: 2153–2158.

Rutland P, Pulleyn LJ, Reardon W, Baraitser M, Hayward R, Jones B, Malcolm S, Winter RM, Oldridge M, Slaney SF (1995) Identical mutations in the FGFR2 gene cause both Pfeiffer and Crouzon syndrome phenotypes. *Nat Genet* 9: 173–176.

Schell U, Hehr A, Feldman GJ, Robin NH, Zackai EH, de Die-Smulders C, Viskochil DH, Stewart JM, Wolff G, Ohashi H (1995) Mutations in FGFR1 and FGFR2 cause familial and sporadic Pfeiffer syndrome. *Hum Mol Genet* 4: 323–328.

Shiang R, Thompson LM, Zhu YZ, Church DM, Fielder TJ, Bocian M, Winokur ST, Wasmuth JJ (1994) Mutations in the transmembrane domain of FGFR3 cause the most common genetic form of dwarfism, achondroplasia. *Cell* 78: 335–342.

69

Shimizu T, Kitamura S, Kinouchi K, Fukumitsu K (1999) A rare case of upper airway obstruction in an infant caused by basal encephalocele complicating facial midline deformity. *Paediatr Anaesth* 9: 73–76.

Slaney SF, Oldridge M, Hurst JA, Moriss-Kay GM, Hall CM, Poole MD, Wilkie AO (1996) Differential effects of FGFR2 mutations on syndactyly and cleft palate in Apert syndrome. *Am J Hum Genet* 58: 923–932.

Steinberger D, Reinhartz T, Unsold R, Muller U (1996) FGFR2 mutation in clinically nonclassifiable autosomal dominant craniosynostosis with pronounced phenotypic variation. *Am J Med Genet* 66: 81–86.

Tartaglia M, Di RC, Lajeunie E, Valeri S, Velardi F, Battaglia PA (1997) Jackson–Weiss syndrome: identification of two novel FGFR2 missense mutations shared with Crouzon and Pfeiffer craniosynostotic disorders. *Hum Genet* 101: 47–50.

Tavormina PL, Shiang R, Thompson LM, Zhu YZ, Wilkin DJ, Lachman RS, Wilcox WR, Rimoin DL, Cohn DH, Wasmuth JJ (1995) Thanatophoric dysplasia (types I and II) caused by distinct mutations in fibroblast growth factor receptor 3. *Nat Genet* 9: 321–328.

Taylor W, Hayward RD, Lasjaunias P, Britto JA, Thompson DN, Jones BM, Evans RD (2001) The enigma of raised intracranial pressure in complex craniosynostosis: the role of abnormal intracranial venous drainage. *J Neurosurg* 94: 377–385.

Thompson LM, Raffioni S, Wasmuth JJ, Bradshaw RA (1997) Chimeras of the native form or achondroplasia mutant (G375C) of human fibroblast growth factor receptor 3 induce ligand-dependent differentiation of PC12 cells. *Mol Cell Biol* 17: 4169–4177.

Tyler MS (1983) Development of the frontal bone and cranial meninges in the embryonic chick: an experimental study of tissue interactions. *Anat Rec* 206: 61–70.

Ueno H, Gunn M, Dell K, Tseng AJ, Williams LT (1992) A truncated form of fibroblast growth factor receptor 1 inhibits signal transduction by multiple types of fibroblast growth factor receptor. *J Biol Chem* 267: 1470–1476.

van Herwerden L, Rose CS, Reardon W, Brueton LA, Weissenbach J, Malcolm S, Winter RM (1994) Evidence for locus heterogeneity in acrocephalosyndactyly: a refined localization for the Saethre–Chotzen syndrome locus on distal chromosome 7p – and exclusion of Jackson–Weiss syndrome from craniosynostosis loci on 7p and 5q. *Am J Hum Genet* 54: 669–674.

Velinov M, Slaugenhaupt SA, Stoilov I, Scott CI Jr, Gusella JF, Tsipouras P (1994) The gene for achondroplasia maps to the telomeric region of chromosome 4p. *Nat Genet* 6: 314–317.

Voronova A, Baltimore D (1990) Mutations that disrupt DNA binding and dimer formation in the E47 helix-loop-helix protein map to distinct domains. *Proc Natl Acad Sci USA* 87: 4722–4726.

Wang F, Kan M, Xu JM, Yan GC, McKeehan WL (1995) Ligand-specific structural domains in the fibroblast growth factor receptor. *J Biol Chem* 270: 10222–10230.

Webster MK, Donoghue DJ (1996) Constitutive activation of fibroblast growth factor receptor 3 by the transmembrane domain point mutation found in achondroplasia. *EMBO J* 15: 520–527.

Webster MK, D'Avis PY, Robertson SC, Donoghue DJ (1996) Profound ligand-independent kinase activation of fibroblast growth factor receptor 3 by the activation loop mutation responsible for a lethal skeletal dysplasia, thanatophoric dysplasia type II. *Mol Cell Biol* 16: 4081–4087.

Wedden SE (1987) Epithelial-mesenchymal interactions in the development of chick facial primordia and the target of retinoid action. *Development* 99: 341–351.

Werner S, Duan DS, de Vries C, Peters KG, Johnson DE, Williams LT (1992) Differential splicing in the extracellular region of fibroblast growth factor receptor 1 generates variants with different ligand-binding specificities. *Mol Cell Biol* 12: 82–88.

Wilcox WR, Tavormina PL, Krakow D, Kitoh H, Lachman RS, Wasmuth JJ, Thompson LM, Rimoin DL (1998) Molecular, radiologic, and histopathologic correlations in thanatophoric dysplasia. *Am J Med Genet* 78: 274–281.

Wilke TA, Gubbels S, Schwartz J, Richman JM (1997) Expression of fibroblast growth factor receptors (FGFR1, FGFR2, FGFR3) in the developing head and face. *Dev Dyn* 210: 41–52.

Wilkes D, Rutland P, Pulleyn LJ, Reardon W, Moss C, Ellis JP, Winter RM, Malcolm S (1996) A recurrent mutation, ala391glu, in the transmembrane region of FGFR3 causes Crouzon syndrome and acanthosis nigricans. *J Med Genet* 33: 744–748.

Wilkie AO (1997) Craniosynostosis: genes and mechanisms. *Hum Mol Genet* 6: 1647–1656.

Wilkie AOM, Slaney SF, Oldridge M, Poole MD, Ashworth GJ, Hockley AD, Hayward RD, David DJ, Pulleyn LJ, Rutland P, Malcolm S, Winter RM, Reardon W (1995) Apert syndrome results from localized mutations of FGFR2 and is allelic with Crouzon syndrome. *Nat Genet* 9: 165–172.

Wilson C (1994) Receptor tyrosine kinase signalling: not so complex after all? *Trends Cell Biol* 4: 409–414.

70

Winter RM, Reardon W (1996) Lumpers, splitters, and FGFRs. *Am J Med Genet* 63: 501–502. (Letter; comment.)

Xu X, Weinstein M, Li C, Naski M, Cohen RI, Ornitz DM, Leder P, Deng C (1998) Fibroblast growth factor receptor 2 (FGFR2)-mediated reciprocal regulation loop between FGF8 and FGF10 is essential for limb induction. *Development* 125: 753–765.

Yamaguchi TP, Harpal K, Henkemeyer M, Rossant J (1994) fgfr-1 is required for embryonic growth and mesodermal patterning during mouse gastrulation. *Genes Dev* 8: 3032–3044.

Yayon A, Zimmer Y, Shen GH, Avivi A, Yarden Y, Givol D (1992) A confined variable region confers ligand specificity on fibroblast growth factor receptors: implications for the origin of the immunoglobulin fold. *EMBO J* 11: 1885–1890.

Yu JC, McClintock JS, Gannon F, Gao XX, Mobasser JP, Sharawy M (1997) Regional differences of dura osteoinduction: squamous dura induces osteogenesis, sutural dura induces chondrogenesis and osteogenesis. *Plast Reconstr Surg* 100: 23–31.

Yu K, Herr AB, Waksman G, Ornitz DM (2000) Loss of fibroblast growth factor receptor 2 ligand-binding specificity in Apert syndrome. *Proc Natl Acad Sci USA* 97: 14536–14541.

Zhou YX, Xu X, Chen L, Li C, Brodie SG, Deng CX (2000) A Pro250Arg substitution in mouse Fgfr1 causes increased expression of Cbfa1 and premature fusion of calvarial sutures. *Hum Mol Genet* 9: 2001–2008.

Zhu H, Anchin J, Ramnarayan K, Zheng J, Kawai T, Mong S, Wolff ME (1997) Analysis of high-affinity binding determinants in the receptor binding epitope of basic fibroblast growth factor. *Protein Eng* 10: 417–421.

4
INCIDENCE AND EPIDEMIOLOGY
OF CRANIOSYNOSTOSIS

Louise C. Wilson

Introduction

For parents of a child with craniosynostosis the condition is usually unexpected, the terminology is complicated and unfamiliar and the most immediate concerns are how it will affect their child and what can be done to help. In time questions about why it happened and about recurrence risks for themselves, their child and members of the wider family usually follow. This chapter aims to answer these latter questions as far as possible and to outline the contribution that molecular genetic testing and the clinical geneticist can make in the management of these families.

Incidence of craniosynostosis

The overall prevalence of craniosynostosis is around 1 in 2500 births although estimates have ranged between 1 in 709 and 1 in 3225 births (Hunter and Rudd 1976, Shuper et al 1985, French et al 1990, Lajeunie et al 1995, Alderman et al 1997, Singer et al 1999). The variation appears to be partly dependent on the rigour of the inclusion criteria.

Syndromic craniosynostosis

COMMON CRANIOSYNOSTOSIS SYNDROMES

The prevalences of Apert syndrome and Crouzon syndrome appear to be similar at around 1 in 65,000 (~15/million), each accounting for 4–6 per cent of all craniosynostosis (Cohen and Kreiborg 1992, Cohen et al 1992, Singer et al 1999), but estimates for Apert syndrome have varied quite widely (Czeizel et al 1993, Tolarova et al 1997). In virtually all patients with Apert syndrome and between 30 and 60 per cent of patients with Crouzon syndrome (al-Qattan and Phillips 1997) the condition has arisen *de novo* and there is a correlation with increasing paternal age. The prevalence of Pfeiffer syndrome is lower than Crouzon but there is currently little data on the individual prevalence for this, FGFR3-related craniosynostosis, and the other syndromic forms.

RARER SINGLE GENE SYNDROMES INCLUDING CRANIOSYNOSTOSIS

For patients in whom craniosynostosis is associated with other malformations or learning disability with a normal karyotype, expert search tools such as the London Dysmorphology Database and Possum are a valuable resource. Over 150 syndromes of which craniosynostosis may be a feature are listed on the London Dysmorphology Database, many of which are rare and some of which have only been reported in single families or sporadic individuals. They are too numerous to detail exhaustively but the more distinctive and the commoner ones are described in Table 4.1. Referral of these patients for assessment by a clinical geneticist is recommended.

TABLE 4.1
Craniosynostosis syndromes for which the aetiology is known

Craniosynostosis syndrome	Commonly associated features	Inheritance	Gene
Adelaide-type craniosynostosis	Brachydactyly, carpal fusions, cone epiphyses, middle phalangeal hypoplasia, hearing loss, developmental delay in some	AD	FGFR3
Apert	Choanal stenosis, midface hypoplasia, mitten hands and feet, osseous syndactyly, proptosis, mental handicap in around 50%	AD	FGFR2
Beare–Stevenson	Cutis gyrata, acanthosis nigricans, proptosis, choanal atresia, abnormal genitalia, anterior anus, umbilical and coccygeal anomalies,	AD	FGFR2
Boston-type craniosynostosis	Variable craniosynostosis, short 1st metatarsal, cleft palate, triphalangeal thumb, seizures	AD	MSX2
Crouzon	Proptosis, midface hypoplasia, beak-shaped nose, small jaw	AD	FGFR2
Crouzon with acanthosis nigricans	Crouzon-like face, acanthosis nigricans	AD	FGFR3
Multiple exostoses–parietal foramina–craniofacial dysostosis (DEFECT 11)	Multiple exostoses, parietal foramina, learning disability/seizures in some	AD	Microdeletion encompassing EXT2 and contiguous genes on 11p
Greigs cephalo-polysyndactyly	Macrocephaly, hypertelorism, pre- and post-axial polydactyly, syndactyly	AD	GLI3
Jackson–Weiss	Variable proptosis, hypertelorism, midface hypoplasia, broad deviated halluces, pre-axial polydactyly, skin syndactyly, tarsal fusions	AD	FGFR2
FGFR3-related (Muenke)	Facies variable from normal to Crouzon/ Pfeiffer- or Saethre–Chotzen-like, short middle phalanges, cone epiphyses, carpal/tarsal/ calcaneo-cuboidal fusions, developmental delay in some	AD	FGFR3
Pfeiffer	Crouzon-like face, broad thumbs and halluces, hallux varus, skin syndactyly	AD	FGFR2; FGFR1
Robinow–Sorauf	Similar to Saethre–Chotzen but with bifid/ duplicated halluces	AD	TWIST
Saethre–Chotzen	Facial asymmetry, ptosis, broad forehead, loss of frontonasal angle, beaked nose, prominent ear crus, broad thumbs and halluces, skin syndactyly, developmental delay in some	AD	TWIST

Craniosynostosis can also be a feature of a number of skeletal dysplasias (including camptomelic dysplasia, hypophosphatasia, osteodysplastic dwarfism, osteoglophonic dwarfism, pyknodysostosis and thanatophoric dysplasia) and may also occur in various metabolic storage disorders (including mannosidosis, the mucolipidoses and mucopolysaccharidoses).

CHROMOSOMAL CAUSES OF CRANIOSYNOSTOSIS
Over 58 chromosomal aberrations of which craniosynostosis may be a feature are listed in the Schinzel catalogue of human chromosomal abnormalities. Karyotyping should be undertaken in any child with craniosynostosis in whom the aetiology is unknown, particularly if they have associated developmental delay. There are a number of chromosomal abnormalities where craniosynostosis has been a frequent finding, in particular deletions (del) of chromosome 9p (Huret et al 1988), del 11q (Lewanda et al 1995, Leegte et al 1999), del 7p (Grebe et al 1992), del 13q (Lajeunie et al 1998, Walsh et al 2001), and duplications (dup) of chromosome 3q (Wilson et al 1985) and dup 15q (Zollino et al 1999).

TERATOGENIC CAUSES OF CRANIOSYNOSTOSIS
Craniosynostosis has been reported in association with a small number of teratogenic agents including anticonvulsants (valproate, hydantoin (Kelly 1984)), cytotoxic agents (methotrexate (Milunsky et al 1968, Friedman and Polifka 1994), cyclophosphamide, cytarabine), abortifacients (aminopterin (Shaw and Steinback 1968, Friedman and Polifka 1994)), nitrosatable drugs (chlorpheniramine, nitrofurantoin, chlordiazepoxide (Gardner et al 1998)) and fluconazole (Aleck and Bartley 1997). The craniosynostosis associated with valproate exposure seems to involve specifically the metopic suture (Ardinger et al 1988, Clayton-Smith and Donnai 1995, Lajeunie et al 2001).

Non-syndromic craniosynostosis
Isolated craniosynostosis is considerably commoner than the syndromic forms and multiple sutures may be involved. In a series from Western Australia, around 85 per cent of all craniosynostosis was found to be non-syndromic (Singer et al 1999). It is likely that the prevalence of lambdoid synostosis has often been overestimated due to the difficulty distinguishing it from posterior deformational plagiocephaly (Wilkie 2000). Taking that into account, sagittal suture involvement appears to be commonest, followed by the coronal sutures, then metopic (Cohen 1979, Lajeunie et al 1995, 1996, 1998, Singer et al 1999). True lambdoid synostosis appears to be relatively rare, accounting for around 3.3 per cent of all craniosynostosis (Wilkie 2000).

ISOLATED SAGITTAL CRANIOSYNOSTOSIS
Sagittal suture involvement accounts for around 55 per cent of all craniosynostosis in most studies; 56 per cent in North American series (Shillito and Matson 1968, Hunter and Rudd 1976); 41 per cent in a Western Australian series (53 per cent if cases with posterior plagiocephaly are excluded) (Singer et al 1999); and 40 per cent in a French series where the ascertainment was estimated at 0.78 (Lajeunie et al 1996). A suggestion for the unusually

TABLE 4.2
Commoner or more distinctive craniosynostosis syndromes for which the aetiology is unknown

Craniosynostosis syndrome	Commonly associated features	Inheritance	Reference
Antley–Bixler	Choanal atresia, radio-humeral synostosis, bowed femurs, joint contractures, rocker-bottom feet, dysplastic ears, genital abnormalities in females, developmental delay. Reported FGFR2 mutations but overlap with severe Pfeiffer	Unknown: some AD FGFR2 mutations; some AR POR mutations ?other genes; possible digenic *in utero* exposure to fluconazole	(Chun et al 1998, Gripp et al 1999, Reardon et al 2000, Kelley et al 2002, Fluck et al 2004)
Baller–Gerold	Radial ray defects, bowed ulna, anal stenosis, renal abnormalities, cardiac defects. TWIST mutations in some	AR; AD if TWIST mutation	(Seto et al 2001)
Berant	Radio-ulnar synostosis	AD	(Berant and Berant 1973)
Blair	Colobomas, microphthalmia, arachnodactyly, post-axial polydactyly, renal agenesis, developmental delay	AR	(Blair et al 2000)
Brachydactyly–craniostenosis–symphalangism	Hip dysplasia, symphalangism, middle and distal phalangeal hypoplasia/aplasia, missing nails, carpal and tarsal fusions	AD	(Ventruto et al 1976)
Carpenter acrocephalopoly–syndactyly type II	Pre-axial polydactyly of feet, syndactyly, radial deviation of thumbs, hypoplastic middle phalanges, cardiac defects, hypogenitalism, umbilical hernias, obesity, ear anomalies	AR	(Cohen et al 1987)
Cerebro-oculo-nasal	Macrocephaly, anophthalmia, bifid nose with dysplastic nares, nasal skin tags, midline brain malformations	Unknown	(Ercal and Say 1998)
Cole	Multiple fractures, dentinogenesis, craniosynostosis, blue sclerae	Unknown	(Amor et al 2000)
Cranioectodermal dysplasia	Sagittal craniosynostosis, short limbs, sparse fine hair, hypodontia, narrow thorax, cardiac abnormalities, epiphyseal dysplasia, renal failure. Resembles Ellis van Creveld/Jeunes	AR	(Savill et al 1997)
Craniofrontonasal dysplasia	Hypertelorism, bifid nasal tip, longitudinal splitting/ridging of nails	XLR	(Saavedra et al 1996)
Craniorhiny	Wide anteverted nares, upper lip cysts and fistulae, aplasia of nasolacrimal ducts	AD	(Mindikoglu et al 1991)
Curry Jones	Colobomas, microphthalmia, scalp defects, broad thumbs, finger syndactyly, pre-axial polydactyly, atrophic streaks, intestinal myofibromas and dysmotility	Unknown	(Temple et al 1995)
Furlong	Marfanoid body habitus, hypospadias, hernias, aortic dissection, mitral valve abnormalities	Unknown	(Megarbane and Hokayem 1998)
Gorlin–Chaudhry–Moss	Midface hypoplasia, eyelid colobomas, microphthalmia, hypermetropia, dental anomalies, genital hypoplasia, short distal phalanges	AR	(Ippel et al 1992)
Opitz C Oberklaid–Danks	Metopic synostosis, forehead haemangioma, additional features poorly defined: short stature, loose skin, post-axial polydactyly, syndactyly, joint contractures, cleft lip/palate, thick alveolar ridges, oral frenulae, midline brain abnormalities	AR; chromo-somal	(Sargent et al 1985, Bohring et al 1999, McGaughran et al 2000)
Philadelphia type	Sagittal craniosynostosis, variable syndactyly of fingers 2–5 and toes 1–5, face unlike Apert	AD	(Robin et al 1996)
Shprintzen–Goldberg	Arachnodactyly, camptodactyly, hernias, exophthalmos, hypotonia, learning disability	Unknown	(Greally et al 1998)

low frequency of sagittal suture involvement reported in Mediterranean populations has been the high frequency of oxycephaly, which is rare elsewhere (Lajeunie et al 1996).

Sagittal synostosis appears to be around three times commoner in males (Shillito and Matson 1968, Hunter and Rudd 1976, Lajeunie et al 1996) and is commoner in twins (Lajeunie et al 1996). Most are sporadic. In a study of 373 children with isolated sagittal synostosis from 366 families, there was a relative with proven scaphocephaly in 6 per cent and a family history of a different suture involvement in around 1 per cent. In the familial cases, the inheritance pattern appeared to be autosomal dominant with a low penetrance of around 38 per cent. In an estimated 72 per cent of patients the sagittal synostosis appeared to be sporadic and no parental age effect was found, suggesting that new autosomal dominant mutations were unlikely to be the cause (Lajeunie et al 1996). In the series of Hunter and Rudd (1976) the percentage of familial cases was around 2 per cent.

ISOLATED CORONAL CRANIOSYNOSTOSIS
Coronal suture involvement accounts for around 20 per cent of isolated non-syndromic craniosynostosis (Lajeunie et al 1995, Singer et al 1999). Coronal synostosis is twice as common in females, and unicoronal involvement is twice as common as bicoronal. Coronal synostosis is more likely to be syndromic than other single suture synsostoses, and is more likely to be familial, particularly when bilateral. There is an association with increased paternal age (Lajeunie et al 1995).

In recent years it has become clear that a significant proportion of patients with isolated coronal synostosis have an underlying FGFR3 P250R mutation. Moloney et al (1997) found the mutation in 6/18 (33 per cent) and 2/8 (25 per cent) patients with bilateral and unilateral coronal craniosynostosis respectively. In six of the patients, the mutation had arisen *de novo*. Gripp et al (1998) found the mutation in 11 per cent of patients with unilateral coronal synostosis. Lajeunie et al (1999) found the FGFR3 mutation in 42 per cent of 62 patients with coronal craniosynostosis overall, 74 per cent where it was familial and 17 per cent where it was sporadic. In the familial cases only 80 per cent of people carrying the mutation had craniosynostosis. Interestingly, females carrying the mutation were more likely to be affected, and were more likely to have bilateral suture involvement than males. Although it has not yet been formally demonstrated, it seems likely that the increased paternal age effect observed in coronal craniosynostosis will be accounted for by a high rate of new FGFR3 P250R mutations in sperm and/or selection for mutant sperm.

ISOLATED METOPIC CRANIOSYNOSTOSIS
In a series of 1713 patients with craniosynostosis reported by Lajeunie et al (1998), 14 per cent had metopic synostosis. However, widely varying figures have been reported, from around 3 per cent to 50 per cent of all craniosynostoses, by Singer et al (1999) and Shuper et al (1985) respectively, and may in part reflect differences in referral criteria. Like sagittal synostosis, it appears to be around twice as common in males and commoner in twins.

Metopic synostosis is clearly aetiologically heterogeneous and is more likely to be associated with additional malformations and learning disability than other single suture craniosynostoses. A significant proportion of those with associated malformations and/or learning disability have an underlying chromosome abnormality detectable on routine karyotyping. Deletions of chromosomes 9p and 11q are particularly associated with trigono-cephaly (Huret et al 1988, Lewanda et al 1995), but many other chromosome aberrations have been reported. It is likely that many will have cryptic chromosome imbalance.

Opitz C (C-trigonocephaly) syndrome has tended to be used as an umbrella diagnosis for patients who have metopic synostosis with associated malformations. A rather wide clinical spectrum has been reported in the literature, such that the underlying aetiology is likely to be heterogeneous (see Table 4.2).

Fetal valproate exposure is increasingly recognised as a cause of metopic craniosyn-ostosis with or without additional abnormalities which include learning disability, behavioural abnormalities, limb defects particularly of the radial ray, neural tube defects, clefting and minor facial, limb and nail anomalies (Ardinger et al 1988, Clayton-Smith and Donnai 1995, Lajeunie et al 2001).

Isolated metopic craniosynostosis, in the absence of developmental delay or teratogenic exposure, is usually sporadic. In the series reported by Lajeunie et al (1998), 5.6 per cent of cases were familial. No parental age effect was observed in the sporadic patients, sug-gesting that new autosomal dominant mutations are unlikely in this group. Consistent with that, Tartaglia et al (1999) found no patients with the FGFR3 P250R mutation in a series of nine newborns with metopic craniosynostosis. They also screened for mutations in FGFR1 and FGFR2 and found a mutation in FGFR2 in a single patient whose phenotype had subsequently evolved to be consistent with Crouzon syndrome.

ISOLATED LAMBDOID CRANIOSYNOSTOSIS

The incidence of posterior plagiocephaly appears to be increasing. The majority appear to be deformational and not associated with craniosynostosis. Risk factors for deformational posterior plagiocephaly include intra-uterine constraint, prematurity, complicated delivery, torticollis and, probably, sleeping babies on their backs (see Littlefield et al 1999). In those series that have sought to distinguish accurately between deformational plagiocephaly and craniosynostosis, the average incidence of true lambdoid synostosis was 2.9 per cent (reviewed: Wilkie 2000). Clearly, distinguishing the two can be difficult but is important given that those without true craniosynostosis generally respond well to conservative management. There is little data about the frequency of familial forms or parental age effects.

SECONDARY CRANIOSYNOSTOSIS

Craniosynostosis may occur secondary to deformation, for example as a result of constraint due to a uterine malformation, twinning or amniotic bands. It is more common in pre-term infants. Craniosynostosis can also occur in children with hyperthyroidism or following maternal hyperthyroidism during pregnancy (Hirano et al 1995, Gardner et al 1998).

Inheritance patterns in craniosynostosis syndromes

AUTOSOMAL DOMINANT

These conditions result from a mutation in one copy of a gene carried on an autosome, for which both males and females have two copies. In many autosomal dominant conditions, differences in severity, known as 'variable expression', are observed between affected members of the same family, despite the fact that they carry the same underlying mutation. In some instances there may be 'non-penetrance', where an individual proven to carry the family mutation is clinically normal. It seems likely that in most instances, variable expression and non-penetrance are the result of the interplay of variations in other 'modifier' genes. However, in the individual in whom the condition first arose in any family, it is possible that a milder phenotype could result from a mixture of mutant and normal cells (known as 'mosaicism') if the underlying mutation arose as a post-zygotic event.

An affected person with an autosomal dominant condition has a 1 in 2 (50 per cent) chance in each pregnancy of passing on their normal allele, in which case their child will be unaffected. Equally there will be a 50 per cent chance that their child will inherit the mutation and hence the condition. The chance the child will be affected to a significant extent will be somewhat lower, depending on the degree of associated penetrance and variable expression. For Apert syndrome penetrance approaches 100 per cent but for the other conditions, particularly the FGFR3-related craniosynostoses and Saethre–Chotzen syndrome, severity may be very variable within a family and non-penetrance has been observed (Marini et al 1991, Robin et al 1998, Lajeunie et al 1999, Dollfus et al 2002).

Autosomal dominant conditions frequently start *de novo* because of new mutations. In the FGFR2- and FGFR3-related craniosynostosis syndromes, a consistent correlation between *de novo* occurrences and increased parental age has been observed. Detailed studies in Apert syndrome (Moloney et al 1996) and in Crouzon/Pfeiffer (Glaser et al 2000) families have shown that new mutations are almost exclusively paternal in origin and have confirmed the correlation with increased paternal age. In females, replication of the genes as a prelude to oogenesis takes place in fetal life and formation of all the oocytes present at birth is believed to involve around 24 cell divisions. In contrast, in males around 36 cell divisions are believed to produce the spermatogonia present by puberty and thereafter the stem cells divide every 16 days (reviewed: Glaser et al 2000). Since replication of the genes must occur prior to every cell division, the likelihood of new mutations would be expected to increase with increasing paternal age; in addition to which, environmental teratogens and other factors may contribute. Nevertheless, the rate of certain mutations in these conditions appears to be exceptionally high (Moloney et al 1996, 1997) and other mechanisms may be involved, such as a selective advantage conferred on male germ cells by specific FGFR2/FGFR3 mutations (Oldridge et al 1997, Tiemann-Boege et al 2002, Glaser et al 2003).

The parents of a child with craniosynostosis should be examined carefully for any evidence of the condition. Childhood photographs and photographs of other family members can be helpful (Marini et al 1991). Where the parents appear to be unaffected clinically, account must be taken of possible non-penetrance and mosaicism affecting their germ-line. Where the specific mutation in their child is known, the parents should be offered testing to exclude non-penetrance. Where neither parent carries the known mutation in their blood, the risk of recurrence is usually quoted at around 1–2 per cent to allow for possible germ-line mosaicism and, despite the relatively small risk, they would still be offered prenatal testing for the family mutation. The non-specialist should note that for parents of an affected child, there is no circumstance where the recurrence risk is zero or even 'one in a million'! Testing of sperm for mosaicism is not currently offered outside a research setting.

AUTOSOMAL RECESSIVE

These conditions result from mutations in both copies of a gene carried on an autosome. Few craniosynostosis syndromes are autosomal recessive and they tend to be the rarer, less well characterised ones. For the majority of autosomal recessive conditions, new mutation rates are very low and it is usually assumed that the unaffected parents of an affected child are carriers, with a 1 in 4 (25 per cent) recurrence risk in each pregnancy. Very rare exceptions occur as a result of uniparental isodisomy (a child inherits both copies of a chromosome from one parent and no copy from the other).

Where parents have separated, recurrence risks will be very low with a new partner, assuming they are unrelated both to each other and the previous partner. For an affected individual and their siblings, offspring risks with an unaffected, unrelated partner are also low.

Where parents are consanguineous and well-recognised craniosynostosis syndromes have been excluded, recurrence risks will be a little higher than for unrelated couples, taking into account the possibility of a rare autosomal recessive syndrome, and the possibility of a low-penetrance autosomal dominant gene passing down through either parent, or both.

X-LINKED

These conditions result from mutation of a gene carried on the X-chromosome for which usually males have just one copy while females have two. This difference in dosage is compensated for in females by inactivation of one of the X-chromosomes in each cell, through a process known as Lyonisation which is usually random. As a result, females with X-linked conditions are usually unaffected or only mildly affected. In rare circumstances females do manifest, examples being those with a Turner syndrome karyotype (45,X) or where Lyonisation has been unfavourable. The commonest X-linked form of craniosyn-ostosis is craniofrontonasal dysplasia which is exceptionally unusual in that males are more mildly affected than females. The gene has been localised to chromosome Xp22 but has not yet been cloned.

Like autosomal dominant syndromes, there is a significant new mutation rate and genetic counselling must take into account the possibility that the mother of an affected boy may not be a carrier.

Female carriers of X-linked conditions must pass on one or other of their X-chromosomes to their offspring. Their sons therefore have a 50 per cent chance of being affected. Their daughters have a 50 per cent chance of being carriers. Where the child's sex is unknown, there is a 25 per cent chance of an affected boy.

Males with an X-linked condition must pass their X-chromosome to their daughters who will all be carriers. They must pass their Y-chromosome to all their sons, none of whom will therefore be affected.

CHROMOSOMAL

Parents of a child in whom an unbalanced chromosome abnormality has been identified should be offered chromosome testing to exclude the possibility that they carry an underlying chromosome rearrangement which predisposed to the imbalance in their offspring. As a general principle, where the parents' chromosomes are normal, recurrence risks will be low in future pregnancies, but antenatal chromosome testing is still available. For a parent who is found to carry a balanced translocation, recurrence risks will be higher (empiric risks are usually of the order of 5–15 per cent), but depend on the nature of the translocation, the sex of the parent and their family history. Chromosome testing should be offered to members of the extended family, usually via the affected parent.

TERATOGENIC

Clearly where a teratogenic cause is identified it is desirable to avoid it in any future pregnancy. In the author's experience the commonest teratogen is maternal valproate. With the help of the prescribing physician or neurologist, consideration should be given to whether anticonvulsant treatment is necessary, minimising the dose and the number of anticonvulsant agents, and changing the particular drug.

UNKNOWN

Where craniosynostosis appears to be isolated it is important to exclude environmental contributors as far as possible. Testing for the FGFR3 P250R mutation is a valuable adjunct since it identifies those individuals with a clear underlying genetic disposition and provides a test to aid accurate counselling for their first-degree relatives. For the remaining individuals where there is no definable aetiology, or those in whom a specific syndrome or chromosomal diagnosis cannot be identified, recurrence risks for their parents, siblings, and their own offspring will be empiric and largely depend on the outcome of careful clinical evaluation.

The genetic clinic

There is a clinical genetics unit based within each health region in the UK, staffed by clinical geneticists and nurse specialists and with affiliated cytogenetic and molecular genetic diagnostic laboratory services.

In most centres, the clinical genetics appointment will last around 45 minutes and ideally involve both parents. There are a number of objectives and areas for discussion.

1 ESTABLISHING A CLINICAL DIAGNOSIS

Accurate diagnosis of a craniosynostosis syndrome is important both for counselling and for directing the molecular genetic analysis cost effectively. It is important to take a careful history, looking particularly for affected relatives, consanguinity, evidence of potential teratogen exposure or fetal constraint. A careful examination of the patient is very important, with particular attention to the facial appearance (e.g. for evidence of asymmetry, proptosis, ptosis, flattening of the forehead, hypertelorism, a bifid nasal tip), the ears (e.g. for dysplastic pinnae, prominent crus), limbs (for broad thumbs and halluces, soft tissue syndactyly, nail ridging, synostoses), flexures (for acanthosis) and sometimes the genitalia. The syndrome diagnosis can often be made without any reference to detailed radiological investigations such as CT.

2 LABORATORY TESTING

In our hospital, given the relative simplicity of testing for the FGFR3 P250R mutation and its frequency and widely varying phenotypic manifestations, it is usually the first mutation to be tested in patients with single suture synostoses (particularly coronal), and in those with suspected FGFR2-, FGFR1- and TWIST-related craniosynostosis. Further screening is directed by the clinical phenotype. Karyotyping should also be undertaken, particularly in those with associated malformations or learning disability.

3 GENETIC COUNSELLING

The family history should be established including whether there is any consanguinity or known relative with similar features. It is usually appropriate to examine the parent or relative involved, and it may be valuable to see childhood photographs of them. The basic genetics underlying the condition can be explained as far as possible, including how it applies to the family. Where the mutation in the proband is known, testing of the parents or other relatives can be undertaken. It is not appropriate to undertake mutation screening in clinically normal individuals if the mutation in the proband cannot be identified. An exception might be if samples from an affected individual from the family are not available. Recurrence risks for future pregnancies can then be discussed and the range of options that would be available for future pregnancies, together with any associated advantages and disadvantages. The aim ultimately is to enable the couple to make informed choices for themselves.

4 PRENATAL TESTING

For couples who do decide to have prenatal testing, the clinical geneticist and genetics nurse specialists are usually involved in liaising between the family, the GP and obstetricians, as well as the laboratories, and in supporting the family both during and after the test.

Where the proband has a known molecular genetic or chromosomal abnormality underlying their craniosynostosis, prenatal testing is straightforward and available from around 11 weeks gestation. Where this is not the case, high-resolution ultrasound should be offered, the sensitivity of which will depend on the form of craniosynostosis and severity. For the milder forms, parents should be aware that the findings may not be detectable or, if so, not until late gestation.

5 ALTERNATIVE REPRODUCTIVE OPTIONS

For individuals known to carry a mutation who wish to avoid having an affected child, for whom termination of pregnancy is not an option, sperm or egg donation may be appropriate.

Pre-implantation genetic diagnosis (PGD) and re-implantation of unaffected embryos has been performed and is increasingly likely to be available in future (Abou-Sleiman et al 2002).

REFERENCES

Abou-Sleiman, PM, Apessos A, Harper JC, Serhal P, Delhanty JD (2002) Pregnancy following preimplantation genetic diagnosis for Crouzon syndrome. *Mol Hum Reprod* 8: 304–309.

Alderman BW, Fernbach SK, Greene C, Mangione EJ, Ferguson SW (1997) Diagnostic practice and the estimated prevalence of craniosynostosis in Colorado. *Arch Pediatr Adolesc Med* 151: 159–164.

Aleck KA, Bartley DL (1997) Multiple malformation syndrome following fluconazole use in pregnancy: report of an additional patient. *Am J Med Genet* 72: 253–256.

al-Qattan MM, Phillips JH (1997) Clinical features of Crouzon's syndrome patients with and without a positive family history of Crouzon's syndrome. *J Craniofac Surg* 8: 11–13.

Amor DJ, Savarirayan R, Schneider AS, Bankier A (2000) New case of Cole–Carpenter syndrome. *Am J Med Genet* 92: 273–277.

Ardinger HH, Atkin JF, Blackston RD, Elsas LJ, Clarren SK, Livingstone S, Flannery DB, Pellock JM, Harrod MJ, Lammer EJ, et al (1988) Verification of the fetal valproate syndrome phenotype. *Am J Med Genet* 29: 171–185.

Berant M, Berant N (1973) Radioulnar synostosis and craniosynostosis in one family. *J Pediatr* 83: 88–90.

Blair EM, Walsh S, Oldridge M, Wall SA, Wilkie AO (2000) Newly recognised craniosynostosis syndrome that does not map to known disease loci. *Am J Med Genet* 95: 4–9.

Bohring A, Silengo M, Lerone M, Superneau DW, Spaich C, Braddock SR, Poss A, Opitz JM (1999) Severe end of Opitz trigonocephaly (C) syndrome or new syndrome? *Am J Med Genet* 85: 438–446.

Chun K, Siegel-Bartelt J, Chitayat D, Phillips J, Ray PN (1998) FGFR2 mutation associated with clinical manifestations consistent with Antley–Bixler syndrome. *Am J Med Genet* 77: 219–224.

Clayton-Smith J, Donnai D (1995) Fetal valproate syndrome. *J Med Genet* 32: 724–727.

Cohen MM Jr (1979) Craniosynostosis and syndromes with craniosynostosis: incidence, genetics, penetrance, variability, and new syndrome updating. *Birth Defects Orig Artic Ser* 15: 13–63.

Cohen MM Jr, Kreiborg S (1992) Birth prevalence studies of the Crouzon syndrome: comparison of direct and indirect methods. *Clin Genet* 41: 12–15.

Cohen DM, Green JG, Miller J, Gorlin RJ, Reed JA (1987) Acrocephalopolysyndactyly type II – Carpenter syndrome: clinical spectrum and an attempt at unification with Goodman and Summit syndromes. *Am J Med Genet* 28: 311–324.

Cohen MM Jr, Kreiborg S, Lammer EJ, Cordero JF, Mastroiacovo P, Erickson JD, Roeper P, Martinez-Frias ML (1992) Birth prevalence study of the Apert syndrome. *Am J Med Genet* 42: 655–659.

Czeizel AE, Elek C, Susanszky E (1993) Birth prevalence study of the Apert syndrome. *Am J Med Genet* 45: 392–393.

Dollfus H, Biswas P, Kumaramanickavel G, Stoetzel C, Quillet R, Biswas J, Lajeunie E, Renier D, Perrin-Schmitt F (2002) Saethre–Chotzen syndrome: notable intrafamilial phenotypic variability in a large family with Q28X TWIST mutation. *Am J Med Genet* 109: 218–225.

Ercal D, Say B (1998) Cerebro-oculo-nasal syndrome: another case and review of the literature. *Clin Dysmorphol* 7: 139–141.

Fluck CE, Tajima T, Pandey AV, Arlt W, Okuhara K, Verge CF, Jabs EW, Mendonca BB, Fujieda K, Miller WL (2004) Mutant P450 oxidoreductase causes disordered steroidogenesis with and without Antley–Bixler syndrome. *Nat Genet* Feb 01 Epub (PMID: 14758361).

French LR, Jackson IT, Melton LJ 3rd (1990) A population-based study of craniosynostosis. *J Clin Epidemiol* 43: 69–73.

Friedman JM, Polifka JE (1994) *Teratogenic Effects of Drugs: A Resource for Clinicians: TERIS*. London: Johns Hopkins Press.

Gardner JS, Guyard-Boileau B, Alderman BW, Fernbach SK, Greene C, Mangione EJ (1998) Maternal exposure to prescription and non-prescription pharmaceuticals or drugs of abuse and risk of craniosynostosis. *Int J Epidemiol* 27: 64–67.

Glaser RL, Jiang W, Boyadjiev SA, Tran AK, Zachary AA, Van Maldergem L, Johnson D, Walsh S, Oldridge M, Wall SA, Wilkie AO, Jabs EW (2000) Paternal origin of FGFR2 mutations in sporadic cases of Crouzon syndrome and Pfeiffer syndrome. *Am J Hum Genet* 66: 768–777.

82

Glaser RL, Broman KW, Schulman RL, Eskenazi B, Wyrobek AJ, Jabs EW (2003) The paternal-age effect in Apert syndrome is due, in part, to the increased frequency of mutations in sperm. *Am J Hum Genet* 73: 939–947.

Greally MT, Carey JC, Milewicz DM, Hudgins L, Goldberg RB, Shprintzen RJ, Cousineau AJ, Smith WL Jr, Judisch GF, Hanson JW (1998) Shprintzen-Goldberg syndrome: a clinical analysis. *Am J Med Genet* 76: 202–212.

Grebe TA, Stevens MA, Byrne-Essif K, Cassidy SB (1992) 7p deletion syndrome: an adult with mild manifestations. *Am J Med Genet* 44: 18–23.

Gripp KW, McDonald-McGinn DM, Gaudenz K, Whitaker LA, Bartlett SP, Glat PM, Cassileth LB, Mayro R, Zackai EH, Muenke M (1998) Identification of a genetic cause for isolated unilateral coronal synostosis: a unique mutation in the fibroblast growth factor receptor 3. *J Pediatr* 132: 714–716.

Gripp KW, Zackai EH, Cohen MM Jr (1999) Not Antley–Bixler syndrome. *Am J Med Genet* 83: 65–68.

Hirano A, Akita S, Fujii T (1995) Craniofacial deformities associated with juvenile hyperthyroidism. *Cleft Palate Craniofac J* 32: 328–333.

Hunter AG, Rudd NL (1976) Craniosynostosis. I. Sagittal synostosis: its genetics and associated clinical findings in 214 patients who lacked involvement of the coronal suture(s). *Teratology* 14: 185–193.

Huret JL, Leonard C, Forestier B, Rethore MO, Lejeune J (1988) Eleven new cases of del(9p) and features from 80 cases. *J Med Genet* 25: 741–749.

Ippel PF, Gorlin RJ, Lenz W, van Doorne JM, Bijlsma JB (1992) Craniofacial dysostosis, hypertrichosis, genital hypoplasia, ocular, dental, and digital defects: confirmation of the Gorlin–Chaudhry–Moss syndrome. *Am J Med Genet* 44: 518–522.

Kelley RI, Kratz LE, Glaser RL, Netzloff ML, Miller Wolf L, Jabs EW (2002) Abnormal sterol metabolism in a patient with Antley–Bixler syndrome and ambiguous genitalia. *Am J Med Genet* 110: 95–102.

Kelly TE (1984) Teratogenicity of anticonvulsant drugs. I: Review of the literature. *Am J Med Genet* 19: 413–434.

Lajeunie E, Le Merrer M, Bonaiti-Pellie C, Marchac D, Renier D (1995) Genetic study of nonsyndromic coronal craniosynostosis. *Am J Med Genet* 55: 500–504.

Lajeunie, E, Le Merrer M, Bonaiti-Pellie C, Marchac D, Renier D (1996) Genetic study of scaphocephaly. *Am J Med Genet* 62: 282–285.

Lajeunie E, Le Merrer M, Marchac D, Renier D (1998) Syndromal and nonsyndromal primary trigonocephaly: analysis of a series of 237 patients. *Am J Med Genet* 75: 211–215.

Lajeunie E, El Ghouzzi V, Le Merrer M, Munnich A, Bonaventure J, Renier D (1999) Sex related expressivity of the phenotype in coronal craniosynostosis caused by the recurrent P250R FGFR3 mutation. *J Med Genet* 36: 9–13.

Lajeunie E, Barcik U, Thorne JA, Ghouzzi VE, Bourgeois M, Renier D (2001) Craniosynostosis and fetal exposure to sodium valproate. *J Neurosurg* 95: 778–782.

Leegte B, Kerstjens-Frederikse WS, Deelstra K, Begeer JH, van Essen AJ (1999) 11q-syndrome: three cases and a review of the literature. *Genet Couns* 10: 305–313.

Lewanda AF, Morsey S, Reid CS, Jabs EW (1995) Two craniosynostotic patients with 11q deletions, and review of 48 cases. *Am J Med Genet* 59: 193–198.

Littlefield TR, Kelly KM, Pomatto JK, Beals SP (1999) Multiple-birth infants at higher risk for development of deformational plagiocephaly. *Pediatrics* 103: 565–569.

McGaughran J, Aftimos S, Oei P (2000) Trisomy of 3pter in a patient with apparent C (trigonocephaly) syndrome. *Am J Med Genet* 94: 311–315.

Marini R, Temple K, Chitty L, Genet S, Baraitser M (1991) Pitfalls in counselling: the craniosynostoses. *J Med Genet* 28: 117–121.

Megarbane A, Hokayem N (1998) Craniosynostosis and marfanoid habitus without mental retardation: report of a third case. *Am J Med Genet* 77: 170–171.

Milunsky A, Graef JW, Gaynor MF Jr (1968) Methotrexate-induced congenital malformations. *J Pediatr* 72: 790–795.

Mindikoglu AN, Erginel A, Cenani A (1991) An unknown syndrome of nose deformity, oxycephaly, aplasia of the nasolacrimal ducts, and symmetrical cyst formation on the upper lip in siblings: craniorhiny. *Plast Reconstr Surg* 88: 699–702.

Moloney DM, Slaney SF, Oldridge M, Wall SA, Sahlin P, Stenman G, Wilkie AO (1996) Exclusive paternal origin of new mutations in Apert syndrome. *Nat Genet* 13: 48–53.

83

Moloney DM, Wall SA, Ashworth GJ, Oldridge M, Glass IA, Francomano CA, Muenke M, Wilkie AO (1997) Prevalence of Pro250Arg mutation of fibroblast growth factor receptor 3 in coronal craniosynostosis. *Lancet* 349: 1059–1062.

Oldridge M, Lunt PW, Zackai EH, McDonald-McGinn DM, Muenke M, Moloney DM, Twigg SR, Heath JK, Howard TD, Hoganson G, Gagnon DM, Jabs EW, Wilkie AO (1997) Genotype–phenotype correlation for nucleotide substitutions in the IgII– IgIII linker of FGFR2. *Hum Mol Genet* 6: 137–143.

Reardon W, Smith A, Honour JW, Hindmarsh P, Das D, Rumsby G, Nelson I, Malcolm S, Ades L, Sillence D, Kumar D, DeLozier-Blanchet C, McKee S, Kelly T, McKeehan WL, Baraitser M, Winter RM (2000) Evidence for digenic inheritance in some cases of Antley–Bixler syndrome? *J Med Genet* 37: 26–32.

Robin NH, Segel B, Carpenter G, Muenke M (1996) Craniosynostosis, Philadelphia type: a new autosomal dominant syndrome with sagittal craniosynostosis and syndactyly of the fingers and toes. *Am J Med Genet* 62: 184–191.

Robin NH, Scott JA, Cohen AR, Goldstein JA (1998) Nonpenetrance in FGFR3-associated coronal synostosis syndrome. *Am J Med Genet* 80: 296–297.

Saavedra D, Richieri-Costa A, Guion-Almeida ML, Cohen MM Jr (1996) Craniofrontonasal syndrome: study of 41 patients. *Am J Med Genet* 61: 147–151.

Sargent C, Burn J, Baraitser M, Pembrey ME (1985) Trigonocephaly and the Opitz C syndrome. *J Med Genet* 22: 39–45.

Savill GA, Young ID, Cunningham RJ, Ansell ID, Evans JH (1997) Chronic tubulo-interstitial nephropathy in children with cranioectodermal dysplasia. *Pediatr Nephrol* 11: 215–217.

Seto ML, Lee SJ, Sze RW, Cunningham ML (2001) Another TWIST on Baller–Gerold syndrome. *Am J Med Genet* 104: 323–330.

Shaw EB, Steinback HL (1968) Aminopterin-induced fetal malformation. Survival of infant after attempted abortion. *Am J Dis Child* 115: 477–482.

Shillito J Jr, Matson DD (1968) Craniosynostosis: a review of 519 surgical patients. *Pediatrics* 41: 829–853.

Shuper A, Merlob P, Grunebaum M, Reisner SH (1985) The incidence of isolated craniosynostosis in the newborn infant. *Am J Dis Child* 139: 85–86.

Singer S, Bower C, Southall P, Goldblatt J (1999) Craniosynostosis in Western Australia, 1980–1994: a population-based study. *Am J Med Genet* 83: 382–387.

Tartaglia M, Bordoni V, Velardi F, Basile RT, Saulle E, Tenconi R, Di Rocco C, Battaglia PA (1999) Fibroblast growth factor receptor mutational screening in newborns affected by metopic synostosis. *Childs Nerv Syst* 15: 389–393; discussion 393–394.

Temple IK, Eccles DM, Winter RM, Baraitser M, Carr SB, Shortland D, Jones MC, Curry C (1995) Craniofacial abnormalities, agenesis of the corpus callosum, polysyndactyly and abnormal skin and gut development – the Curry Jones syndrome. *Clin Dysmorphol* 4: 116–129.

Tiemann-Boege I, Navidi W, Grewal R, Cohn D, Eskenazi B, Wyrobek AJ, Arnheim N (2002) The observed human sperm mutation frequency cannot explain the achondroplasia paternal age effect. *PNAS* 99: 14952–14957.

Tolarova MM, Harris JA, Ordway DE, Vargervik K (1997) Birth prevalence, mutation rate, sex ratio, parents' age, and ethnicity in Apert syndrome. *Am J Med Genet* 72: 394–398.

Ventruto V, Di Girlamo R, Festa B, Romano A, Sebastio G, Sebastio L (1976) Family study of inherited syndrome with multiple congenital deformities: symphalangism, carpal and tarsal fusion, brachydactyly, craniosynostosis, strabismus, hip osteochondritis. *J Med Genet* 13: 394–398.

Walsh LE, Vance GH, Weaver DD (2001) Distal 13q deletion syndrome and the VACTERL association: case report, literature review, and possible implications. *Am J Med Genet* 98: 137–144.

Wilkie AO (2000) Epidemiology and genetics of craniosynostosis. *Am J Med Genet* 90: 82–84.

Wilson GN, Dasouki M, Barr M Jr (1985) Further delineation of the dup(3q) syndrome. *Am J Med Genet* 22: 117–123.

Zollino M, Tiziano F, Di Stefano C, Neri G (1999) Partial duplication of the long arm of chromosome 15: confirmation of a causative role in craniosynostosis and definition of a 15q25-qter trisomy syndrome. *Am J Med Genet* 87: 391–394.

5
PRENATAL DIAGNOSIS OF CRANIOSYNOSTOSIS

Olav B. Petersen and Lyn S. Chitty

Introduction

The prenatal diagnosis of craniosynostosis can be approached from two angles. The first concerns diagnosis in families at known increased risk because of a relevant family history. The second is often more complicated, and addresses the diagnostic approach following the unexpected finding of an abnormal head shape at the time of a routine fetal anomaly scan in families at no prior risk. In the last few years advances in molecular genetics have seen the identification of the molecular basis of many of the craniosynostosis syndromes (see Chapter 3), thereby permitting early prenatal diagnosis, using invasive techniques, for families at increased risk. At the same time progress in ultrasound technology and the more widespread use of routine fetal anomaly scanning in the western world have resulted in an increasing number of reports describing the sonographic diagnosis of a variety of syndromes with associated craniosynostosis. However, these syndromes are rare (see Chapter 4) and so there is still a relative paucity of literature in these areas.

In this chapter the molecular and sonographic diagnosis of craniosynostosis will be discussed. The diagnosis of individual syndromes will be covered, and then the approach to the management of a fetus with an unexpected finding of craniosynostosis will be described. The literature will be reviewed and examples of cases seen in the Fetal Medicine Unit at University College London Hospital (UCLH) will be used to illustrate points where appropriate.

Routine scanning

Fetal ultrasound is now an established part of standard obstetric care in many countries. It can be performed in early gestation and in the first, second and third trimester, as part of routine obstetric care, or as a targeted investigation in women at increased risk for a particular problem. In many countries fetal ultrasound is offered routinely both in the first trimester of pregnancy to establish the gestation and viability and again later (around 20 weeks) to examine the anatomy in more detail. Scanning earlier and later in pregnancy in most units tends to be performed on clinical indication rather than routinely. As part of any fetal ultrasound examination the head is visualised and would usually be measured to determine the biparietal diameter and head circumference. These measurements are useful, both as an indicator of gestational age (before 24 weeks' gestation) and later as a marker of fetal growth. The fetal head is usually oval, or 'rugby football'-shaped (Fig. 5.1(a)).

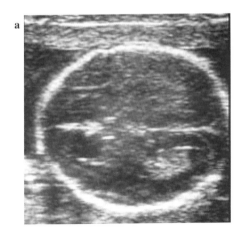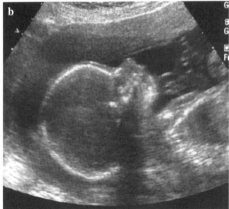

Fig. 5.1 (a) Axial view of a normal fetal head at 20 weeks' gestation and (b) the parasagittal view showing a normal fetal profile.

Variation in this appearance can either be because the sonographer has angled the transducer wrongly, or because there is some predisposing factor (e.g. dolicocephaly is seen more commonly in the presence of oligohydramnios or when the fetus is in the breech position) or underlying pathology (Tables 5.1 and 5.2). The fetal profile (Fig. 5.1(b)) can also be seen at the time of a routine scan, although this view is often only obtained when other anomalies have been detected or when there is another risk factor present.

Prenatal diagnosis in families at increased risk
There are over 160 syndromes listed on the London Dysmorphology Database which may have craniosynostosis as a feature. Many are very rare and some have only been reported in single families or sporadic cases (Winter and Baraitser 2000). Some have associated features that can be sought using fetal ultrasound, while for others the specific gene defect is known. The aids to prenatal diagnosis for those with potential sonographic features, and other methods of prenatal diagnosis for the commoner ones, are summarised in Table 5.1.

INVASIVE TESTING
In those families where there is a known genetic mutation and the parents request prenatal diagnosis (Table 5.1; see also Chapters 3 and 4), invasive testing using either chorionic villus sampling or amniocentesis should be discussed. Chorionic villus sampling (CVS) can be done from around 11 weeks' gestation onwards and carries a risk of miscarriage of around 1–2 per cent. The chorionic villi collected provide a good source of fetal DNA and results of the molecular analysis are usually available within a week of the procedure in syndromes where the precise mutation is known. When molecular diagnosis is dependent on linkage analysis, the results are usually available around two weeks after the CVS.

Amniocentesis is a slightly safer procedure, carrying a risk of procedural-related loss of around 1 per cent, but it cannot be done until about 15 weeks' gestation. The yield of fetal

TABLE 5.1

Aids to prenatal diagnosis: summary of the syndromes commonly associated with craniosynostosis

Syndrome	Associated features in addition to craniosynostosis which may aid sonographic diagnosis	Inheritance	Gene location/ defect
Adelaide-type craniosynostosis		AD	FGFR3
Antley–Bixler	Bowing of long bones, radio-humeral synostosis	AR	
Apert	mitten hands and feet, osseous syndactyly, proptosis, polyhydramnios	AD	FGFR2
Baller–Gerold	Radial anomalies	AR	
Beare–Stevenson	Abnormal genitalia, umbilical anomalies	AD	FGFR2
Boston-type craniosynostosis		AD	MSX2
Carpenter	Polysyndactyly of hands and feet, cardiac anomalies	AR	?
Cerebro-oculo-nasal	Anophthalmia, midline brain defects	?	?
Cranio-frontonasal dysplasia	Severe hypertelorism, neck webbing, facial cleft	?	Xp2.2
Crouzon	Hypertelorism, proptosis	AD	FGFR2
Elejalde (acrocephalopoly-dactylous dysplasia)	Short limbs and ribs, polydactyly, renal anomalies, hygromata, hydrops	AD	?
Greigs cephalo-polysyndactyly	Macrocephaly, hypertelorism, pre- and post-axial polydactyly, syndactyly	AD	GLI3
Jackson–Weiss	Abnormal great toes	AD	FGFR2
Muenke		AD	FGFR3
Multiple exostoses–parietal foramina–craniofacial dysostosis (DEFECT 11)	Parietal foramina	AD	11p.1.2 (ALX4)
Pfeiffer	Broad thumbs	AD	FGFR2; FGFR1
Robinow–Sorauf	Bifid great toe	AD	TWIST
Saethre–Chotzen		AD	TWIST
Thanatophoric dysplasia	Short limbs, small chest, trident hands, frontal bossing, polyhydramnios	AD	FGFR3

cells for molecular testing following amniocentesis is smaller, and frequently culturing is required before analysis. This means the result may not be available for 2–3 weeks. However, when the precise disease-causing mutation is known, polymerase chain reaction (PCR) may be used for molecular diagnosis directly on the cells obtained at amniocentesis, and then the results may be available within the week. In all situations where parents are seeking prenatal diagnosis of a craniosynostosis syndrome, it is advisable to liaise closely both with the clinical genetics team and with the fetal medicine team who will be undertaking the testing.

SONOGRAPHIC DIAGNOSIS

The *in utero* sonographic findings of craniosynostosis are occasionally described, and have recently been reviewed by Miller et al (2002). There are several reports of the *Kleeblattschadel* seen in type II thanatophoric dysplasia, and a few reports of the sonographic findings in Crouzon, Apert, Saethre–Chotzen, Antley–Bixler, Pfeiffer and Carpenter syndromes, as well as some non-syndromic cases. While *Kleeblattschadel* is not uncommonly detected in the second trimester of pregnancy (or, rarely, earlier), many of the other reports describe the identification of an abnormal skull shape in the third trimester (Table 5.2). It is unclear in most reports whether this is due to the late development of sonographically detectable features, or whether the fetuses were not scanned earlier in pregnancy, although the late diagnosis of Apert syndrome at 28 and 33 weeks' gestation, after normal second trimester scans, has been reported (Filkins et al 1997, Kaufmann et al 1997) and we have recently observed the later presentation of skull anomalies in a fetus with Muenke craniosynostosis (Fig. 5.2).

TABLE 5.2
Gestation at diagnosis for cases reported with craniosynostosis syndromes

Diagnosis	Gestation at diagnosis	Authors
Crouzon syndrome	19–35 weeks	Leo et al 1991, Gollin et al 1993, Sergi et al 1997, Miller et al 2002
Apert syndrome	19, 20, 24, 28, 31, 33	Hill et al 1987, Narayan and Scott 1991, Parent et al 1994, Filkins et al 1997, Kaufmann et al 1997, Chang et al 1998, Boog et al 1999, Pooh et al 1999, Lyu and Ko 2000, Mahieu-Caputo et al 2001
Pfeiffer syndrome	27, 35	Hill and Grzybek 1994, Martinelli et al 1997, Miller et al 2002
Kleeblattschadel (with thanatophoric dysplasia)	15, 17, 27, 31	Chervenak et al 1983, Burrows et al 1984, Weiner et al 1986, Corsello et al 1992, Chen et al 2001, Kalache et al 2002, Miller et al 2002
Kleeblattschadel	20, 29, 30, 32, 34	Brahman et al 1979, Salvo 1981, Fischer et al 1982, Stamm et al 1987, Krepelova et al 1998, Hsu et al 2001, Miller et al 2002
Antley–Bixler	17, 20	Savoldelli and Schinzel 1982, Schinzel et al 1983, LeHeup et al 1995, Chen et al 2001, Machado et al 2001
Saethre–Chotzen	19, 21	Miller et al 2002
Carpenter syndrome	20, 27, 34	Ashby et al 1994, Balci et al 1997, Martinelli et al 1997
Non-syndromic	17–42, 31, 33	van der Ham et al 1995, Huang et al 2001, Miller et al 2002
Muenke	29	Chitty and Petersen 2004

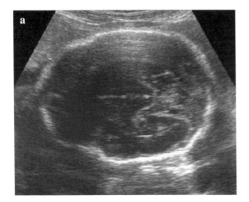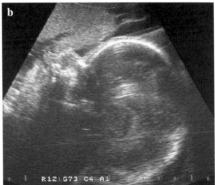

Fig. 5.2 (a) View through the head in the axial plane at 29 weeks' gestation in a fetus with Meunke's craniosynostosis. Note the prominent parietal area and the slight depression over the coronal sutures. (b) View of the profile showing the marked degree of frontal bossing. This fetus was also scanned at 14, 16 and 22 weeks' gestation, but detailed sonography at those times failed to demonstrate any abnormality of skull shape or profile.

In pregnancies at risk of a craniosynostosis syndrome with a known genetic abnormality, but not associated with other major anomalies, parents who want a definitive prenatal diagnosis should be advised to have an invasive prenatal diagnosis. This will, however, only determine the genetic status of the fetus, and, particularly when expressivity is variable (e.g. Crouzon, Saethre–Chotzen, Muenke), will not give a good indication of the prognosis for the fetus. In these conditions, where parents are only likely to consider pregnancy interruption if there are signs of significant structural abnormality, serial scanning (with no guarantees of detecting problems even when the neonate will have obvious clinical signs) should be considered.

Many craniosynostosis syndromes have a reasonably predictable phenotype with associated abnormalities amenable to detection using fetal ultrasound examination (Table 5.1). In these conditions – e.g. Apert, Carpenter – prenatal diagnosis can reliably depend upon fetal ultrasound. This is obviously helpful in families at high risk of recurrence with no known mutation (e.g. Carpenter syndrome), or where the risks are small (e.g. previous pregnancy complicated by *de novo* Apert syndrome) and parents would like to avoid the risks of invasive testing. In conditions associated with significant digital and limb anomalies, sonographic diagnosis from 13 weeks' gestation may be possible as scanning at this gestation, either using the transabdominal route or, preferably, transvaginally, usually allows good definition of limbs and extremities. Filkins et al (1997) reported the detection of the mitten-like hands in the early second trimester in a fetus subsequently found to have Apert syndrome. The abnormalities in skull shape in this case were not seen until 33 weeks when the mother was referred for another scan because of polyhydramnios. Detection of the skull anomalies in Apert syndrome in the third trimester is frequently reported (Kim et al 1986, Hill et al 1987, Parent et al 1994, Kaufmann et al 1997), although earlier diagnosis is possible (Fig. 5.3) and has been reported at 16 (Narayan and Scott 1991) and 19 weeks (Pooh et al 1999). In

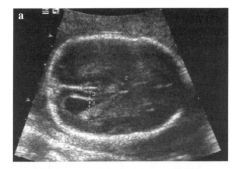

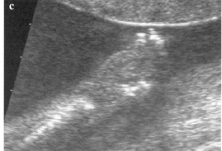

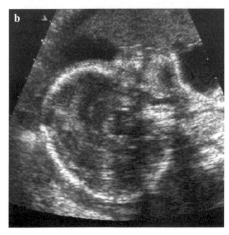

Fig. 5.3 (a) Axial view through the fetal head at 22 weeks' gestation in a fetus with Apert syndrome showing the mild dilatation of the lateral cerebral ventricle. The profile (b) demonstrates the turricephaly. Detection of the limb anomalies, mitten hands (c) and feet suggested the diagnosis in this *de novo* case. Amniocentesis and identification of the mutation in the FGFR2 gene enabled informed counselling for the parents. The mild dilatation of the lateral cerebral ventricles in this case was noted at 16 weeks' gestation. Detailed scanning in a tertiary referral centre at 22 weeks identified the other anomalies.

other conditions, e.g. Greigs cephalo-polysyndactyly, the associated features may be a more consistent finding, thus making a more reliable sonographic diagnostic tool (Fig. 5.4).

Occasionally it is the detection of the abnormal head shape that aids diagnosis of syndromes that may be associated with craniosynostosis but have limited other sonographic findings. Fig. 5.5 shows the abnormal head shape in a fetus at 25 per cent risk of I-cell disease. The parents had declined invasive testing as they did not want to face the procedural-related risk of miscarriage, but did want forewarning of a recurrence if possible. Scanning at 21 weeks revealed an unusual head shape and, as I-cell disease has been reported in association with craniosynostosis, this raised the suspicion of a recurrence. Later in pregnancy, when the fetal limbs were slightly short, concern increased. The diagnosis was confirmed after birth at term.

The majority of cases with isolated craniosynostosis have a non-syndromic form. These tend to have a low recurrence risk and, while a proportion will have a detectable mutation (see Chapter 4 for details), prenatal detection of a recurrence will rely on fetal ultrasound. There are a number of cases reported in the literature, but, as with other forms of craniosynostosis, sonographic presentation tends to be in the third trimester when scanning is performed because of polyhydramnios (Table 5.2) (Meilstrup et al 1995, van der Ham et al 1995, Huang et al 2001).

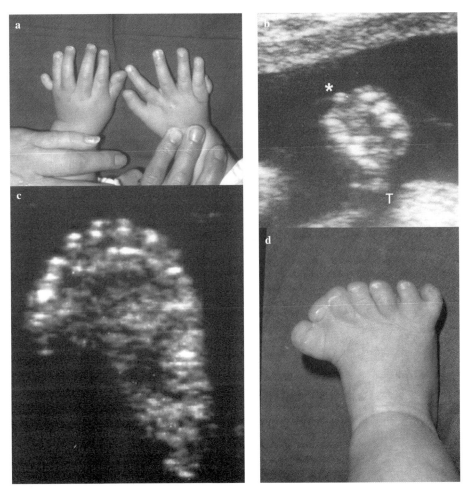

Fig. 5.4 Image demonstrating the polydactyly of hands (a) at 20 weeks' gestation with (b) postnatal view in this fetus with Greigs cephalo-polysyndactyly (T thumb; * extra digit). Views of the feet (c, d) are also shown. The mother was known be a gene carrier, and detailed examination of the fetal extremities revealed these anomalies. The head shape remained within normal limits throughout pregnancy. (Image reproduced courtesy of David Griffin.)

COUNSELLING

All parents at risk of having a child with a craniosynostosis syndrome should be referred for counselling with a geneticist and/or fetal medicine specialist (who should liaise with his/her genetics colleagues). There are rapid advances in the molecular aspects of prenatal diagnosis and geneticists are best placed to be aware of the most appropriate tests on offer in these circumstances. Many craniosynostosis syndromes are inherited in an autosomal dominant fashion with a high degree of penetrance but variable expressivity, with some family members having minimal features and others being severely affected (Marini et al

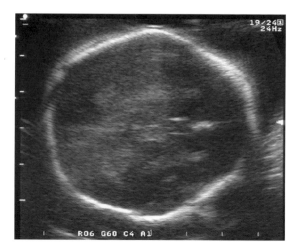

Fig. 5.5 Abnormal head shape seen at 21 weeks in a fetus at 25 per cent risk of I-cell disease. Views of the head at 13 weeks' gestation had been normal.

1991). However, while prenatal diagnosis is possible using chorionic villus sampling or amniocentesis for molecular analysis in families at high risk if the mutation causing the syndrome in that family has been identified, when expression is so variable knowledge of carrier status is not sufficient to predict outcome. We have recently reported a case where early analysis of amniocytes demonstrated that the fetus carried the FGFR3-P250R mutation responsible for Muenke syndrome, but serial ultrasound in a tertiary unit failed to demonstrate any significant abnormality until the third trimester (Fig. 5.2).

Parents also need to be aware of the variability in expression found in many of these syndromes and thus of the limitations of dependence on molecular prenatal diagnosis alone. Discussion with a fetal medicine specialist is also valuable, as they are best placed to discuss the limitations of fetal ultrasound. It must be remembered that the accuracy of sonographic diagnosis will vary depending on the timing of development of the abnormality, as well as on the extent of the deformity. Many seemingly severe pathologies presenting after birth are not amenable to prenatal sonographic diagnosis.

Diagnosis in the low-risk population

MANAGEMENT FOLLOWING THE DIAGNOSIS OF AN UNEXPECTED
ABNORMAL HEAD SHAPE
An abnormal head shape is found at the time of a routine scan in around 2–3 per cent of pregnancies. A variety of shapes are seen with varied aetiologies (Table 5.3). True craniosynostosis is rarely seen in the second trimester and probably the most common presentation is a cloverleaf skull seen in association with thanatophoric dysplasia (Fig. 5.6), although severe manifestations of other craniosynostosis syndromes do occasionally present around the time of the routine second trimester anomaly scan (Fig. 5.7).

TABLE 5.3
**Classification and diagnosis in 277 cases with an abnormal
head shape scanned in a tertiary fetal medicine unit**

	Aneuploidy	NTD	Syndrome	Oligo/breech	Other
Bracycephaly	7		1	2	19
Dolicocephaly	1		1	32/6	10
Microcephaly	9		2		19
Prominent forehead		1	3		4
Prominent occiput			1	2	
Lemon-shaped		77			9
Cloverleaf skull			6		2
Strawberry-shaped	29	1	2	1	4
Macrocephaly					4
Other		9	7	1	5

NTD: neural tube defect; oligo: oligohydramnios.

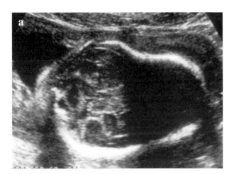
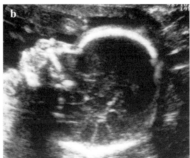

Fig. 5.6 (a) Axial view of the fetal head at 18 weeks' gestation in a case with thanatophoric dysplasia and a clover leaf skull. The profile (b) demonstrates the classical frontal bossing. The presence of short limbs, trident fingers and a small chest indicated the underlying pathology which was confirmed by postnatal radiology and identification of the FGFR3 mutation.

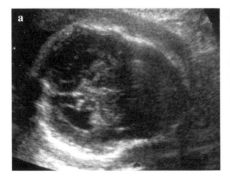
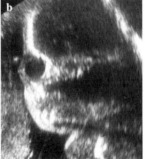

Fig. 5.7 Images of the fetal head (a) and view of the face (b) of a fetus in the second trimester diagnosed after birth as having Antley–Bixler syndrome. Note the prominent orbits seen in the view of the face. Contractures at the elbows and choanal atresia were also found after birth.

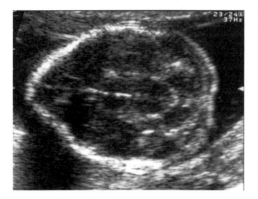

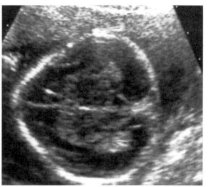

Fig. 5.8 A fetus scanned at 19 weeks' gestation with the classical 'lemon-shaped' head seen in 99 per cent of fetuses with spina bifida scanned before 26 weeks' gestation. This unusual head resolves in the majority of affected fetuses by the end of the second trimester, and can be seen as an incidental finding in 1 per cent of normal fetuses.

Fig. 5.9 An axial view through the head of a fetus with trisomy 18, demonstrating the classical 'strawberry' shape.

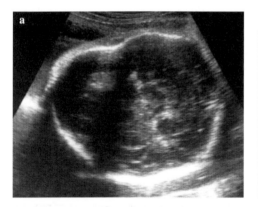

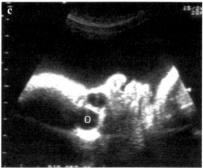

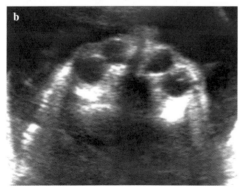

Fig. 5.10 (a) Axial view through the fetal head at 34 weeks' gestation demonstrating the unusual skull shape in this fetus found to have craniofrontonasal dysplasia after birth. The axial view (b) at the level of the orbits showing the orbits (o) and cystic structures (dacrocystocoeles) lying medial to the orbits. The parasagittal view (c) shows the profile. Note the unusual skull shape, with turricephaly, and the cystic structure lying inferior and medial to the orbit (o).

A retrospective search of the computerised database analysis in the Fetal Medicine Unit at UCLH revealed a total of 297 fetuses with an abnormal head shape seen in the last 10 years. Only 11 of these had craniosynostosis (Table 5.3). The most common association with an abnormal head shape was spina bifida seen in fetuses with a 'lemon'-shaped head (Fig. 5.8), then trisomy 18 seen in conjunction with 'strawberry'-shaped heads (Fig. 5.9) (Table 5.3). Given these relatively common associations, it is essential to perform a detailed anomaly scan searching for other anomalies once an unusual head shape is identified.

Karyotyping should be considered, as, in addition to trisomy 18, a number of abnormal karyotypes have been reported in association with craniosynostosis (see Chapter 4 for details). Careful attention must be paid to the examination of the fetal extremities, as it is in this area that clues to the underlying pathology (aneuploidy or genetic syndrome) may lie (Figs 5.3 and 5.4, Table 5.1). Referral for detailed scanning in these cases is recommended, as associated features may be subtle and a good knowledge of possible syndromes is required if the examination is to be helpful. Where this is not possible, discussion of the findings with the local geneticist may give clues as to other findings to look for. Identification of features such as mitten hands and feet may allow for invasive testing with targeted molecular analysis and confirmation of diagnosis. The case shown in Fig. 5.10 is an example of where this team approach to diagnosis was helpful. A referral for detailed scanning and a genetic opinion was made by the local unit when an unusual facial appearance was detected at 34 weeks' gestation. Severe polyhydramnios was noted in conjunction with an abnormal skull shape and cystic structures medial to the orbits thought to represent dacrocystocoeles. The polyhydramnios was considered to be secondary to choanal atresia as colour Doppler could not identify any flow through the nose during fetal breathing. Discussion with the geneticists suggested the possibility of Saethre–Chotzen as this has been reported in association with lacrimal duct cysts, but parental examination and review of their early photographs failed to show any indication that either was a gene carrier. On postnatal examination the diagnosis was thought more likely to be craniofrontonasal dysplasia in view of the significant degree of ocular hypertelorism. This had not been detected prenatally as the lacrimal duct cysts precluded accurate measurement of orbital diameters.

COUNSELLING

In all cases with the unexpected finding of craniosynostosis parents should be referred for a genetic consultation, as careful examination of parental features and their early photographs may suggest a dominantly inherited condition. Once a diagnosis of craniosynostosis in a fetus has been made, regardless of whether the underlying aetiology is known, parents should be referred to a craniofacial unit specialising in congenital disorders for discussion of prognosis and postnatal management. It may be helpful to review images or a video of the fetus before the consultation, or for the expert involved to attend a scan if possible. In these rare situations, the health professionals experienced in the management of children with these conditions are best placed to give parents the accurate information they need upon which to base difficult decisions.

Conclusions

Craniosynostosis is only occasionally seen in the prenatal period. Whether dealing with the family at increased risk, or when confronted with an unexpected finding in a low-risk family, a team approach to the management of these rare cases is essential. The fetal medicine specialist, geneticist and neurosurgeons need to work together in order to offer the best service to parents in these difficult circumstances.

REFERENCES

Ashby T, Rouse GA, De Lange M (1994) Prenatal sonographic diagnosis of Carpenter syndrome. *J Ultrasound Med* 13: 905–909.

Balci S, Onol B, Eryilmaz M, Haytoglu T (1997) A case of Carpenter syndrome diagnosed in a 20-week-old fetus with postmortem examination. *Clin Genet* 51: 412–416.

Boog G, Le Vaillant C, Winer N, David A, Quere MP, Nomballais MF (1999) Contribution of tridimensional sonography and magnetic resonance imaging to prenatal diagnosis of Apert syndrome at mid-trimester. *Fetal Diagn Ther* 14: 20–23.

Brahman S, Jenna R, Wittenauer HJ (1979) Sonographic in utero appearance of Kleeblattschadel syndrome. *J Clin Ultrasound* 7: 481–484.

Burrows PE, Stannard MW, Pearrow J, Sutterfield S, Baker ML (1984) Early antenatal sonographic recognition of thanatophoric dysplasia with cloverleaf skull deformity. *Am J Roentgenol* 143: 841–843.

Chang CC, Tsai FJ, Tsai HD, Tsai CH, Hseih YY, Lee CC, Yang TC, Wu JY (1998) Prenatal diagnosis of Apert syndrome. *Prenat Diagn* 18: 621–625.

Chen CP, Chern SR, Shih JC, Wang W, Yeh LF, Chang TY, Tzen CY (2001) Prenatal diagnosis and genetic analysis of type I and type II thanatophoric dysplasia. *Prenat Diagn* 21: 89–95.

Chervenak FA, Blakemore KJ, Isaacson G, Mayden K, Hobbins JC (1983) Antenatal sonographic findings of thanatophoric dysplasia with cloverleaf skull. *Am J Obstet Gynecol* 146: 984–985.

Chitty L, Petersen OB (2004) Prenatal diagnosis of craniosynostosis: sonographic features of Muenke syndrome. *Prenat Diagn* (submitted for publication).

Corsello G, Maresi E, Rossi C, Giuffre L, Cittadini E (1992) Thanatophoric dysplasia in monozygotic twins discordant for cloverleaf skull: prenatal diagnosis, clinical and pathological findings. *Am J Med Genet* 42: 122–126.

Filkins K, Russo JF, Boehmer S, Camous M, Przylepa KA, Jiang W, Jabs EW (1997) Prenatal ultrasonographic and molecular diagnosis of Apert syndrome. *Prenat Diagn* 17: 1081–1084.

Fischer G, Hori A, Ulbrich R, Rath W (1982) [Early stage of a cloverleaf skull malformation]. *Rontgenblatter* 35: 438–443.

Gollin YG, Abuhamad AZ, Inati MN, Shaffer WK, Copel JA, Hobbins JC (1993) Sonographic appearance of craniofacial dysostosis (Crouzon syndrome) in the second trimester. *J Ultrasound Med* 12: 625–628.

Hill LM, Grzybek PC (1994) Sonographic findings with Pfeiffer syndrome. *Prenat Diagn* 14: 47–49.

Hill LM, Thomas ML, Peterson CS (1987) The ultrasonic detection of Apert syndrome. *J Ultrasound Med* 6: 601–604.

Hsu TY, Chang SY, Wang TJ, Ou CY, Chen ZH, Hsu PH (2001) Prenatal sonographic appearance of Beare–Stevenson cutis gyrata syndrome: two- and three-dimensional ultrasonographic findings. *Prenat Diagn* 21: 665–667.

Huang HW, Lin H, Chang SY, Hsu YH, Hsu TY (2001) Isolated craniosynostosis: prenatal ultrasound of scaphocephaly with polyhydramnios. *Chang Gung Med J* 24: 816–819.

Kalache KD, Lehmann K, Chaoui R, Kivelitz DE, Mundlos S, Bollmann R (2002) Prenatal diagnosis of partial agenesis of the corpus callosum in a fetus with thanatophoric dysplasia type 2. *Prenat Diagn* 22: 404–407.

Kaufmann K, Baldinger S, Pratt L (1997) Ultrasound detection of Apert syndrome: a case report and literature review. *Am J Perinatol* 14: 427–430.

Kim H, Uppal V, Wallach R (1986) Apert syndrome and fetal hydrocephaly. *Hum Genet* 73: 93–95.

Krepelova A, Baxova A, Calda P, Plavka R, Kapras J (1998) FGFR2 gene mutation (Tyr375Cys) in a new case of Beare–Stevenson syndrome. *Am J Med Genet* 76: 362–364.

LeHeup BP, Masutti JP, Droulle P, Tisserand J (1995) The Antley–Bixler syndrome: report of two familial cases with severe renal and anal anomalies. *Eur J Pediatr* 154: 130–133.

Leo MV, Suslak L, Ganesh VL, Adhate A, Apuzzio JJ (1991) Crouzon syndrome: prenatal ultrasound diagnosis by binocular diameters. *Obstet Gynecol* 78: 906–908.

Lyu KJ, Ko TM (2000) Prenatal diagnosis of Apert syndrome with widely separated cranial sutures. *Prenat Diagn* 20: 254–256.

Machado LE, Osborne NG, Bonilla-Musoles F (2001) Antley–Bixler syndrome: report of a case. *J Ultrasound Med* 20: 73–77.

Mahieu-Caputo D, Sonigo P, Amiel J, Simon I, Aubry MC, Lemerrer M, Delezoide AL, Gigarel N, Dommergues M, Dumez Y (2001) Prenatal diagnosis of sporadic Apert syndrome: a sequential diagnostic approach combining three-dimensional computed tomography and molecular biology. *Fetal Diagn Ther* 16: 10–12.

Marini R, Temple K, Chitty L, Genet S, Baraitser M (1991) Pitfalls in counselling: the craniosynostoses. *J Med Genet* 28: 117–121.

Martinelli P, Paladini D, D'Armiento M, Scarano G (1997) Prenatal diagnosis of cloverleaf skull in the subtype 2 Pfeiffer syndrome. *Clin Dysmorphol* 6: 89–90.

Meilstrup JW, Botti JJ, MacKay DR, Johnson DL (1995) Prenatal sonographic appearance of asymmetric craniosynostosis: a case report. *J Ultrasound Med* 14: 307–310.

Miller C, Losken HW, Towbin R, Bowen A, Mooney MP, Towbin A, Faix RS (2002) Ultrasound diagnosis of craniosynostosis. *Cleft Palate Craniofac J* 39: 73–80.

Narayan H, Scott IV (1991) Prenatal ultrasound diagnosis of Apert's syndrome. *Prenat Diagn* 11: 187–192.

Parent P, Le Guern H, Munck MR, Thoma M (1994) Apert syndrome, an antenatal ultrasound detected case. *Genet Couns* 5: 297–301.

Pooh RK, Nakagawa Y, Pooh KH, Nakagawa Y, Nagamachi N (1999) Fetal craniofacial structure and intracranial morphology in a case of Apert syndrome. *Ultrasound Obstet Gynecol* 13: 274–280.

Salvo AF (1981) In utero diagnosis of Kleeblattschadel (cloverleaf skull). *Prenat Diagn* 1: 141–145.

Savoldelli G, Schinzel A (1982) Prenatal ultrasound detection of humero-radial synostosis in a case of Antley–Bixler syndrome. *Prenat Diagn* 2: 219–223.

Schinzel A, Savoldelli G, Briner J, Sigg P, Massini C (1983) Antley–Bixler syndrome in sisters: a term newborn and a prenatally diagnosed fetus. *Am J Med Genet* 14: 139–147.

Sergi C, Stein H, Heep JG, Otto HF (1997) A 19-week-old fetus with craniosynostosis, renal agenesis and gastroschisis: case report and differential diagnosis. *Pathol Res Pract* 193: 579–585.

Stamm ER, Pretorius DH, Rumack CM, Manco-Johnson ML (1987) Kleeblattschadel anomaly. In utero sonographic appearance. *J Ultrasound Med* 6: 319–324.

van der Ham LI, Cohen-Overbeek TE, Geuze HD, Vermeij-Keers C (1995) The ultrasonic detection of an isolated craniosynostosis. *Prenat Diagn* 15: 1189–1192.

Weiner CP, Williamson RA, Bonsib SM (1986) Sonographic diagnosis of cloverleaf skull and thanatophoric dysplasia in the second trimester. *J Clin Ultrasound* 14: 463–465.

Winter RM, Baraitser M (2000) *London Dysmorphology Database*. Oxford: Oxford University Press.

6
IMAGING THE PATIENT WITH CRANIOSYNOSTOSIS

R.I. Aviv, D. Armstrong and W.K. Chong

Introduction

There are several radiological modalities and techniques available to the craniofacial surgeon to assist in the diagnosis and management of craniosynostosis. The aim of this chapter is to outline the modalities available and discuss their role in the pre- and post-operative setting. Emphasis will be on plain films and computed tomography (CT), as these two modalities are usually all that is required to manage these patients effectively. The utility of MRI and transcranial ultrasound will be discussed briefly. Radionuclide imaging is no longer utilised in our practice and will not be discussed. The primary and secondary radiological features of craniosynostosis and the associated intracranial, orbital and nasopharyngeal abnormalities will be illustrated. The role of imaging in the detection of complications of craniosynostosis and its surgery will be presented.

In clinical practice an unusual head shape, diagnosed at or shortly after birth, triggers a series of investigations including skull radiographs and computed tomography. Hand, feet and cervical radiographs are also performed. It is very important that an appropriate clinical history, including birth and family history, and a head circumference measurement are provided, together with the pertinent clinical findings on the request form. The referring clinician requests the above investigations to confirm his or her clinical suspicion. The two modalities together will confirm whether the suspicion is founded by demonstrating primary and secondary features of craniosynostosis, or provide the alternative reason for the abnormal head shape, e.g. fibrous dysplasia and positional plagiocephaly.

Plain films

Skull radiographs of antero-posterior (AP), lateral and Towne's views are obtained in most centres. Tangential views and submentovertical (SMV) views of the affected sutures need not be performed where CT is available. The AP view allows assessment of the coronal, sagittal, lambdoid and metopic suture. The Towne's view visualises the lambdoid and sagittal sutures while the lateral projection demonstrates the coronal and lambdoid sutures. The lateral view also affords a good view of the upper cervical spine, which is assessed for abnormalities of segmentation or formation (Campbell 1979). The posterior nasopharyngeal space may be noted but if specific radiological assessment of this is required, CT or magnetic resonance imaging (MRI) provides better information.

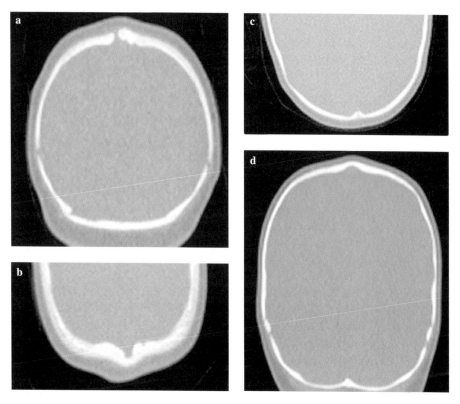

Fig. 6.1 Primary features of craniosynostosis. Patient with sagittal synostosis demonstrating bone heaping, sclerosis, bridging and enostosis on axial CT.

The primary features of sutural synostosis are identified by direct inspection of the suture involved. Findings include: sutural absence, loss of sutural clarity, parasutural sclerosis/bridging, sutural narrowing and heaping up or beaking of bone (enostosis) (Figs 6.1(a–d), 6.3(b), 6.5(a)). The plain film findings may affect the entire suture or a very short (1–2 mm) portion of the suture. In the latter case, the primary features may be missed and the suture reported as normal. It is important to appreciate that the suture may have a fibrous union which will not be identified on plain films.

The secondary radiological features include the alteration in head shape, facial appearance, foramen magnum and fontanelles as well as distortion of the subarachnoid cerebrospinal fluid (CSF) spaces and ventricles (Fig. 6.2). Timing of closure of the fontanelles may also be affected.

The traditional approach to the plain film diagnosis of craniosynostosis is to examine the appearance of the sutures, carefully identifying the recognised primary features of sutural synostosis, followed by the identification of supportive secondary features.

In our practice, we find it is usually much simpler and more reliable to make the diagnosis of sutural synostosis by the patterned alteration in skull shape and facial appearances,

Fig. 6.2 T2-weighted coronal MRI: left uni-coronal synostosis. Restriction of vault growth on the left produces effacement of subarachnoid space and ventricles. Forward displacement of the ipsilateral petrous bone accounts for post-fossa asymmetry.

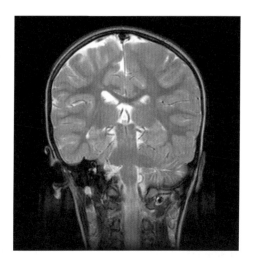

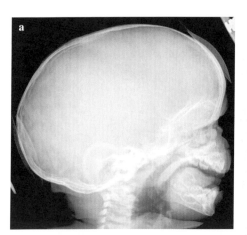

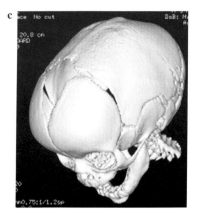

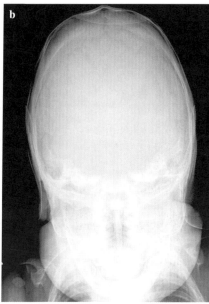

Fig. 6.3 Scaphocephaly in a 3-month-old male. (a) There is antero-posterior elongation of the calvarium with sclerosis of the midportion of the sagittal suture. No indentation is present in this patient. (b) Towne's view. There is sclerosis, bone heaping and bridging with prominent ridge formation. The most posterior portion of the suture is patent. (c) These features are easily appreciated on the 3D CT.

100

i.e. by using these so-called 'secondary features' in the first instance. The 'primary features' thereby play more of a supportive role in the final diagnosis.

Plain film appearances of craniosynostosis

The following is a summary of the key radiological features that are most helpful in the diagnosis of various types of craniosynostosis.

Sagittal synostosis (Fig. 6.3(a–c)) produces an elongated or scaphocephalic/olichocephalic head shape best appreciated on the lateral view. There may be a focal depression

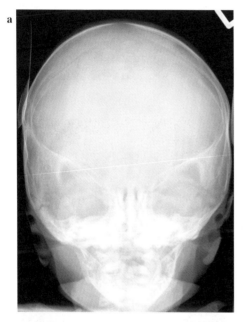

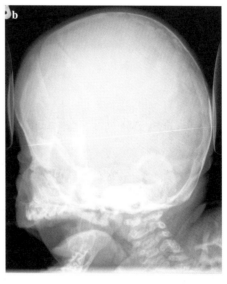

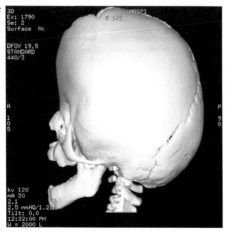

Fig. 6.4 Apert skull in a 3-month-old female. (a) There is a bilateral harlequin deformity. Perisutural sclerosis is evident along the coronal sutures bilaterally. The cribriform plate is inferiorly displaced and there is subtle upward tilt of the petrous bones. (b, c) Plain film and 3D CT lateral view confirm sutural sclerosis and anterior bowing with the superior portions of the suture patent. Note how the surface shaded image overestimates the degree of sutural synostosis. Brachycephaly with frontal bossing and a small anterior cranial fossa is present. The greater wings of the sphenoid are displaced forwards and downwards and assume a vertical configuration reducing the orbital volume and producing temporal bossing best appreciated on the 3D CT. The maxilla is hypoplastic and the nasopharynx is narrow. The pituitary fossa lies below the level of the cribriform plate.

over the convexity indicative of the initial synostosis site. The AP projection demonstrates transverse skull narrowing. Towne's view demonstrates the primary features best.

Brachycephaly, or foreshortening in the antero-posterior direction, is seen with *bicoronal synostosis* (Fig. 6.4(a–c)). The lesser wing of the sphenoid is elevated laterally resulting in the harlequin deformity. Hypertelorism, prolapse of the cribriform plate and upward slanting of the petrous apices are demonstrated on the AP view. The lateral radiograph confirms bilateral flattening of the frontal eminences, a shallow anterior cranial fossa and downward and forward displacement of the greater wing of the sphenoid with deepening of the middle cranial fossa (Mafee and Valvassori 1981). Turricephaly or oxicephaly implies growth in the superior-inferior direction often due to concomitant *bicoronal and sagittal craniosynostosis.*

Unicoronal synostosis shares many of the features of bicoronal synostosis except that the appearances are unilateral (Fig. 6.5(a, c)). Compensatory growth on the opposite side results in contralateral frontal and parietal bossing, with deviation of the metopic and sagittal suture towards the opposite side with the apex centred on the anterior fontanelle producing anterior plagiocephaly. These features are appreciated on the AP view, but best seen on three-dimensional (3D) CT (Fig. 6.5(b)).

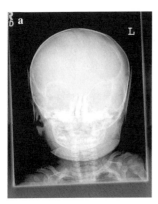 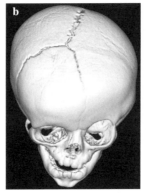 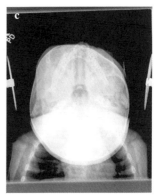

Fig. 6.5 Left unicoronal synostosis. (a) The left coronal suture is absent. Sclerosis is present. The lesser wing of the sphenoid and superior orbital roof are elevated producing a harlequin deformity. There is ipsilateral deviation of the nasal root, crista gali and fovea ethmoidalis. Note angulation of the patent metopic and sagittal sutures about a fulcrum centred on the anterior fontanelle which is deviated contralaterally. (b, c) There is ridging of the fused left coronal suture. Flattening of the ipsilateral frontal eminence with compensatory growth contralaterally and parietal bossing gives a trapezium-shaped configuration from above. The sagittal and metopic sutures converge upon the anterior fontanelles which are deviated contralaterally. The left superior orbital rim is elevated and recessed and the zygomatic buttress is posteriorly deviated. The ipsilateral deviation of the nasal root and contralateral deviation of the left maxilla and chin are characteristic and important in the distinction from anterior deformational plagiocephaly. The greater wing of the sphenoid bulges forward limiting the orbital capacity and causing prominence of the temporal fossa. The flattening of the left frontal eminence, temporomandibular joint fossa and petrous bone results in foreshortening the anterior cranial fossa. The nasal root and ethmoid air cells are displaced towards the left with the mandible deviated contralaterally. The changes are eloquently demonstrated on the 3D surface-shaded reconstruction.

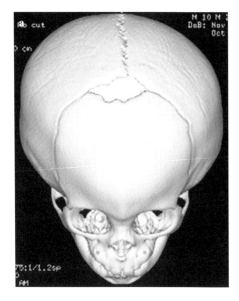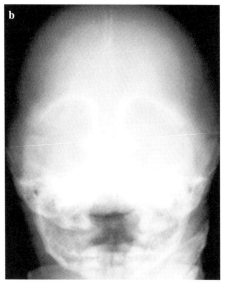

Fig. 6.6 Metopic synostosis. (a) 3D surface projection image. There is ridging of the fused metopic suture and bifrontal eminence flattening producing trigonencephaly. The coronal sutures bow anteriorly. (b) Antero-posterior skull view demonstrates absence of the inferior portion of the metopic suture with parasutural sclerosis within the upper aspect. There is hypotelorism (less than 15 mm under 1 year) with medial canting of the orbits, resulting in a 'quizzical' look. A line drawn along the vertical long axis of the orbits intersects in the midline a short distance above. The ethmoid air cell complex is hypoplastic.

Posterior plagiocephaly occurs in *unilambdoid synostosis*. The head shape is distinctly different and also differs from anterior and posterior deformational plagiocephaly or non-synostotic plagiocephaly, which will be discussed more fully later (see below).

Trigonocephaly or a keel-deformity occurs in *metopic synostosis* (Fig. 6.6(a)). The ensuing deformity results in hypotelorism with tall parallel medial orbital margins due to orbital canting as well as ethmoidal hypoplasia on the AP projection (Fig. 6.6(b)). The lateral projection demonstrates thickening of the vertical plate of the frontal bone and anterior curving of the coronal sutures (Dominguez et al 1981).

Multisutural synostosis results in complex skull shapes including the Kleeblattschadel or cloverleaf deformity.

The radiographic assessment of raised intracranial pressure (ICP) is complex and will be discussed together with the CT features of raised ICP. Abnormalities better assessed on CT include maxillary hypoplasia, palatal abnormalities, dental malocclusion and orbital apex abnormalities.

Syndromic craniosynostoses, for practical purposes, are always bilateral or multisutural. Review of the spine in syndromic craniosynostosis may reveal a failure of segmentation with fusion of vertebral bodies and/or posterior elements. This finding has been reported in 70 per cent of Apert syndrome cases, usually affecting the fifth and sixth cervical vertebrae, but has also been described with Pfeiffer and Crouzon syndromes. Atlanto-occipital assimilation, basilar impression and basilar kyphosis are seen in Apert and Crouzon syndromes. Lumbar fusion may also occur (Taybi and Lachman 1996).

Limb abnormalities are common in the syndromic craniosynostoses, with the exception of Crouzon syndrome, and are often clinically obvious. Radiographs elucidate the extent and nature of the bone abnormality. Commonly occurring abnormalities include bone syndactyly which is more commonly distal (i.e. carpal/tarsal, metacarpal/tarsal and phalangeal) but may involve more proximal joints such as the elbow. Phalangeal, carpal, tarsal and metacarpal/tarsal abnormalities are common. Brachydactyly or broadening, symphalangism (fusion along the longitudinal axis), duplication especially of the hallices and thumb phalanges, with or without notching, and varus deformity occur. Patterns of involvement help formulate likely differential diagnoses: Apert syndrome usually has a symmetric hand deformity with soft tissue and bone syndactyly producing a mitten or glove deformity (Fig. 6.7(a, b)). Pfeiffer syndrome has less severely affected limbs with predominantly soft tissue syndactyly. Broad hallices/thumbs with medial deviation (varus deformity) are seen, whereas Saethre–Chotzen has broad, bifid hallices that are laterally deviated. Crouzon syndrome usually spares the hands and feet. Other skeletal abnormalities described include an associated multiple epiphyseal dysplasia and glenoid dysplasia in Apert syndrome and delay in postnatal ossification centres (Cohen and Kreiborg 1993).

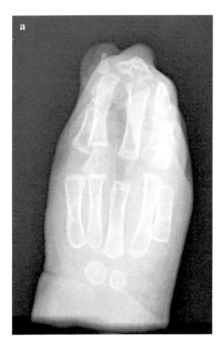
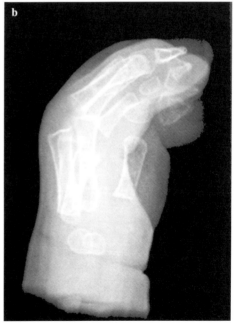

Fig. 6.7 Antero-posterior and lateral views of the left hand in a child with Apert syndrome. There is soft tissue syndactyly producing a mitten deformity. There is symphalangism of the first to fourth proximal and middle phalanges though less complete in the index finger. There is syndactyly of the second to fourth distal phalanges. The fifth finger is normal.

Computed tomography (CT)

CT is currently the modality of choice for the imaging of patients with craniosynostosis. The use of 3D CT significantly improves diagnostic performance when compared to plain CT and radiography (Vannier et al 1989). The sensitivity and specificity for craniosynostosis detection of 3D CT are estimated at 96.4 per cent and 100 per cent respectively, as opposed to 80 per cent and 95 per cent for plain films (Vannier et al 1994).

It is worth noting, however, that for simple (non-syndromic) single suture craniosynostosis, an experienced clinician can achieve a diagnosis without imaging support in virtually all cases (Cerovac et al 2002). CT may then be reserved for purposes other than diagnosis. In practice, the role of imaging in simple craniosynostosis may be reserved for diagnostic uncertainty or surgical planning (Cerovac et al 2002).

Despite the availability of multislice CT with rapid acquisition times, patient movement needs to be avoided. Most patients referred for craniosynostosis assessment are under 2 years of age and sedation or general anaesthesia (where there are concomitant airway concerns) are invariably required. CT is a robust modality, readily available with few contraindications. It is useful in the preoperative scenario to confirm the clinical diagnosis by eloquently demonstrating underlying sutural synostosis and skull base morphology. In contradistinction to plain films CT allows the entire suture and skull base to be evaluated. Essential information about the brain, ventricles and subarachnoid CSF spaces is obtained. The CT dataset is acquired using both bone and soft tissue algorithms for evaluation of the sutures and intracranial contents respectively. Intravenous iodinated contrast medium is not routinely administered. A CT venogram may be performed if there are questions concerning patency or variations of drainage of the venous sinus. CT provides information on foraminal stenosis, extent of bone involvement of sinus pericranii and venous sinus patency. MR angiography (MRA) or venography (MRV) may also be considered; however, cerebral angiography remains the criterion standard for demonstrating venous sinus anatomy (Thompson et al 1995). Multiplanar image reformats and 3D reconstruction are useful adjuncts to the examination. The appropriately acquired dataset can be transferred for 3D model (milling, stereolithography) (Klein et al 1992, Sailer et al 1998) or computer assisted (CAD) model production (Mommaerts et al 2001). These techniques enhance the surgeon's understanding of the effects of the sutural synostosis (Marsh et al 1991) and guide treatment strategy. In the early postoperative period CT enables assessment of complications such as subdural and parenchymal haemorrhage, hydrocephalus, venous sinus thrombosis and infection. Later, the functional result of the surgery can be demonstrated and a baseline obtained of the CSF spaces for future follow-up.

The radiation dose delivered to the patient and in particular to the lens of the eyes is not insubstantial and should always be considered. This is especially true as these patients are young and frequently have multiple repeat studies. There are three strategies for data acquisition in the preoperative period. The first technique involves scanning the head twice: first with a low mA (20–50 mA) and fine slice thickness (usually 1 mm), obtaining the dataset for 3D reconstruction but with such attenuation of the X-ray beam that brain imaging is precluded. The second scan involves conventional kV and mA and slice parameters (5 mm and 10 mm transaxial slices through the posterior fossa and supratentorium respectively) for brain imaging. This approach attempts to reduce the radiation dose by using the lowest mA possible during the acquisition involving the greatest number of slices (the 3D dataset) where only the bone detail is of interest and the orbits are irradiated. The summation of the dose from the two scans should then be lower than the second approach which involves a single thin-slice (1 mm) acquisition with a standard kV and mA. A third approach involves a modest reduction in the mA with one thin-slice acquisition through the cranium. The first and third approaches are both reasonable and widely practised.

Once the dataset has been acquired, postprocessing can be performed with thresholding of the model to display either bone or overlying soft tissue. The model can be manipulated and viewed from any angle. The display technique most commonly employed is surfaces shaded display (SSD) (Vannier et al 1994); other approaches advocated include 3D-volumetric reconstruction and maximum intensity projection (MIP) (Medina 2000). SSD has some limitations whereby an open suture may blend with adjacent bone giving the false impression of synostosis. Heaping up of bone and perisutural sclerosis may also not be identified. These limitations are rarely of importance in the clinical setting where both the 2D and the 3D data are reviewed.

The morphology on plain film of the head shape resulting from sutural synostosis has been discussed above. CT provides further information concerning the craniofacial proportions, skull base (Carmel et al 1981) and petrous bone. Multiplanar reformatting enables visualisation of the sagittal suture and the palate in the coronal plane. The cervical spine may be reformatted in both the coronal and sagittal plane.

Bicoronal synostosis in the context of the acrocephalosyndactyly group of syndromic craniosynostoses produces hypertelorism (Fig. 6.8(a)) and shallow anterior cranial fossa

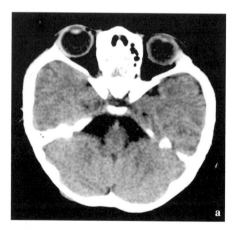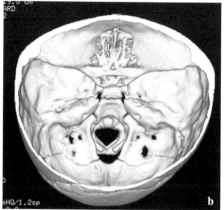

Fig. 6.8 (a) Axial CT at the level of the middle cranial fossa and orbits demonstrates brachycephaly with forward deviation of the greater wings of the sphenoid to assume a more coronal alignment. Together with expansion of ethmoidal air cells and downward slanting of the orbital roof (not shown), there is restriction of orbital volume. Note the prominent temporal fossa bulge. (b) 3D CT in a 12-month-old child with Apert syndrome. There is brachycephaly with small anterior cranial fossa. The middle cranial fossae are deepened bilaterally with temporal bossing.

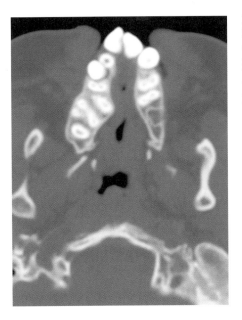

Fig. 6.9 Apert syndrome. There is maxillary hypoplasia, a narrow v-shaped jaw and dental crowding. The excessive lateral palatal soft tissue produces a pseudocleft or deep median groove. There is obliteration of the nasopharyngeal airway by a combination of basilar kyphosis and maxillary hypoplasia.

(Fig. 6.8(b)). The superior orbital rims are flattened, elevated and superolaterally canted. The ethmoidal air cells are enlarged in Crouzon syndrome and the cribriform plate is inferiorly displaced in both Apert and Crouzon syndromes. The inferior orbital rim is recessed due to maxillary hypoplasia. The above factors together with forward displacement of the greater wing of the sphenoid reduce the orbital dimensions, which in Crouzon may lead to herniation of the globe. Similar appearances occur in Apert although frontal sinus hypoplasia is more common. There is varying degree of midface hypoplasia, most severe in Crouzon syndrome where there may be airway compromise. The palate may be high-arched (exaggerated by the accumulation of soft tissue on the palatine processes), more severe in Apert than Crouzon syndrome with or without a cleft. There may be choanal atresia or stenosis in Pfeiffer syndrome. Relative mandibular prognathism, maxillary dental crowding (Fig. 6.9) in Crouzon and Apert syndromes and supernumerary teeth in Pfeiffer syndrome are described.

Upward tilting of the apices of the petrous is common in Apert and Crouzon. The external auditory meatus may be atretic in Pfeiffer and Crouzon syndromes. Middle ear opacification due to Eustachian tube obstruction is seen in Crouzon where deformity of the semicircular canals and ossicular chain is described. The stapes may be fixed in Apert syndrome.

CT illustrates the primary features of synostosis eloquently and also the effect on the underlying brain and subarachnoid CSF space. The ability to view the CT dataset in many ways allows easy distinction between posterior positional and synostotic (lambdoid) plagiocephaly (Fig. 6.10(a, b)). As for plain film analysis, it is often much easier to distinguish the various patterns of craniosynostosis and its mimics from the shape of the skull than from the direct examination of the sutures themselves, the latter playing a more supportive role.

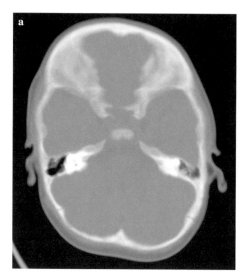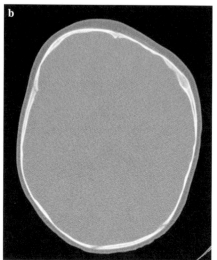

Fig. 6.10 (a) Right posterior deformational plagiocephaly. There is right occipital flattening with ipsilateral frontal bossing. The ipsilateral petrous and ear are anteriorly displaced. The right lambdoid suture is patent. The head has a parallelogram appearance. (b) Left unicoronal synostosis: flattening of the left frontal eminence and bulging of the right frontal eminence in combination with right parietal bossing produce a trapezium appearance from above.

Lambdoid synostosis produces ipsilateral occipitoparietal flattening with ipsilateral postero-inferior ear displacement and contralateral parietal bossing. The skull base is tilted downwards ipsilaterally with resultant compensatory cervical spine deviation. There may be contralateral frontal bossing, producing a trapezium-shaped head when viewed from above but parallelogram appearance from behind due to the ipsilateral occipitomastoid bulge and contralateral parietal bulge. Deformational posterior plagiocephaly causes ipsilateral frontal bossing, anterior ear displacement (without supero-inferior deviation) and contralateral occipital rather than parietal bossing, producing a parallelogram-shaped head when viewed from above. The skull base and the cervical spine are unaffected (Hansen and Mulliken 1994, Huang et al 1996).

Frontal plagiocephaly can be similarly differentiated. In positional plagiocephaly the ipsilateral cheek, forehead and ear are posteriorly deviated with ipsilateral chin but no nasal root deviation, producing a parallelogram-shaped head when viewed from above. Frontal (unicoronal) synostosis elevates the superior orbital rim, deviates the nasal root towards the synostosis, and the ipsilateral cheek and ear are deviated anteriorly. The chin and anterior fontanelles are deviated contralaterally (Hansen and Mulliken 1994).

In practice, the various types of craniosynostosis are recognisable and distinguishable from their mimics in the clinical setting alone. Radiological examinations add a further level of diagnostic refinement usually by supporting the clinical suspicions and only occasionally offering an alternative definitive diagnosis.

The application of non-invasive imaging is therefore greatest in the identification of craniosynostosis complications and potential surgical hazards and in the monitoring of cases during the course of their treatment. The following sections review some of these important roles.

Assessment of the intracranial structures

Intracranial abnormalities may occur as part of a syndromic craniosynostosis and these may have an influence on clinical outcome. Abnormalities such as agenesis of the corpus callosum or distortion of the intracranial contents by the secondary effects of the synostosis – e.g. venous sinus stenosis, tonsillar ectopia (Chiari I malformation), ventricular asymmetry, sulcal and cisternal effacement – may be seen.

CT will detect the major intracranial abnormalities and is sufficient in most cases. These include gross structural changes such as hydrocephalus, abnormalities of the corpus callosum and absence of the septum pellucidum (Fig. 6.11). MRI provides better soft tissue contrast and multiplanar abilities over CT with the added advantage of not requiring the use of ionising radiation. As a result, MRI easily demonstrates more subtle intracranial abnormalities including limbic system abnormalities, subtle heterotopia, Chiari malformations and syringomyelia. Despite this, MRI is infrequently required in our practice and is usually only applied if there are clinical findings which raise concern of a possible underlying neurological disorder or complication.

Tonsillar herniation is most commonly seen in Crouzon and Pfeiffer syndromes. Herniaton is due to a combination of raised ICP and craniocerebral disproportion of the posterior fossa (Kreiborg et al 1993). The presence of tonsillar herniation is one factor in the development of hydrocephalus. Venous hypertension is another important factor and is discussed below. Tonsillar herniation and alteration of CSF dynamics at the craniocervical junction may be studied with phase-contrast MRI techniques. This has been applied in patients with achondroplasia but not specifically in patients with craniosynostosis (Hofmann et al 2000, Rollins et al 2000b). We do not find this to be a useful technique on our practice.

In Apert syndrome, dygenesis of the corpus callosum, malformation of the limbic system (septum pellucidum and hippocampus), megalencephaly, asymmetry of the brain,

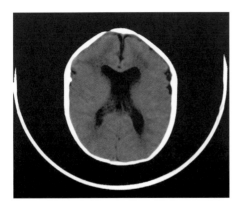

Fig. 6.11 Apert syndrome post-surgical repair. The ventricles are enlarged with a small anterior recess of the third ventricle and temporal horns (not shown) consistent with ventriculomegaly. The cavum septum pellucidum is absent.

and a non-progressive ventricular dilatation with normal temporal horns have been described (Noetzel et al 1985), but are rare in our practice. Gyral and pyramidal tract abnormalities, frontal/occipital encephalocoele, heterotopic grey matter and hypoplasia of white matter have also been described (Cohen and Kreiborg 1990). Crouzon syndrome is reported as not having central nervous system anomalies, although agenesis of the corpus callosum has been described.

Raised intracranial pressure (ICP): radiological assessment

The radiologist is frequently asked to opine on whether the ICP is raised in both preoperative and postoperative patients. The surgeon prefers to avoid pressure monitoring due to its invasiveness and potential complications.

Plain films and CT have been the most used for this, because of easy accessibility. Predicting raised ICP is notoriously difficult and there is a difference of opinion regarding the significance of many of the radiological signs such as copper beating (Fig. 6.12). A consensus view is that there are no radiological indicators of raised intracranial pressure that can be said to be consistently both useful and reliable.

Transcranial ultrasound has been used to calculate brain compliance using the arterial pulsatile (PI) and resistive index (RI) (Westra et al 2001). Arterial PI and RI indices are reported as showing direct correlation with ICP in hydrocephalus (Goh and Minns 1995). The technique has also been applied to the intracranial veins with pre- and postoperative compliance monitoring (Mursch et al 1999). Limitations of this technique include the effect of a multitude of factors (cardiac output, arterial resistance and general anaesthesia or hyperventilation) on the Doppler results as well as the inability to find a suitable acoustic window in older patients.

Hydrocephalus is reported in 4–25 per cent of craniosynostosis (Cinalli et al 1988) and is a relatively common finding in syndromic synostosis. Hydrocephalus is the most sensitive radiological indicator of raised ICP, but only detects 40 per cent of patients with this complication (Tuite et al 1996). Tuite et al found that the specificity is high, ranging from

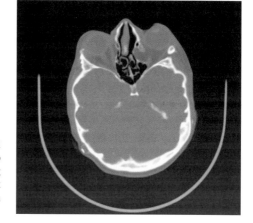

Fig. 6.12 Crouzon syndrome post-total calvarial remodelling and right occipital shunt. Follow-up CT demonstrates progressive diffuse scalloping of the inner table of the calvarium. The patient had intracranial pressure monitoring which confirmed elevated ICP.

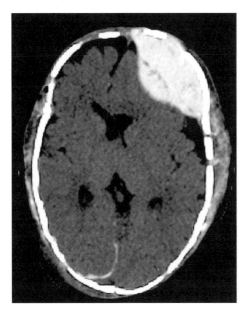

Fig. 6.13 Seven-month-old infant with sagittal synostosis post-total calvarial remodelling. There is a large left epidural haemorrhage causing mass effect on the underlying frontal lobe and frontal horn of the lateral ventricle. There is midline shift to the right with subfalcine herniation. A small right-sided parafalcine subdural is also present. Soft tissue swelling and a subgaleal haematoma are present. The epidural was evacuated.

100 per cent in children aged between 18 months and 4 years to 75 per cent in children younger than 18 months, with an overall specificity of 80 per cent. The authors concluded that diffuse copper beating, obliteration of the anterior sulci and effacement of the basal cisterns in a child less than 18 months were predictors for elevated ICP in over 95 per cent of cases, but the specificity dropped in older children. Erosion of the dorsum sella and sutural diastasis was 90 per cent specific for raised ICP in all age groups.

Venous hypertension may be an important and under-appreciated co-contributor to intracranial hypertension. Abnormal intracranial venous drainage secondary to jugular foraminal stenosis causes outflow restriction (Rich et al 2003). Several collateral pathways develop, most notably stylomastoid venous collaterals (Taylor et al 2001). MRV demonstrates the collateral circulation and occlusion of the sigmoid sinus–jugular vein complex (Rollins et al 2000a). MRV is under-utilised in the context of craniosynostosis but the clinician should remember that it is flow and not vessel size that is being demonstrated. Frequent artifacts may be present such as arachnoid granulations (Mamourian and Towfighi 1995), focal non-continuity of the transverse sinuses (Ayanzen et al 2000), and slow flow resulting in misinterpretation of sinus patency.

Postoperative complications

Complications may be divided into early and late. Early complications include haemorrhage (Fig. 6.13), contusion, infection and venous sinus damage/occlusion. The latter may lead to hydrocephalus and raised intracranial pressure. Late complications include infection, granuloma formation secondary to bone paste and leptomeningeal cyst or growing fracture.

CT is the modality of choice in the follow-up of symptomatic post-surgical patients. Within the first few days of surgery, imaging may demonstrate extensive soft tissue swelling and oedema. Many of these changes are transient and reversible. Extradural air and/or blood are often present. No intradural or intra-axial air or blood should be evident. Intra-axial blood could signify contusion or cortical vein or venous sinus damage/occlusion. Intravenous contrast should be administered during the acquisition of a CT venogram, with careful inspection of venous sinus patency. The dataset can be presented as a maximum intensity projection (MIP) or as coronal and sagittal reformats. Hyperdensity of a vein precontrast and the 'empty delta sign', or focal non-filling of the venous sinus with surrounding enhancement due to venous collaterals and dural spaces, suggest thrombotic venous occlusion.

Infection may manifest as a ventriculitis, abscess, empyema, meningitis or osteomyelitis. Intravenous contrast may reveal ependymal and leptomeningeal enhancement respectively. Stranding and encysting of the ventricles may occur, leading to hydrocephalus. More commonly infection occurs within the extradural or subcutaneous compartment as an abscess with or without associated osteomyelitis (Fig. 6.14). CT has advantages over MRI in the demonstration of the lytic and destructive bone changes of osteomyelitis.

Following surgery in patients with Apert and Crouzon syndromes, the ventricles and subarachnoid spaces may be seen to increase. In Apert syndrome ventricular enlargement is often non-progressive (Fig. 6.11) and seldom requires shunting, whereas in Crouzon syndrome shunting is usual. The presumed aetiology is venous hypertension, which in the context of prematurely fused sutures results in higher CSF pressures required to maintain CSF outflow balance. Once reconstructive surgery is performed the ventricle and subarachnoid CSF spaces increase until a new balance is achieved. Careful follow-up of these patients is required both radiologically and clinically to detect raised ICP.

Granuloma formation secondary to methylmethacrylate results in an inflammatory response with an increase in soft tissue thickening in the overlying subcutaneous tissues.

Damage to the dura at the time of surgery may lead to the formation of a leptomeningeal cyst. The characteristic enlarging or 'growing' defect of the calvarium is due to the

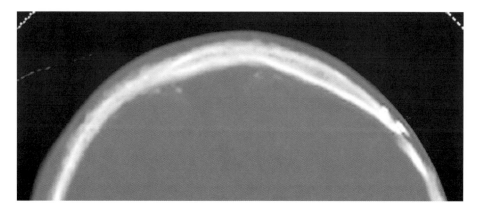

Fig. 6.14 Right frontal osteomyelitis. A permeative pattern is present within the right frontal bone in a patient with pyrexia three weeks post-surgery, consistent with an osteomyelitis.

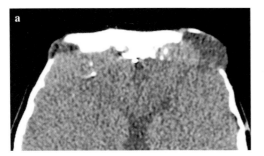

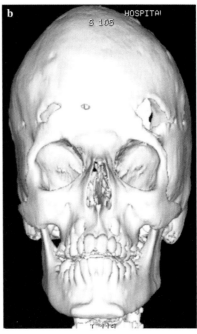

Fig. 6.15 Ten-year-old female with Crouzon syndrome, post-total calvarial remodelling. Expanding bone defects are present bifrontally with herniation of CSF density collections consistent with leptomeningeal cysts.

effect of the pulsatile CSF on the overlying bone, producing progressive thinning and enlargement of the bone defect (Fig. 6.15(a, b)).

Orbital considerations of craniosynostosis

Alterations in the orbital configuration resulting in shallow orbits, hypertelorism and exopthalmos in Apert and Crouzon syndromes have been discussed above. Absence of the extraocular muscles has been described in Apert syndrome, including superior, inferior and superior oblique muscles. The orbit may also undergo rotation of the normally vertical superior–inferior axis (Fig. 6.16). Vision may be impaired by strabismus, amblyopia, exposure keratopathy or optic nerve atrophy. Optic neuropathy is no longer considered a result of optic canal narrowing (Kreiborg and Pruzansky 1981) but rather secondary to transmission of raised ICP or, rarely, a complication of surgery.

Imaging of the airway

Assessment of the airway is possible on the unenhanced CT performed for craniofacial assessment, although administration of contrast does more easily delineate vascular structures. Sagittal and coronal reformatted images are useful adjuncts to axial imaging. Midface hypoplasia is a feature of both Apert and Crouzon syndromes. Basilar kyphosis results in a reduced distance between the soft palate and adenoids, producing nasopharyngeal obstruction (Fig. 6.9(a, b)). Oropharyngeal narrowing occurs in combination with a small high-arched maxilla, dental overcrowding and thickening of the alveolar process, hard and soft palates. Nasal septal deviation and choanal atresia further aggravate airway patency.

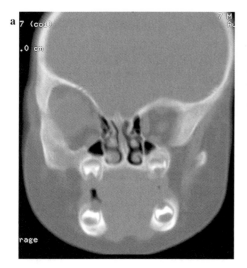 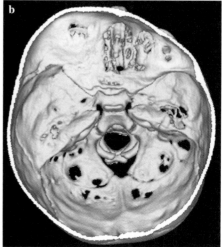

Fig. 6.16 Right unicoronal synostosis: harlequin appearance due to elevation of orbital roof. The long axis of the right orbit is rotated relative to that on the left.

Asymmetrical descent of the palate antero-posteriorly results in an anterior open bite. Anterior and posterior crossbite are also frequent.

REFERENCES

Ayanzen RH, Bird CR, Keller PJ, McCully FJ, Theobald MR, Heiserman JE (2000) Cerebral MR venography: normal anatomy and potential pitfalls. *AJNR* 21: 74–78.

Campbell JA (1979) Craniofacial anomalies. In: Newton TH, Potts DG, editors. *Radiology of the Skull Base and Brain*. St Louis: Mosby, pp 207–221.

Carmel PW, Luken MG 3rd, Ascherl GF (1981) Craniosynostosis: computed tomographic evaluation of skull base and calvarial deformities and associated intracranial changes. *Neurosurgery* 9: 367–372.

Cerovac S, Neil-Dwyer JG, Rich P, Jones BM, Hayward RD (2002) Are routine preoperative CT scans necessary in the management of single suture craniosynostosis? *Br J Neurosurg* 16: 348–354.

Cinalli G, Sainte-Rose C, Kollar EM, Zerah M, Brunelle F, Chumas P, Arnaud E, Marchac D, Pierre-Kahn A, Renier D (1988) Hydrocephalus and craniosynostosis. *J Neurosurg* 88: 209–214.

Cohen MM Jr, Kreiborg S (1990) The central nervous system in the Apert syndrome. *Am J Med Genet* 35(1): 36–45.

Cohen MM Jr, Kreiborg S (1993) Skeletal abnormalities in the Apert syndrome. *Am J Med Genet* 47(5): 624–632.

Dominguez R, Sang Oh K, Bender T, Girdany BR (1981) Uncomplicated trigonencephaly. A radiographic affirmation of conservative therapy. *Radiology* 140: 681–688.

Goh D, Minns RA (1995) Intracranial pressure and cerebral artery flow velocity indices in childhood hydrocephalus: current review. *Childs Nerv Syst* 11: 392–396.

Hansen M, Mulliken JB (1994) Frontal plagiocephaly diagnosis and treatment. *Clin Plast Surg* 21: 543–553.

Hofmann E, Warmuth-Metz M, Bendszus M, Solymosi L (2000) Phase-contrast MR imaging of the cervical CSF and spinal cord: volumetric motion analysis in patients with Chiari malformation. *AJNR* 21: 151–158.

Huang MHS, Gruss J, Clarren SK, Mouradian WE, Cunningham ML, Roberts TS, Loeser JD, Cornell CJ (1996) The differential diagnosis of posterior plagiocephaly: true lambdoid synostosis versus positional moulding. *Plast Reconstr Surg* 98: 765–774.

Klein HM, Schneider W, Alzen G, Voy ED, Gunther RW (1992) Pediatric craniofacial surgery: comparison of milling and stereolithography for 3D model manufacturing. *Pediatr Radiol* 22(6): 458–460.

Kreiborg S, Pruzansky S (1981) Craniofacial growth in premature craniofacial synostosis. *Scand J Plast Reconstr Hand Surg* 15: 171–186.

Kreiborg S, Marsh JL, Cohen MM, Liversage M, Pedersen H, Skovby F, Borgesen SE, Vannier MW (1993) Comparative three-dimensional analysis of the calvaria and skull base in Apert and Crouzon syndromes. *J Craniomaxillofac Surg* 21: 181–188.

Mafee MF, Valvassori GE (1981) Radiology of craniofacial anomalies. *Otolaryngol Clin North Am* 14(4): 930–988.

Mamourian AC, Towfighi J (1995) MR of giant arachnoid granulation, a normal variant presenting as a mass within the dural venous sinus. *AJNR* 16(4 suppl): 901–904.

Marsh JL, Galic M, Vannier MW (1991) The craniofacial anatomy of Apert syndrome. *Clin Plast Surg* 18(2): 237–249.

Medina LS (2000) Three-dimensional CT maximum intensity projections of the calvaria: a new approach for diagnosis of craniosynostosis and fractures. *AJNR* 21: 1951–1954.

Mommaerts MY, Jans G, Vander Sloten J, Staels PF, Van der Perre G, Gobin R (2001) On the assets of CAD planning for craniosynostosis surgery. *J Craniofac Surg* 12(6): 547–554.

Mursch K, Enk T, Christen HJ, Markakis E, Behnke-Mursch J (1999) Venous intracranial haemodynamics in children undergoing operative treatment for the repair of craniosynostosis. *Childs Nerv Syst* 15: 110–118.

Noetzel MJ, Marsch JL, Palkes H, Gado M (1985) Hydrocephalus and mental retardation in craniosynostosis. *J Paediatr* 107: 885–892.

Rich PM, Cox TCS, Hayward RD (2003) The jugular foramen in complex and syndromic craniosynostosis and its relationship to raised intracranial pressure. *Am J Neuroradiol* 24: 45–51.

Rollins N, Booth T, Shapiro K (2000a) MR venography in children with complex craniosynostosis. *Paediatr Neurosurg* 32: 308–315.

Rollins N, Booth T, Shapiro K (2000b) The use of gated cine phase contrast and MR venography in achondroplasia. *Childs Nerv Syst* 16: 569–577.

Sailer HF, Haers PE, Zollikofer CP, Warnke T, Carls FR, Stucki P (1998) The value of stereolithographic models for preoperative diagnosis of craniofacial deformities and planning of surgical corrections. *Int J Oral Maxillofac Surg* 27(5): 327–333.

Taybi H, Lachman RS (1996) *Radiology of Syndromes, Metabolic Disorders, and Skeletal Dysplasias*, 4th edn. St Louis: Mosby, pp 383–384.

Taylor WJ, Hayward RD, Lasjaunias P, Britto JA, Thompson DNP, Jones BM, Evans RD (2001) Enigma of raised intracranial pressure in patients with complex craniosynostosis: the role of abnormal intracranial venous drainage. *J Neurosurg* 94: 377–385.

Thompson DNP, Hayward RD, Harkness WJ (1995) Lessons from a case of Kleeblattschadel. Case report. *J Neurosurg* 82: 1071–1074.

Tuite GF, Evanson J, Chong WK, Thompson DP, Harkness WF, Jones BM, Hayward RD (1996) The copper beaten skull: a correlation between intracranial pressure, skull radiographs and CT scans in children with craniosynostosis. *Neurosurgery* 39: 691–699.

Vannier MW, Hildebolt CF, Marsh JL, Pilgram TK, McAlister WH, Shackelford GD, Offutt CJ, Knapp RH (1989) Craniosynostosis: diagnostic value of three-dimensional CT reconstruction. *Radiology* 173: 669–673.

Vannier MW, Pilgram TK, Marsh JL, Kraemer BB, Rayne SC, Mokhtar HG, Moran JM, McAlister WH, Shackleford GD, Hardesty RA (1994) Craniosynostosis: diagnostic imaging with three-dimensional CT presentation. *AJNR* 15: 1861–1869.

Westra SJ, Stotland MA, Lazareff J, Anderson CTM, Sayre JW, Kawamoto H (2001) Perioperative transcranial doppler to evaluate intracranial compliance in young children undergoing craniosynostosis repair surgery. *Radiology* 218: 816–823.

7
PRINCIPLES OF MANAGEMENT OF THE CHILD WITH CRANIOSYNOSTOSIS

Richard Hayward and Barry Jones

Introduction

It requires only a glance at the chapter headings of this book to appreciate that the proper management of children with craniosynostosis can be complex and involves the input of many different specialists. Each of these specialties' chapters surveys a particular problem that these children may develop and discusses its management. Exclusive reliance upon this 'independent specialty' approach as a guide to overall management would, however, leave the care of affected children fragmented in a way that does not accord with clinical practice. It is therefore the purpose of this chapter to focus on the overall approach to the care of children with craniosynostosis rather than treating them as no more than the sum of the individual problems they may run into. This approach requires first an account of our philosophy of management as it has evolved over the last 15 years or so. We shall then describe how that philosophy translates to our care first of children with syndromic craniosynostosis and then of those with single suture involvement. Readers will find themselves frequently referred on to those chapters where each particular subject has been dealt with in more detail – and inevitably there will be a degree of overlap.

Summary of our management philosophy

Craniosynostosis, with the possible exception of the milder forms of unisutural synostosis, is a dynamic process. In the syndromic forms the reasons for this are now well known – there are mutations in a gene (usually of the *fibroblast growth factor receptor* – FGFR – series) which has a particular role in the growth of the skull and facial skeleton (see Chapter 2). It would not be surprising therefore if such an abnormal gene continued to exert its effects for as long as the child's skull and facial skeleton are growing – a process that can be seen in, for example, the phenomenon of progressive fusion of previously open sutures (Reddy et al 1990), the possibly increasing interference with intracranial venous drainage with age (see Chapter 8), and, of particular importance to those planning reconstructive operations, the apparent relapse – or reversion – of children towards their preoperative appearances from what appeared at the time of surgery to have been a satisfactory cosmetic result. Indeed, Mullikan has written (in an article confined to fronto-orbital and forehead surgery), 'In the final analysis, the expression of the underlying genetic defect probably is the major determinant of the final fronto-orbital position despite our best surgical efforts' (Wong et al 2000). This is a sentiment with which we would most whole-heartedly agree – and not for the fronto-orbital region alone, but for all those structures, including particularly the maxilla, affected by the genetic aberrations underlying syndromic craniosynostosis.

Although this phenomenon of relapse is seen dramatically in those children most severely affected by one or another of the various craniofacial-associated syndromes, it is not confined to them. Even a child with the more severe forms of 'simple' unicoronal, metopic or sagittal synostosis, for which no genetic mutation has been identified at the time of writing, may show some evidence of reversion towards their original appearance (often referred to as relapse) when viewed a few years after surgery performed when the skull vault was expanding most rapidly – in particular during the first six months (Wall et al 1994).

These observations can be summarised as follows. All surgery for craniosynostosis carries with it the potential for later reversion (or relapse) and the degree of this process is related to the severity of the syndrome responsible for the craniosynostosis in the first place and the age at which surgery has been performed. Or, put another way, for as long as the child is growing there will be a tendency for that growth to continue along the abnormal lines dictated by the underlying genetic defect (known or putative) responsible for the condition in the first place.

Clearly this has implications for the management of children with craniosynostosis of whatever type and severity. Reconstructive surgery, if the result is to be stable in terms of its potential for relapse, should ideally be postponed until the most active growth phase for the anatomical area being operated upon is over. For cases of unisutural synostosis in which facial deformity is not usually a major issue the timing will be dependent upon the growth characteristics of the skull vault (which a glance at a head circumference chart will confirm has completed its most rapid expansion by the age of 1 year), while for the management of the various craniosynostosis-associated syndromes it is necessary to take into account the growth characteristics of the face and jaws, with particular emphasis on the child's dentition. This means that some aspects of surgical treatment, if they are to be definitive, should not be undertaken until the patient is 17 or 18 years old. (The subject of facial and skull vault growth is dealt with in detail in Chapter 1.) It is important to bear in mind also that definitive (or 'final') surgery is made no easier and the results may be compromised by the scarring etc. produced by earlier operations.

Because of the difference in management between children with 'simple' unisutural synostosis and those with the more complex syndromic forms, the two groups will now be discussed separately.

Management of syndromic forms of craniosynostosis

As has already been described in Chapters 2 and 3, the syndromic forms of craniosynostosis affect both the skull vault and the facial skeleton to produce functional disabilities in addition to any cosmetic effects. These result in affected children being at risk from a variety of complications of their primary condition, each of which may have a serious effect upon both their developmental progress and the degree of their final disability.

These complications include:

1 Raised intracranial pressure (ICP)
2 Airway obstruction
3 Feeding difficulties
4 Ophthalmic problems
5 Cognitive and behavioural problems
6 Disorders of dental occlusion
7 Psychological problems

Each of these topics will be discussed in more detail in their own chapters, but in summary it can be stated that if a lasting result is to be achieved by reconstructive surgery then the definitive operation(s) should be delayed until at least the period of maximum growth for that particular structure being operated upon is over *unless a particular functional problem or complication demands earlier intervention*. This means that in practice a majority of children with, say, Apert, Pfeiffer and Crouzon syndromes will require a series of procedures of one sort or another during their early years for, among other functional problems, raised ICP, exorbitism of a degree to threaten the eyes through exposure, and respiratory problems secondary to airway obstruction.

Our policy therefore is to encourage referral to a formally established craniofacial unit at as early an age as possible so that the correct diagnosis can be made (supported when possible by genetic analysis), the child's risk of various complications predicted as accurately as possible, and a management plan decided upon. It may be suspected that, for example, raised ICP (if not already present) is highly likely to occur and therefore a particular regime of scanning and clinical (including in particular ophthalmological) examinations should be initiated. For milder cases – those children with Crouzon syndrome in whom the only abnormality appears to be a modest degree of maxillary hypoplasia, for example – a less intensive regime might be recommended and early surgery would be less likely to be required. In other words, a management plan tailored to each child's likely needs can be made and the necessary monitoring instituted.

Some general principles of management of the syndromic forms of craniosynostosis will now be described before dealing with each particular condition in turn.

Details of the surgical procedures referred to can be found in Chapter 18.

ALL CASES OF COMPLEX/SYNDROMIC CRANIOSYNOSTOSIS
The general management of children with the syndromic forms of craniosynostosis will be described under the following headings:

1 Timing of first referral
2 Initial assessment
3 Initial management policy
4 Follow-up

Timing of first referral

The recognition by obstetricians and paediatricians that a newborn child has one of the more severe forms of craniofacial disorder is not usually difficult even if the precise diagnosis is unknown – the combination of an abnormal head shape combined perhaps with maxillary hypoplasia, exorbitism and digital anomalies being obvious at birth (and may even have been suspected on the basis of antenatal ultrasound examinations – see Chapter 5). In some cases there may be a significant family history and, as the majority of syndromic forms of craniosynostosis have an autosomal dominant inheritance (Carpenter syndrome – autosomal recessive – is an exception to this), each child of an affected parent will have a one-in-two chance of exhibiting the disorder. However, not all cases are so obvious. Some children with Crouzon syndrome, for example (where digital anomalies are not part of the syndrome), may have a normal appearance at birth – or exhibit only mild exorbitism – and yet one year later as progressive suture fusions occur may have developed a quite characteristic appearance.

As a general rule, therefore, any child suspected of having a craniosynostosis-related syndrome should be referred to a specialised multi-specialty craniofacial unit as soon as possible. For the majority of children there may be no acute clinical urgency, apart of course from parental anxiety, but in a significant minority an urgent assessment will be needed because of immediate concerns about, in particular, corneal exposure, respiratory obstruction, raised intracranial pressure and difficulties with feeding.

Initial assessment

It is our policy when possible to admit all children newly referred to us with a craniosynostosis-related syndrome for a period of assessment that lasts usually from three to four days. An in-patient stay, using a patient 'hotel' facility where available, can be a more efficient way of accommodating the various specialist investigations and reviews needed to make a diagnosis and evaluate the current condition of the child, particularly when the family lives a long way away – something that is almost inevitable given the rarity of the conditions we are dealing with and therefore the large size of the catchment areas of the few specialist units needed to look after them.

The aims of the initial assessment (which may vary according to the age and condition of the child) can be summarised as follows:

1 *To make the diagnosis* – clinically, genetically and radiologically (see Chapters 2, 3 and 6).
2 *To assess the current clinical situation* – the details of each aspect of this and subsequent assessments are given in the appropriate chapters. However, the initial assessment is likely to involve the following specialties:

   a *'Reconstructive cranio-maxillo-facial surgery'* – a term used here to include both plastic surgery and maxillofacial surgery
   b *Neurosurgery*

119

c   *Ophthalmology* – which should ideally include photography of the fundi and visual evoked potentials (Chapter 10)
d   *ENT (ear, nose and throat)/respiratory paediatrics* – for the assessment of the airway and respiratory status (Chapter 9).
e   *'Developmental paediatrics'* – which in this context includes psychology (Chapter 12), neurology (Chapter 13), speech and language (Chapter 14)
f   *Audiology* (Chapter 15).
g   *Orthodontic/dental* (Chapter 11)
h   *Feeding and nutrition* (Chapter 16)

3   *Radiological assessment* (Chapter 6) – with the aim of identifying the sutures involved, the size of the ventricles, any evidence of raised ICP (such as lacunae in the skull vault bone and absence of CSF in the cortical sulci) and any associated cerebral malformations (for details see Chapters 2 and 3).

Initial management strategy
The initial assessment should achieve the following:

1   *A diagnosis*
2   *An initial craniofacial management strategy*

As has already been explained, our general strategy for children newly diagnosed with the syndromic forms of craniosynostosis is not to proceed automatically to early reconstructive surgery but to concentrate upon those functional problems (present or predicted) identified by the initial assessment that if left untreated are likely to compromise a child's developmental progress. These include, in particular, raised ICP (Chapter 8), respiratory problems due to airway obstruction (Chapter 9) and, for the very young child, feeding difficulties (Chapter 16).

Some of these may require urgent attention – for example, the provision of a nasopharyngeal airway in a child with breathing difficulties, or some form of cerebrospinal fluid (CSF) diversion when raised ICP is due to hydrocephalus. For the majority of children, however, the initial assessment will result not in any immediate interventions but in the craniofacial team being in a position to decide the intensity of follow-up that is required, and which specialists need to see the child at which particular intervals.

Our policy is for the results of the initial assessment to be discussed at the craniofacial unit's combined specialty meeting, which is held weekly, and for the appropriate strategy to be agreed upon then – including the optimum timing of any elective craniofacial reconstructions. The results are then transmitted to the child's family (and their local medical team) and a clinic visit is arranged to allow discussion of all relevant issues with a senior member of the team. Other clinic visits and their timing are also decided at this meeting.

Many families will have arrived for their assessment believing – certainly hoping – that all their child's problems can be put right by surgery – preferably by one early and no doubt major procedure. It is part of the educational responsibility of the craniofacial team to explain how the management of each child's problems will probably not consist of a one-off operation but will more likely involve many operations until he or she is well into their adolescence.

3   A policy for non-primary craniofacial problems

Children with craniosynostosis-related syndromes may have a variety of problems whose management may or may not fall directly within the remit of the primary members of the craniofacial team. Such problems might include the management of syndactyly in children with Apert syndrome, for example, and ptosis in Saethre–Chotzen syndrome. The expertise needed to manage the cleft palate so frequently seen in children with Apert syndrome is likely to be available in most craniofacial units.

4   Liaison/communication

Many of these children live far from the craniofacial unit and the major part of their general paediatric care will therefore be undertaken by local paediatric and other services. It is of the greatest importance that local paediatricians and family doctors are kept up to date with the policies decided upon by the craniofacial unit and that there is a clear understanding between all parties as to where responsibility for the management of particular problems begins and ends.

Follow-up

The organisation (and communication) of an agreed follow-up strategy is most important for the proper care of these children with their complex needs involving so many different specialties. We have found the input of a clinical nurse specialist to be invaluable in this respect and the reader is directed to Chapter 17 where the strategies most frequently employed by us are described.

The patient will then continue with follow-up visits and repeat assessments punctuated by surgery on an elective and/or urgent basis as dictated by events. For example, children with the cloverleaf skull deformity are likely to require frequent assessments of, among other features, their vision and airway, and the need for several surgical interventions performed by a variety of specialists in the craniofacial team can be confidently predicted. In contrast, a child with craniofrontonasal dysplasia may have no immediately complicating features at all and will therefore need only intermittent contact with the craniofacial team until he or she is old enough to be suitable for surgery to correct their hypertelorism (see Chapters 1 and 19).

Although dealt with in detail elsewhere, the management of the various complications that these children may develop can be summarised as follows:

1   Raised intracranial pressure

Raised ICP can be due to hydrocephalus, venous hypertension, respiratory obstruction and cranio-cerebral disproportion – or a mixture of all four. Hydrocephalus requires a

CSF-diversion procedure – either an endoscopic third ventriculostomy or a ventriculo-peritoneal shunt. Venous hypertension is effectively treated by a vault-expanding operation that can be posterior (parieto-occipital), bilateral (biparietal) or anterior (a fronto-orbital advance).

The question of whether all children with syndromic forms of craniosynostosis should have some form of vault expansion procedure performed at an early age regardless of whether or not they are showing signs of raised ICP is discussed in the following chapter. Our policy at present is not to do so, but this raises the question of whether or not a future rise in ICP can be predicted. Some crude predictions can be made on the basis of the syndrome alone – a child with Saethre–Chotzen syndrome, for example, is much less likely to run into raised ICP problems than one with, say, Pfeiffer or Crouzon syndrome. The phenotypic severity of the syndrome and the presence or absence of airway obstruction are also likely to be relevant. There is no evidence available at present to tell us if a particular degree of abnormal venous drainage as assessed by magnetic resonance venography (MRV) in a child with syndromic synostosis and (at present) normal ICP will translate to raised ICP in the years to come. For this reason and because there is at the moment no specific vein-to-vein reconstruction procedure available for these children, we do not routinely investigate them either with digital subtraction angiography or MRV, but clearly this situation will change as further information becomes available.

Some craniofacial units do indeed advise a fronto-orbital advance for all children with syndromic craniosynostosis regardless of the status of their ICP. In a recent analysis of the results of such a policy it was pointed out that the re-operation rate (for forehead and fronto-orbital surgery alone) was 100 per cent for Apert, 26 per cent for Crouzon, about 40 per cent for Pfeiffer and 65 per cent for Saethre–Chotzen syndrome (Wong et al 2000). The case for selectivity in both the performance and the timing of such surgery would thus appear to be well supported.

Respiratory obstruction of a degree that is contributing to raised ICP may need any of the interventions listed in Chapter 9.

2   *Airway obstruction*

In addition to the interventions listed in Chapter 9, some children (particularly those who are older) may benefit from surgery designed to open up the naso- and oro-pharynx by advancing the maxilla, either on its own (as an extracranial midfacial osteotomy (or Le Fort procedure)) or combined with the supraorbital and frontal regions (as a monobloc advance).

3   *Exorbitism*

Exorbitism of a degree that leaves the eyes in danger from exposure (often preceded by episodes of anterior subluxation of the globes in front of the eyelids) can be treated either by advancing the supraorbital/frontal region on its own, or preferably by combining this with an advance of the maxilla (a monobloc procedure).

As has already been explained, for both a cosmetically and functionally effective cranio-facial reconstruction to be free from the risk of relapse/reversion it is necessary to delay surgery until that part of the face or skull vault being operated upon has passed its period of most rapid growth. For many children and their families the burden of going through perhaps their entire schooling with a significant cosmetic disability may be unacceptable – particularly for those children whose 'hold' upon a place in the regular schooling system is most precarious. For them early surgery for cosmetic purposes may be essential, but it is important that the family (and the patient) recognise that all or part of an operation performed at a less than ideal age may need to be repeated. However, this may well be an acceptable compromise if the quality of the child's social interactions both in and out of school is to be as optimal as possible (not to mention providing a counter to teasing and bullying). In this respect, it should never be forgotten that any cosmetic disability has the potential to be as great a functional disadvantage for the child as those apparently more urgent problems such as raised intracranial pressure (see Chapter 12).

At this point it is important to consider – albeit briefly – the ethical implications involved in such decision making. What is the place of major surgical procedures that are being carried out for primarily cosmetic indications for those children whose cognitive, learning and communication abilities are so severely affected by their syndrome that they may never be able to enjoy an independent life? From a purely practical point of view, a significant degree of co-operation (which includes the capacity to cope with what can be the severe discomfort involved) is required from the older child undergoing, say, a monobloc or bipartition procedure, particularly when distraction is being used. There will therefore always be some particularly severely affected children who will not be suitable candidates for purely cosmetic reconstructive surgery (as opposed to operations needed to deal with some reversible functional problem such as raised ICP or airway obstruction). But to what extent should the decision to carry out such a procedure for primarily cosmetic reasons (most 'purely' functional issues are likely to have been dealt with by this age) on a teenager with significant learning difficulties be dependent upon their informed consent?

This opens up the question of whether children with learning difficulties should be subjected to surgery for primarily cosmetic reasons at all. As has already been mentioned, severe learning difficulties, particularly in older children, may impose technical restrictions upon some procedures, rendering them impossible to perform. But what about a child of a year or so who is predicted as unlikely ever to lead an independent life but whose appearance could undoubtedly be improved by an operation for which their co-operation would not be required – a fronto-orbital reconstruction in a child with metopic synostosis and a chromosomal disorder, for example? Although it is not our intention here to set out rules for such decision making, the problem can perhaps be best summarised by describing the two extremes of the range of opinions parents express to us – from, on the one hand, 'It would be an unjustified assault to subject such children with all their other problems to the risks and disturbances of a cosmetic procedure whose advantages they will never be able to appreciate' to 'These children already have severe problems, yet they will still to some extent be out in the world so why not at least render them physically less remarkable.' Clearly it requires both open-mindedness and sensitivity, not to mention a dispassionate appreciation of what craniofacial surgery can and cannot deliver, on the part of the specialists involved in order to come to a decision that is primarily in the best interests of the child – and no one else.

(Details of the various operations listed in this section – including distraction – can be found in Chapter 19.)

THE MANAGEMENT OF THE MORE COMMONLY ENCOUNTERED SYNDROMES

Crouzon syndrome

Affected children can have a very variable expression of their phenotype – ranging from those with no significant cranial problems at all but severe maxillary retrusion to those who run into early problems with raised ICP and exorbitism and airway obstruction. Perhaps this variability reflects the many different FGFR2 mutations responsible for this condition (Chapter 3). What most patients with Crouzon syndrome do have in common, however, is shallowness of the orbits. Their cognitive development may well be normal and it therefore becomes of extreme importance to ensure that none of the complications listed above interferes with that potential. Regular contact with the craniofacial team is essential while the child is growing up, even for those with no obvious functional problems, so that adjustments to whatever long-term strategy was decided upon when the child was first assessed can be made as necessary and, if surgery at a particular date has been planned, the necessary orthodontic preparation can be started at the appropriate time (which may be as long as one or two years before the definitive surgical procedure).

In general, however, the management policy for children with Crouzon syndrome follows much along the lines of the 'general' policy described above. Their definitive 'final' surgery may consist either of a monobloc frontofacial advance (for those whose maxillary and supraorbital hypoplasia balance each other), or of a supraorbital and frontal reconstruction and an extracranial Le Fort III maxillary advance. Where the latter has failed to restore satisfactory dental occlusion (or when early surgery has allowed a gradual reversion to a class III malocclusion), a Le Fort I advance of the lower third (tooth-bearing) section of the maxilla may be needed when the patient is aged 17 or 18. All these procedures may be carried out using a variety of bone distraction devices. Those with a marked laterally down-turning slant to their orbits and hypertelorism will benefit from a facial bipartition. A rhinoplasty may also be required as part of the final refinement (or 'tidying-up') of the correction of the facial deformity of the child with Crouzon syndrome, and in some cases mandibular surgery (genioplasty) will be needed as well.

Apert syndrome

Although children with Apert syndrome may differ from each other in several ways (in the degree of their facial deformity and in the complexity of their syndactyly, for example), they form on the whole a very homogeneous group with regard to their appearance and their

124

impaired cognitive development, and a great deal of input from a wide variety of specialists is required in their management.

In addition to the complications already listed, children with Apert syndrome have a high incidence of cleft palate (Slaney et al 1996) (which may be of the submucosal type), premature closure of which may further obstruct an already compromised airway.

The infant with Apert syndrome has a characteristic appearance, which has already been illustrated in Chapter 2. Airway obstruction is common and this can make assessment of the child's intracranial pressure difficult, as with each laboured breath there is a tense bulging of the large anterior fontanelle region – an area that in Apert syndrome often extends downwards to just above the glabella anteriorly and may extend posteriorly along a widened sagittal suture.

The combination of cleft palate and breathing difficulties can make these children difficult to feed and particular attention must be paid to this at their initial assessment. From a management point of view, priority must be given to the provision of an adequate airway (see Chapter 9), but even when this has been done, nasogastric feeding may still be required in a significant proportion of children.

Children with Apert syndrome can develop raised intracranial pressure, which is more likely to be due to venous hypertension aggravated by the effects of airway obstruction than progressive hydrocephalus, which is a less frequent complication than in Crouzon and Pfeiffer syndromes – perhaps because the early fusion of the lambdoid sutures that is a feature of those conditions is seen less in Apert syndrome (Cinalli et al 1995).

The rather stereotypical cognitive and communication problems of children with Apert syndrome demand particular attention (Shipster et al 2002). Most affected children are likely to start their education in mainstream schooling, usually with some assistance, but with age their placement within the regular school system becomes more precarious and some form of special education is often required. However, a large study from France (Renier et al 1996) has shown that there is a distinct correlation between the IQ of these children and whether or not they have spent part of their life in an 'institution', a fact that emphasises the vulnerability of their learning potential to the stimulation – or lack of it – provided by their environment.

Of all the children with syndromic craniosynostosis it is those with Apert syndrome (and some with Pfeiffer syndrome) who are most likely to demonstrate a laterally down-turning slant to their orbits, and with it a typical see-saw disorder of eye movements (on looking to the right, the right eye travels outwards and down, and the left travels inwards and up). The only surgical procedure which has the ability to correct this basic abnormality of their facial anatomy is the bipartition (see Chapter 19) – an operation that is best reserved until a child has developed his or her secondary dentition, and preferably until as late an age as possible if the necessity for further reconstructive surgery is to be kept to a minimum.

Management of the syndactyly in Apert syndrome does not fall within the remit of this book but the interested reader is referred to the chapter on congenital problems of the hand in Paul Smith's fourth edition of *Lister's The Hand – Diagnosis and Indications* (Smith 2002).

Pfeiffer syndrome

Pfeiffer syndrome has been classified into three groups (see Chapter 2) which for simplicity can be summarised as: *type 1* – (the least severe form) in which bicoronal synostosis may exist with only modest maxillary hypoplasia; *type 2* – a severe form in which marked maxillary hypoplasia and frontal recession (due to the bicoronal synostosis) combine with hydrocephalus to produce a cloverleaf skull deformity; and *type 3* – which is as severe a form as type 2 but without the cloverleaf skull deformity. All types have bicoronal synostosis combined with maxillary hypoplasia and a variety of digital abnormalities, which although characteristic are never as functionally severe as the syndactyly seen in Apert syndrome.

It is the type 2 form of Pfeiffer syndrome that is most commonly responsible for the cloverleaf skull deformity (which can occasionally also complicate Apert and Crouzon syndromes). In it a constricting band of bone runs horizontally backwards across the head from the outer limit of the sphenoid ridge towards the occiput. Below this is a patent squamous-temporal suture and above it a usually widely patent sagittal suture and anterior fontanelle region. Hydrocephalus is common and its effect is to expand the head upwards and laterally, the result of the constriction band being to 'pinch' the calvarium so that when viewed from in front the head has a typical cloverleaf shape. Maxillary hypoplasia is usually severe in these children and they are often suffering from marked exorbitism, raised ICP and airway obstruction by the time they are first presented to the craniofacial unit.

Few other conditions associated with craniosynostosis demonstrate so graphically as the child with Pfeiffer syndrome and the cloverleaf deformity the disappointing results of early surgery in terms of the potential for relapse. This is not to argue against recommending whatever surgical procedures are necessary to keep the child's ICP normal (the majority of children are likely to require not only some form of CSF diversion but also one or more vault expansion procedures to achieve this), to prevent damage due to exposure of the eyes and to maintain a functional airway, but it must be recognised that even if a satisfactory result (particularly in aesthetic terms) has been achieved in a child of under 4 years of age, the next 4 years will see the gradual re-emergence of some if not all of the previously abnormal features.

In type 1 Pfeiffer syndrome the cosmetic effects upon the face and skull may be comparatively mild. This unfortunately does not mean that the risk of raised ICP is similarly reduced, and these children need monitoring every bit as closely as those more severely affected.

Cloverleaf skull syndrome

The cloverleaf skull syndrome is most commonly seen in association with Pfeiffer syndrome (for details see above) but it does occur occasionally as a complication of Crouzon or Apert syndrome.

Saethre–Chotzen syndrome

Of all the individual syndromes discussed in this chapter, Saethre–Chotzen syndrome and craniofrontonasal dysplasia are associated with the lowest incidence not only of cognitive and learning difficulties but also of such complications as exorbitism, raised ICP and airway obstruction. Some prediction of the expression of the genotype in the individual child can often be made by assessing its effects in first-degree relatives, in some of whom there may be little more to find than a mild ptosis or a characteristic shape to the nose.

Craniofacial surgery is therefore more likely to be needed, if at all, for aesthetic rather than strictly functional reasons and should be delayed (if practical from a psychological point of view) until the risk of relapse/reversion is low. In fact, significant maxillary hypoplasia is unusual in these children who tend to be most concerned by their supraorbital recession (which may be very asymmetrical) and their ptosis.

Muenke syndrome

The syndromes discussed so far in this section were all first described (and named eponymously) on the basis of a clinician recording the conjunction of a particular set of physical abnormalities with or without effects on learning and cognition. The recent spectacular advance of knowledge of the molecular genetic basis of these disorders was hailed at first as a way of 'tidying-up' this rather unscientific situation – each child could now, it was hoped, be described not by the name of that initial observer but by the results of DNA analysis. Unfortunately this has not proved to be the case. Apart from Apert syndrome, in which only two mutations cover the great majority of children (who are still labelled clinically as *Apert syndrome*), DNA analysis has raised as many contradictions as it has answered – 30 or more different mutations in Crouzon syndrome, and identical mutations of FGFR2 associated with both Crouzon and Pfeiffer syndromes, for example (Rutland et al 1995).

Muenke syndrome is of special interest because its 'discovery' came not primarily from clinical observations but from the laboratories of the molecular geneticist (Muenke et al 1997). At first the *pro250arg* mutation of the FGFR3 gene was thought to be responsible only for those children with a particularly severe form of unicoronal synostosis, who also had a positive family history and were likely to suffer from significant learning difficulties; but we now find that an increasing number of children previously labelled as having 'non-syndromic' synostosis (single suture and bicoronal) may also have the relevant FGFR3 mutation (Reardon et al 1997).

As in Saethre–Chotzen syndrome, associated functional complications such as raised ICP, exorbitism, maxillary hypoplasia and airway obstruction are rare and most craniofacial procedures are performed to correct the cosmetic effects of unilateral or bilateral supraorbital ridge recession – operations best postponed until children are around (or over) 18 months of age if the effects of relapse are to be kept to a minimum.

Craniofrontonasal dysplasia

The effects of craniofrontonasal dysplasia are confined almost exclusively to the orbits (both vertical and horizontal dystopia – hypertelorism) and frontal region (usually an asymmetrical coronal synostosis). Maxillary problems are rare and, although the frontal and supraorbital problems can be addressed from the age of 18 months or so onwards, correction of the hypertelorism is best reserved until the patient is 12 years of age. The operations that can be used for this correction are described in Chapter 19 – a 'box-type' procedure or a facial bipartition.

Multiple suture, 'non-syndromic' craniosynostosis

With the advent of testing for specific genetic abnormalities (particularly the *pro250arg* mutation – for Muenke syndrome (Muenke et al 1997)), the proportion of children still labelled as 'non-syndromic' is falling. However there are still children with combinations of premature suture fusion who cannot as yet be fitted into any classification system – except in purely descriptive terms. Examples include children with bicoronal synostosis but no other syndromic features, sagittal synostosis combined with one or – more usually – both lambdoids, and sagittal combined with a single coronal synostosis.

Such cases should – at least with regard to their initial assessment – be treated in the same way as children with recognised syndromes, and the same care should be taken to look for indications of, for example, raised ICP. If such complications have been excluded then surgery may well be needed on cosmetic grounds, but as a general rule the element of relapse is likely to be greater for these children than might be expected for those with the individual suture involvements alone (see below) – an important reason for not proceeding too early with whatever reconstructive procedure is required.

(For an alternative overview of the management of syndromic craniosynostosis, the reader is referred to a review by Renier (Renier et al 2000).)

SIMPLE/SINGLE SUTURE CRANIOSYNOSTOSIS

Introduction

Although the single suture synostoses (sagittal, coronal, metopic and – extremely rarely – unilateral lambdoid) may overlap with the syndromic forms (an example is Muenke syndrome – see above), it is convenient to consider them as a separate group because of the differences in the implications of the diagnosis and hence the requirements for assessment, treatment and continuing surveillance.

The question of what constitutes 'raised' intracranial pressure will be discussed in the following chapter but suffice it to say here that, as a general rule, raised ICP in the sense of a complication likely to compromise vision is sufficiently rare in the single suture synostoses to make it unnecessary to recommend surgical treatment routinely for every affected child in order to prevent it. Indeed in the only single suture synostosis group in whom raised ICP is sometimes detected (some older children with sagittal synostosis presenting with cognitive and behavioural problems), ophthalmic morbidity is extremely rare.

Airway obstruction and exorbitism are also rare and this means that the primary indication for surgical treatment of these conditions is cosmetic – an indication not to be belittled when an operation can make the difference between a child being teased at school or not, but also one against which the never-absent risks of the craniofacial procedure required need to be considered. Putting this more succinctly, for the milder cases, surgery may represent more of a risk to the child than a conservative approach. An alternative approach has been advanced by Jimenez and colleagues (Jimenez et al 2002). For the young child, they advise a 'simple' excision of the fused suture (carried out endoscopically), and then, for the subsequent moulding of the head shape, the child wears an orthotic helmet for several months.

Our own policy for these children, therefore, is not to submit them to the formal craniofacial assessment we recommend for our syndromic cases but to refer cases to appropriate specialists in the craniofacial team on an individual basis as indicated by their particular problems – the child with unicoronal synostosis being in particular need of an ophthalmological assessment, for example (see below).

The degree to which children with a single suture synostosis are – or should be – submitted to radiological investigations is a matter of some debate. Our own studies (Cerovac et al 2002) have confirmed what every experienced craniofacial specialist already knew – that the diagnosis of each of the single suture synostoses can usually be made clinically on the basis of the child's appearance alone, and that once the child has been seen by such a specialist and the diagnosis has been made in this way, further investigations ('plain' X-rays, CT with or without 3D reconstructions and MRI) are unnecessary. Our present policy therefore is to omit such investigations unless there is an indication separate to the diagnosis of the abnormal head shape alone (such as developmental delay, for example) to support them.

This leaves unanswered the question of what – if any – radiological investigations the 'non-craniofacial doctor' presented with a child with an abnormal head shape and who is considering referral to a specialist craniofacial unit should undertake. The most frequent differential diagnostic confusion these days is between 'positional posterior plagiocephaly' and unilateral lambdoid synostosis (see below) – both conditions for which there are few if any indications for surgical intervention. Skull X-rays may indeed provide a correct diagnosis but are often misinterpreted by non-neuroradiologists, particularly in the very young, resulting sometimes in inappropriate referrals and unnecessary anxiety for the family. Our advice is to be guided by the child's appearance, and the best way of recording that is by obtaining good quality clinical photographs. These (together with any plain X-rays that may already have been taken) can then be sent to the craniofacial unit for their opinion as to whether the child needs to be seen or not. It is difficult to support submitting children with no problems other than their unusual head shape to the sedation or general anaesthesia that may be required for CT or MRI if neither investigation is needed to make the diagnosis.

The decision to operate or not for otherwise uncomplicated cases of single suture synostosis (the majority of such children) needs to be made on cosmetic grounds. This clearly places a grave responsibility upon the parents who have to choose whether or not to submit their child to an operation which although in experienced hands carries an extremely low complication rate still involves major surgery to the head in a patient who may be below 1 year of age – and which carries risks (of neurological disability or even death) that are never zero. The piece of information all parents therefore need to know before making this decision is what will be the consequences of *not* proceeding to surgery – will their child's head become even more unusual in appearance, will 'pressure on the brain' build up?

For reasons already explained the second question can be answered in the negative. The effect of time upon the untreated head shape is harder to predict but as a general rule most children presenting in infancy will, if seen again after two or three years, have a head shape that is largely unchanged, although those with sagittal synostosis can show an increase in the bossing of the forehead, and in those with metopic synostosis the ridge down the centre of the forehead may become a little more prominent.

As for the operations themselves, at one time all single suture synostoses were treated – if treated at all – by a simple excision of the fused suture sometimes combined with a manoeuvre designed to prevent the now separated bones from joining together again (wrapping the cut bone edges in silastic sheeting, for example). As experience accumulated over the years, it became apparent that these operations were largely ineffective (except perhaps in the very mildest cases where the indications to operate at all also were at their weakest), and nowadays most craniofacial surgeons will either carry out a more extensive craniectomy (in young children with sagittal synostosis, for example) or – more usually – add some form of active reconstruction to the suture excision.

It is interesting in this context to discuss parents' attitudes towards cosmetic skull vault surgery for their infant children. Even though the abnormality of head shape associated with, say, sagittal or unicoronal synostosis may be mild, once parents have had the diagnosis of craniosynostosis confirmed ('The bones of my child's head have stuck together too early'), they usually opt for an operation despite a frank description of the potential dangers of surgery and the benign nature of the condition. However, for 'positional' plagiocephaly – when the initial deformity may be a great deal more obvious – the response tends to be entirely different. Once parents have been reassured that there is no craniosynostosis, it is extremely unusual for a surgical reconstruction to be requested.

Details of the various operations employed in the management of single suture synostosis can be found in Chapter 19.

Sagittal synostosis
Sagittal synostosis is the commonest form of synostosis, simple or complex, and the degree of abnormality it produces varies from little more than a palpable ridge down the line of the fused suture to obvious scaphocephaly.

Most children with sagittal synostosis are presented for possible treatment within the first few months of life, a period during which raised intracranial pressure (and other functional problems) is extremely rare. Decisions at this age therefore need to be made on cosmetic grounds alone – and along the lines described above.

There is however a particular cognitive problem that children with sagittal synostosis may develop and that is the delay in speech and language development described in Chapter 14 (and see Arnaud et al 1995, Shipster et al 2003). Its cause is unknown. It is not related to raised intracranial pressure and does not seem to be affected by whether or not the child has had surgery. It does however make it important that the parents of children with sagittal synostosis (and those professionals caring for them) are warned of the possibility so that remedial therapy can be started as soon as the problem is recognised, ideally at around the age of 3 years.

There are a large number of operative procedures recommended for the young (under 6 months) child with sagittal synostosis – a fact that suggests that none shines above the others. Our own preference is to perform a wide (7 cm) sagittal craniectomy and combine this with a manoeuvre designed both to shorten the antero-posterior diameter and widen the biparietal diameter of the head. This can take the form of a plication of the parietal bones after they have been divided vertically, or a so-called *pi* procedure (or a modification of it) in which a midline (sagittal) strut of bone is used to pull the front and back of the head closer together while multiple vertical cuts through each parietal bone allow these areas to bulge wider and thus prevent the intracranial pressure from rising.

Both procedures are effective at broadening the head and reducing the antero-posterior diameter although the cosmetic effects of the latter are seen mainly at the occiput – prominent bossing (and particularly narrowing) of the forehead being less dramatically improved. In brief, however, these early operations even if they do not always abolish all traces of scaphocephaly are successful in restoring a sufficiently regular shape to the head to make it unusual for further reconstructive surgery to be requested at a later date.

Surgery for the older child with cosmetically unacceptable scaphocephaly due to sagittal synostosis involves significantly more major procedures – usually a formal reconstruction of either all or at least the anterior two-thirds of the calvarium. The reason for limiting the extent of the reconstruction is that, apart from the desire to reduce the overall scale of the operation, the major cosmetic disability for these older children ('Peanut head' is a typical description used by those teasing them at school) is usually the combination of frontal bossing and narrowing – the prominence of the occiput often being disguised by hair.

Metopic synostosis
Metopic synostosis produces the characteristic trigonocephalic abnormality of head shape described in Chapter 2. Although no responsible gene mutation has yet been discovered, it is of all the various forms of craniosynostosis the one most often associated with chromosomal abnormalities – for example, deletions of 1q, 13q and 16q. It also forms part of the fetal valproate syndrome (Lajeunie et al 2001).

Cognitive and developmental problems are common in these 'complex' forms of metopic synostosis, but learning difficulties may complicate a proportion of children with the 'simple' forms – particularly those in which the degree of narrowing of the frontal region is greatest. This has led to the hypothesis that it is constriction of the developing frontal lobes that is responsible for such cognitive problems and that early (below the age of 1 year) reconstructive surgery (whose effect is to restore a normal contour to the forehead) will result in a reduction in the degree of any eventual disability. Unfortunately the only study that has addressed this question with a large number of children (Bottero et al 1998) has a variety of methodological flaws that leave the case unproven (Hayward et al 1999).

Like all forms of single suture synostosis, metopic synostosis can manifest itself in mild and severe forms and at any point along the spectrum between the two. At its most minimal there may be little more to see than a slight ridge along the line of the fused suture with no associated trigonocephaly. The parents of such children need no more than reassurance. However when there is obvious trigonocephaly with hypotelorism and prominent epicanthic folds, reconstructive surgery (which involves the restructuring of the supraorbital ridges and the entire forehead) is very successful at restoring a more normal contour to the front of the head. Of interest is the way the associated hypotelorism may also improve with time even though no specific attempt has been made to deal with it during the operation.

When children are reviewed years later it is not unusual to find that there has been a degree of reversion involving the extreme lateral part of the lower forehead – not usually the central 'metopic' area – but it is extremely rare in our experience for this to be sufficiently obvious for further surgery to be requested.

Recommendations for the timing of surgery depend very much upon the craniofacial surgeon's opinion of the effect of early surgery on improving the child's cognitive outcome set against a reduced degree of relapse for the child operated upon later. Our present policy (having started by advising surgery at as young an age as possible and then gradually advancing this age as we surveyed the long-term results) is to operate when children are about 15 to 18 months of age.

The question of whether or not children with severe cognitive and learning problems (those with chromosome deletions, for example) should be operated upon or not has been discussed earlier in this chapter.

Details of the surgery are given in Chapter 19.

Unicoronal synostosis
With the exception of those children with Muenke syndrome (Muenke et al 1997, Reardon et al 1997) (see above and Chapter 2), which may be associated with both unicoronal and bicoronal synostosis, unicoronal synostosis is the single suture synostosis least often associated with significant other problems – raised intracranial pressure, airway problems and learning difficulties, for example.

The description of affected children as having unicoronal synostosis carries the implication that it is the premature closure of this suture and the effects spreading from this that are responsible for the resulting deformity. This view is too simplistic. It needs experience of only a few cases to see that the abnormality of head shape is more complex and that children have a curvature of the skull and face that can be appreciated in two planes. Viewed from in front there is a facial 'scoliosis' whose line runs from the centre of the forehead down to the tip of the mandible and which is convex to the affected side. It is this that is responsible for the bridge of the nose being angled towards the side of the closed suture. Axial CT shows how there is a similar process affecting the skull base with a marked curvature concave towards the affected side that runs from the nose back through the foramen magnum to the occiput.

The abnormal bony anatomy of the orbital roof that these children have can be responsible for an aberrant placement of the trochlea and in turn a complex interference with eye movement. The diagnosis and management of this are discussed in Chapter 10.

Parents can be reassured of the benign nature of the condition, and the surgery for those who opt for reconstruction can be timed according to the protocols developed by the craniofacial unit involved. Our own policy, as outlined above, is to carry out such surgery at between 15 and 18 months of age.

Relapse following technically successful surgery tends to be related to the severity of the initial deformity. Operating later and exaggerating the extent of the correction – leaving the child with an element of the reconstruction to 'grow into' – can reduce its incidence and degree.

Lambdoid synostosis

Unilateral lambdoid synostosis is the rarest of the single suture synostoses. It produces, as one would expect, flattening of the affected parieto-occipital region (posterior plagio-cephaly) but it is greatly outnumbered as a cause of this asymmetry of head shape by the so-called 'postural' or 'positional' plagiocephaly described in Chapter 1.

It can be differentiated from positional plagiocephaly by the clinical history (it is always present from birth while approximately two-thirds of children with positional posterior plagiocephaly have a normal head shape at birth) and by an examination of the child's head shape when it is viewed from above. In positional plagiocephaly there is a shortening of the distance between the eye and the ear on the side with the flattened occiput and this gives the skull base a parallelogram shape. In unilateral lambdoid synostosis this shortening does not occur – although there is also ipsilateral flattening and contralateral posterior bossing, the shape of the skull base is that of a trapezium (Huang et al 1998) with bossing on the affected side (see Fig. 7.1). In lambdoid synostosis, when viewed from behind, the ear on the affected side is lower, while in positional plagiocephaly the ears are on the same plane.

Unilateral lambdoid synostosis is of no significance in terms of brain compression and decisions concerning surgery need to be made entirely on cosmetic grounds. A reconstructive procedure must inevitably involve the removal and then reshaping of a large proportion of the back of the skull (with the lateral and the posterior part of the sagittal venous sinuses in close proximity) and therefore, for an area that is going to be hidden by hair, the number of parents opting for surgery is in our experience extremely small.

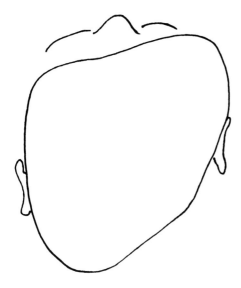

Fig. 7.1 The head of a child with posterior positional moulding viewed from above, showing how the ear–eye distance on the affected side is less than that on the other side, and how the apparent advance of the face on the affected side leaves the overall head shape that of a parallelogram.

'Positional' posterior plagiocephaly

Although not associated with premature fusion of any suture (the sclerosis often seen along the line of the lambdoid suture on the flattened side is probably a secondary rather than a primary process), children with this condition are frequently referred to craniofacial units with a diagnosis (often on the basis of poor quality radiographs) of craniosynostosis. It would seem appropriate therefore to say something here about its management.

If it is accepted that the condition is due to a combination of deforming forces acting upon the young and malleable perinatal skull (an asymmetry of head turning with or without frank torticollis, the increased use of the supine position for nursing the young infant and the popularity of firm mattresses with no pillows), and that the process of deformation ceases as the child becomes more mobile and any asymmetry of head turning resolves, it follows that the process of spontaneous improvement in head shape that can then be observed (and which is usually both slow and incomplete) should be susceptible to acceleration if some opposing (correctional) deforming force could be applied. With such logic in mind a variety of orthotic devices have been devised. Their use, however, remains controversial and there have been to our knowledge no randomised controlled clinical trials to demonstrate their effectiveness. It is not our purpose in a book devoted to craniosynostosis to argue the merits or demerits of such devices here, but the following points would appear relevant in any discussion concerning their use:

1   The age range during which they are likely to have any chance of success.
2   Do orthoses actually do what they claim to do when compared with the natural history?
3   Hair growth – when first seen the child may have little hair; how visible will the shape of the back of the child's head be in a year or two's time?
4   Alternative methods – including physiotherapy for the asymmetry of head turning, encouragement for the child to lie off the flattened side, etc.
5   The psychological implications (for all members of the family) of the child wearing a very visible orthosis.
6   The 'medical culture' of the community and in particular its attitude towards what represents a condition needing treatment and what does not.
7   Expense.

Having said all this, however, it is the responsibility of the paediatric community to consider all the implications of its policy of proscribing the prone position for nursing infants. While it is clearly important to continue with a recommendation that has had a significant effect in lowering the incidence of cot-death (Sudden Infant Death Syndrome – SIDS), the significance of any alteration in head shape (particularly if associated with even the slightest tendency for the child to sleep with his or her head turned preferentially in just one direction) should be pointed out to all parents so that the condition can be recognised earlier than it usually is now and measures taken to correct it that will have a greater chance of success if undertaken while the skull is still malleable.

Summary

The general policy of the craniofacial unit at Great Ormond Street Hospital for Children for the management of children with craniosynostosis can be summarised as follows:

1   The abnormalities of skull and facial growth associated with both the syndromic and the single suture forms of craniosynostosis should be considered as just that – disorders of growth and not just the 'simple' mechanical effects of the early fusion of one or more skull sutures.
2   While the primarily affected areas continue to grow they will exhibit a tendency to grow to the shape genetically determined for them.
3   If surgery is carried out before growth has ceased there will be a tendency for some of the advantage derived from the operation to be lost (reversion or relapse). This is most obvious in syndromic cases.
4   The most effective ways of reducing this process are to postpone surgery until the major period of growth of the affected area is over, and to exaggerate any correction attempted.
5   The major functional problems complicating the syndromic forms of craniosynostosis (raised ICP, respiratory obstruction and exorbitism) all have the potential to restrict the affected child's neurocognitive development. They must be detected early and treated effectively.
6   Affected children should be managed only in conjunction with an established craniofacial unit that can field the proper combination of specialists experienced in the management of these complex cases.
7   The decisions involved in surgery for purely cosmetic reasons raise complex practical and ethical issues that demand that decisions are reached only as the result of a consensus between the family, the craniofacial team and of course – where practical – the patient.

REFERENCES

Arnaud E, Renier D, Marchac D (1995) Prognosis for mental function in scaphocephaly. *J Neurosurg* 83(3): 476-479.

Bottero L, Lajeunie E, Arnaud E, Marchac D, Renier D (1998) Functional outcome after surgery for trigonocephaly. *Plast Reconstr Surg* 102(4): 952–958.

Cerovac S, Neil-Dwyer JG, Rich P, Jones BM, Hayward RD (2002) Are routine preoperative CT scans necessary in the management of single suture craniosynostosis? 1. *Br J Neurosurg* 16(4): 348–354.

Cinalli G, Renier D, Sebag G, Sainte-Rose C, Arnaud E, Pierre-Kahn A (1995) Chronic tonsillar herniation in Crouzon's and Apert's syndromes: the role of premature synostosis of the lambdoid suture. *J Neurosurg* 83(4): 575–582.

Hayward R, Jones BMJ, Evans R (1999) Functional outcome after surgery for trigonocephaly. *Plast Reconstr Surg* 104(2): 582–583.

Huang MHS, Mouradian WE, Cohen SR, Gruss JS (1998) The differential diagnosis of abnormal head shapes: separating craniosynostosis from positional deformities and normal variants. *Cleft Palate Craniofac J* 35(3): 204–211.

Jimenez DF, Barone CM, Cartwright CC, Baker L (2002) Early management of craniosynostosis using endoscopic-assisted strip craniectomies and cranial orthotic molding therapy. *Pediatrics* 110(1 pt 1): 97–104.

Lajeunie E, Barcik U, Thorne JA, Ghouzzi VE, Bourgeois M, Renier D (2001) Craniosynostosis and fetal exposure to sodium valproate. *J Neurosurg* 95(5): 778–782.

Muenke M, Gripp KW, McDonald-McGinn DM, Gaudenz K, Whitaker LA, Bartlett SP, Markowitz RI, Robin NH, Nwokoro N, Mulvihill JJ, Losken HW, Mulliken JB, Guttmacher AE, Wilroy RS, Clarke LA, Hollway G, Ades LC, Haan EA, Mulley JC, Cohen MM Jr, Bellus GA, Francomano CA, Moloney DM, Wall SA, Wilkie AO (1997) A unique point mutation in the fibroblast growth factor receptor 3 gene (FGFR3) defines a new craniosynostosis syndrome 1. *Am J Hum Genet* 60(3): 555–564.

Reardon W, Wilkes D, Rutland P, Pulleyn LJ, Malcolm S, Dean JC, Evans RD, Jones BM, Hayward R, Hall CM, Nevin NC, Baraister M, Winter RM (1997) Craniosynostosis associated with FGFR3 pro250arg mutation results in a range of clinical presentations including unisutural sporadic craniosynostosis. *J Med Genet* 34(8): 632–636.

Reddy K, Hoffman H, Armstrong D (1990) Delayed and progressive multiple suture craniosynostosis 2. *Neurosurgery* 26(3): 442–448.

Renier D, Arnaud E, Cinalli G, Sebag G, Zerah M, Marchac D (1996) Prognosis for mental function in Apert's syndrome. *J Neurosurg* 85(1): 66–72.

Renier D, Lajeunie E, Arnaud E, Marchac D (2000) Management of craniosynostoses. *Childs Nerv Syst* 16(10–11): 645–658.

Rutland P, Pulleyn LJ, Reardon W, Baraitser M, Hayward R, Jones B, Malcolm S, Winter RM, Oldridge M, Slaney SF (1995) Identical mutations in the FGFR2 gene cause both Pfeiffer and Crouzon syndrome phenotypes. *Nat Genet* 9(2): 173–176.

Shipster C, Hearst D, Dockrell JE, Kilby E, Hayward R (2002) Speech and language skills and cognitive functioning in children with Apert syndrome: a pilot study 1. *Int J Lang Commun Disord* 37(3): 325–343.

Shipster C, Hearst D, Somerville A, Stackhouse J, Hayward R, Wade A (2003) Speech, language and cognitive development in children with isolated sagittal synostosis. *Dev Med Child Neurol* 45: 34–43.

Slaney SF, Oldridge M, Hurst JA, Morriss-Kay GM, Hall CM, Poole MD, Wilkie AO (1996) Differential effects of FGFR2 mutations on syndactyly and cleft palate in Apert syndrome. *Am J Hum Genet* 58(5): 923–932.

Smith P (2002) Congenital abnormalities. In: Smith P, editor. *Lister's The Hand – Diagnosis and Indications*, 4th edn. London: Churchill Livingstone, pp 457–522.

Wall SA, Goldin JH, Hockley AD, Wake MJ, Poole MD, Briggs M (1994) Fronto-orbital re-operation in craniosynostosis. *Br J Plast Surg* 47(3): 180–184.

Wong GB, Kakulis EG, Mulliken JB (2000) Analysis of fronto-orbital advancement for Apert, Crouzon, Pfeiffer, and Saethre–Chotzen syndromes. *Plast Reconstr Surg* 105(7): 2314–2323.

8
MANAGEMENT OF RAISED INTRACRANIAL PRESSURE

Richard Hayward and Ken K. Nischal

In the previous chapter (which discussed in general terms the management of children with craniosynostosis) it was pointed out that as the beneficial effects of reconstructive procedures can be lost during a child's subsequent growth – such reversion (or relapse) being a problem affecting particularly those with syndromic forms of craniosynostosis – the emphasis of early intervention should be on the management of the various complications that can affect the development of these children. The most serious of these complications are raised intracranial pressure (ICP), airway obstruction and visual failure (which itself may be due to a combination of exorbitism, leading to corneal exposure, and raised intracranial pressure).

In this chapter it is proposed to discuss the causes of raised ICP in craniosynostosis, its incidence, the problems it may cause, how to investigate and monitor for it and, of course, how best to treat it.

An introduction to intracranial pressure
The traditional view of ICP was very simple – the skull represented (in those with closed vault sutures) a non-expandable box within which there were effectively three non-compressible compartments containing, respectively, brain, blood and cerebrospinal fluid (CSF). As long as these components existed in a state of physiological balance with each other, the ICP would remain normal. Everyday fluctuations of the sort that might occur with transient rises (during coughing or straining, for example) were damped by the temporary egress of CSF through the foramen magnum or a reduction in intracranial venous blood volume. However, although excess of one of these constituents or the addition of a space-taking mass such as a tumour or haematoma might be compensated for in the short term by alterations in the CSF and vascular volumes, a rise in ICP would soon occur. This in turn would manifest itself with a classic set of symptoms and signs – headache, vomiting, papilloedema and, with increasing compromise of the brainstem, drowsiness leading to coma, respiratory failure and eventually death. (For a review of this subject the interested reader is referred to Lee and Hoff 2000.)

The inadequacies of this traditional view are well demonstrated by the problems associated with raised ICP complicating craniosynostosis. Here the clinical picture is more similar to that of benign intracranial hypertension (BIH – often referred to more accurately as idiopathic intracranial hypertension (IIH)) than to that associated with the presence of mass lesions in the head when the dominant pathological processes are as much related to brain distortion as to any actual rise in ICP, offset by the fact that the brain is not of course incompressible but capable of absorbing the effects of significant local pressures, provided these are applied slowly enough.

Another inadequacy that should also be borne in mind relates to the lack of certainty with which we know what the *normal* ICP is. For children it can probably be stated with some confidence that no parent has yet submitted their entirely normal, asymptomatic child to the insertion of, say, an ICP monitoring device (which involves passing a probe or catheter through the skull) or even to more indirect monitoring using a lumbar CSF catheter. All the measurements that we accept as normal are really no more than intuitive guesswork based on studies in which the intracranial pressure was considered unlikely to be raised and which produced readings consistent with what was considered most likely to be normal. The figures quoted below are now widely accepted as normal for each age group but it should be recognised that there is little accurate information about, for example, the standard deviations for each subgroup or the normal differences during quiet and active (REM) sleep (ICP rises during REM sleep).

For a discussion of intracranial pressure in childhood (including normal pressures) the reader is referred to Minns' textbook on this topic (Minns 1991).

NORMAL INTRACRANIAL PRESSURE

It is not surprising given the different constricting effects of the maturing skull upon the intracranial contents that normal ICP values vary with age. Generally accepted values are:

Infants <2 years	<5 mmHg
Children 2–5 years	5–10 mmHg
Children >5 years	<10 mmHg
'Adults'	<15 mmHg
	(Welch 1980)

For most of the published articles on ICP in craniosynostosis the following simplified scale has been used:

<10 mmHg	Normal
10–15 mmHg	Borderline
>15 mmHg	Raised

These figures apply to the baseline ICP. Superimposed upon it in the normal child, however, are transient – and harmless – peaks of raised ICP associated with, in particular, changes in intrathoracic pressure during coughing, straining, etc. There is also a modest rise in ICP during active (or REM) sleep which probably reflects increased cerebral blood flow and volume during these times.

MEASURING ICP

There is a variety of methods for assessing ICP – directly and indirectly, quantitatively and qualitatively, clinically and radiologically.

The criterion standard remains direct ICP monitoring using a probe (or ventricular catheter) passed through the skull to allow the continuous recording of ICP over a period that should include a minimum of one night. This is to allow measurements during quiet and active sleep, and – of great importance for children with syndromic craniosynostosis – during periods of nocturnal respiratory difficulty. Such procedures are of course invasive and carry small but never absent risks of infection, haemorrhage, CSF leakage and epilepsy (Thompson et al 1995a). Measuring ICP at lumbar puncture (or, better still, via a lumbar CSF catheter for an hour or two) in an often sedated child is less invasive but makes for a less accurate – and complete – assessment compared to direct ICP recordings.

Both methods do however provide quantitative (as opposed to qualitative) data which no other system does – at least not in a universally accepted way. Qualitative methods of assessment include transcranial Doppler (Pople et al 1991), fontenometers (Minns 1991) (for the very young) and tympanic membrane displacement (Samuel et al 1998).

Even more indirect methods can be divided into the *clinical* and the *radiological*. The *clinical* symptom most suggestive of raised ICP is of course headache, but the causes of headache are many and varied, and its difficulty of detection in very young children (plus the fact that many children with craniosynostosis with objectively proven raised ICP do not complain of headache) makes it an unreliable indicator – particularly if major cranial surgery is going to be advocated (or denied) on its presence (or absence) alone.

Papilloedema – or its absence – is also not as diagnostic as experience in other clinical conditions would suggest. In our own study of 122 children with all forms of craniosynostosis (Tuite et al 1996a) we concluded that if the normal values for ICP as given above were accepted, papilloedema was 98 per cent specific as an indication of raised ICP but that its sensitivity was age-dependent. It was 100 per cent sensitive in children older than 8 years but only 22 per cent in younger children. The role of repeated, specialised ophthalmological examinations of the state of the optic discs and visual evoked potentials (VEPs) in the monitoring of raised ICP in children with craniosynostosis is described later in this chapter and in Chapters 7 and 10. It should be noted, however, that monitoring of the appearance of the optic discs represents a purely qualitative assessment and that although VEPs are sensitive to an increase in ICP, their usefulness depends largely upon the ease with which they can be repeated, the condition of the child (tired or rested, co-operative or not) and any alterations in peak heights or latencies detected early (Mursch et al 1998).

Palpation of a still open anterior fontanelle (usually widely open in infants with Apert syndrome) can also be used to assess ICP but its tension is affected also by respiratory obstruction – a common accompanying problem in children with syndromic craniosynostosis.

Radiological methods of assessing ICP include the appearances of the skull vault on 'plain' radiographs, and information derived from the various cranial scanning techniques.

139

Raised ICP in children can produce a 'copper-beaten' appearance of part or all of the skull vault. The phenomenon is due to the imprinting of the brain's gyral pattern upon the inner surface of the skull as the vault gradually expands by a mixture of (internal) resorption and (external) deposition of bone. Where the bone is in close apposition to the inner surface of the skull, digital markings may appear. It can be seen in a localised form when one or more adjacent sutures are fused but can be generalised when all vault sutures have fused (craniostenosis) (see Fig. 8.10(c) for an extreme example of this phenomenon). Our own study (Tuite et al 1996b) of the reliability of this as an indicator of raised ICP in 123 children with all forms of craniosynostosis concluded that although copper-beating of the whole of the skull vault can indeed be an indicator of raised ICP, its sensitivity and specificity are so low that it should be used as no more than an indication that more reliable assessments of ICP may be required before any important management decisions are made. No current imaging techniques actually measure ICP. However some indirect and often low-specifity information can be obtained from such changes as an increase in ventricular size compared to a previous study (possibly indicating progressive hydrocephalus), an absence of CSF in the cortical sulci, and herniation of the cerebellar tonsils through the foramen magnum (Chiari 1 malformation).

SUMMARY

As has already been explained, it is unusual for the raised ICP that can complicate the syndromic forms of craniosynostosis to manifest itself clinically with the symptoms and signs one might associate with, say, a cerebral tumour (or other mass). This is not to say that headache should not be properly investigated – with careful examination of the fundi and ICP monitoring when necessary – but in the majority of affected children the diagnosis will be made by ICP monitoring (carried out either as a screening procedure or because of ophthalmological concerns) or clinically – the feel of the anterior fontanelle, for example, when airway obstruction is either absent or has been successfully treated.

Incidence of raised ICP in craniosynostosis

Before discussing this topic it is important to state that there are two components to raised ICP – the baseline pressure and, superimposed upon it, pathological plateaux waves of even higher pressure – and that one or both of these processes has the potential to affect cerebral (including optic pathway) function.

During raised ICP, due to whatever cause, there can occur more dramatic and sustained waves or plateaux of pressure which have been described by Lundberg as A, B and C waves (Lundberg 1960). These can be summarised as follows: A waves are plateaux that may rise to 100 mmHg and last from 5 to 20 minutes; B waves have a frequency of 0.5–2 per minute and can rise to 50 mmHg; C waves show a frequency of 4–8 per minute and pressures up to 20 mmHg. The plateaux waves seen so frequently in children with craniosynostosis and raised ICP (and referred to as such in this chapter) correspond most closely to Lundberg A waves. They consist of a rapid escalation of pressure, sometimes to more than double the baseline pressure (occasionally as high as 50–60 mmHg), which is sustained for 10 or 20 minutes and during which the amplitude of the pulse wave also increases. In children with

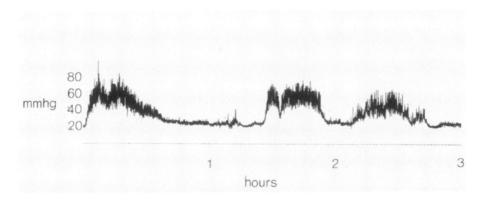

Fig. 8.1 ICP monitoring trace (sleeping) of a child with Crouzon syndrome and intermittent airway obstruction. Baseline pressures around 20–25 mmHg, rising to plateaux (Lundberg A waves) of 45–60 mmHg that coincided with episodes of snoring (airway compromise).

airway problems these plateaux usually coincide with episodes of obstruction and they occur particularly during active sleep (Fig. 8.1).

A recent analysis of the importance of plateaux waves in children with craniosynostosis has been provided by Eide and his colleagues (Eide et al 2002).

Raised ICP complicates the syndromic forms of craniosynostosis a great deal more frequently than the single suture or simple forms. In our own study investigating the uses of ICP monitoring in 136 unoperated children with craniosynostosis of all types (Thompson et al 1995a), raised ICP (pressures >15 mmHg) was demonstrated in 35 per cent – 28/53 of the syndromic children and 20/80 children with single suture involvement (Fig. 8.2). Plateaux waves were recorded in significantly more syndromic than non-syndromic children. In a more detailed study of 74 children (which overlapped with the previous study) with just single suture synostosis (Thompson et al 1995d), raised ICP was demonstrated in 17 per cent – more commonly in sagittal and metopic synostosis than in unicoronal synostosis (Fig 8.2(a)). Plateaux waves were seen in 19 children, only two of whom had a normal baseline pressure. No pressures above 25 mmHg were recorded and only four children had pressures that exceeded 20 mmHg. This raises the question of the relevance of these findings, a topic that is discussed later in the section on the harmful effects of raised ICP.

To investigate the incidence of raised ICP in syndromic craniosynostosis, we re-analysed data that we have previously published on ICP in craniosynostosis and extracted what further information we could from series presented by other authors (Hayward et al 2001).

A total of 259 (Renier et al 1982, Whittle et al 1984, Renier 1989, Siddiqi et al 1995, Thompson et al 1995a, Tuite et al 1996a, Taylor et al 2001) cases of syndromic cranio-synostosis who had had some form of ICP investigation are reported in the five series dealing particularly with ICP that were analysed – although it must be appreciated that some patients appear in more than one series and the majority of the cases come from just two

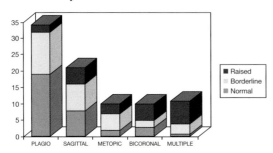

a ICP Profile in Non-Syndromic Craniosynostosis

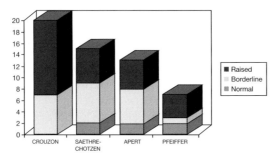

b ICP Profile in Syndromic Craniosynostosis

Fig. 8.2 (a) ICP profile (baseline pressures) of Great Ormond Street Hospital children with non-syndromic forms of craniosynostosis (plagiocephaly = unicoronal synostosis). (b) ICP profile (baseline pressures) of Great Ormond Street Hospital children with syndromic forms of craniosynostosis.

craniofacial centres – those of Paris (Renier et al 1982, Renier 1989) and London (Thompson et al 1995a, Tuite et al 1996a, Taylor et al 2001). The two Paris series also contain a large proportion of children with 'North African' oxycephaly (23/31 in the 1982 series and 66/91 in the 1989 series) – in addition to the more 'usual' selection of children with Apert, Crouzon and Pfeiffer syndromes, for example.

Of these 259 children, 140 are reported as having raised intracranial pressure – either a raised baseline ICP, or plateaux waves, or both – an incidence of about 54 per cent (and in our review of 60 of our own cases the incidence was approximately 70 per cent (Hayward et al 2001)).

Before this incidence is accepted at face value, it should be pointed out that the ICP recordings were not all undertaken for the same reasons. For example, in our own series the indications varied with age – those children studied young were more likely to be being 'screened' for the presence of raised ICP in the absence of other (clinical) indicators, while the older children were more likely to have presented with symptoms and signs suggesting but not necessarily confirming this diagnosis.

The incidence is, nevertheless, high and this accords with our own data showing that the ophthalmological morbidity affecting this group of children is also higher than previously thought (see below).

What about the actual pressures that we and others have recorded? Baseline pressures range from 15 to 30 mmHg (averaging around 20 mmHg) while plateaux waves in our own series ranged in height from 25 to 60 mmHg. (See Figs 8.1 and 8.11.)

Is there a 'natural history' to the raised ICP that can complicate syndromic craniosyn-ostosis? When is it most likely to occur? At what age can its absence mean that it is unlikely to crop up as a future complication? Does it represent a static or a dynamic process – one that is either present (until successfully treated) or, if not present now, will never occur? All available data confirm that it can be present from an early age – it may even exist antenatally (an hypothesis based on the appearance of the optic discs in very young children with phenotypically severe forms of syndromic craniosynostosis (Nischal 2002)) – but, untreated, does it continue indefinitely or does it 'burn itself out', as happens with the raised ICP sometimes seen in young children with achondroplasia? It is impossible to give a definitive answer to this question, although our clinical experience, coupled with the age distribution of the cases we have studied (accepting the provisos given above) and the limited data both on the age of children with visual deterioration (Stavrou et al 2002) and on the age of those re-presenting with ICP despite previous vault-expanding surgical procedures (Siddiqi et al 1995), does suggest that the particular danger period is from the time of the closure of the anterior fontanelle (if present) at around 1 year of age, to around 7 years of age. There are, however, occasional but definite cases presenting later than this with visual deterioration and raised ICP demonstrated by formal ICP monitoring.

Causes of raised ICP in craniosynostosis
There are four important contributors to the raised ICP that can complicate, in particular, the syndromic forms of craniosynostosis. Although dealt with individually here, it must be appreciated that they interact with each other in a variety of complex ways, not all of which are entirely understood. They are:

1   Cranio-cerebral disproportion
2   Hydrocephalus
3   Airway obstruction
4   Intracranial venous hypertension

CRANIO-CEREBRAL DISPROPORTION
Common sense* would suggest that if several sutures of the skull vault have fused prema-turely there should be a consequent failure of the skull to expand to accommodate the growing brain, that this relative disproportion should result in a rise in ICP and that this should in turn have a deleterious effect upon the child's development. Useful confirmation of such a hypothesis would come from demonstrating that the affected child's head was small for its age – small in terms of the intracranial volume (as reflected clinically in the

___

* 'Common sense is the metaphysic of savages', Bertrand Russell.

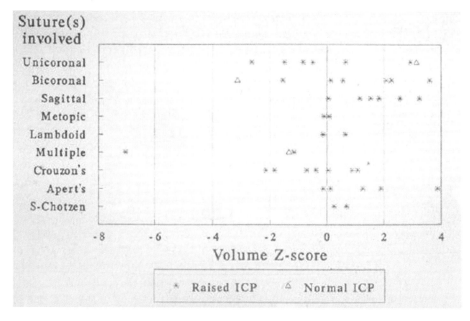

Fig. 8.3 Distribution of raised and normal intracranial pressure according to intracranial volume in children with various forms of craniosynostosis.

child's head circumference falling away from the centile lines as it grows). As with so many problems associated with craniosynostosis, cranio-cerebral disproportion turns out to be a more complex issue. Studies from this hospital (Fok et al 1992) and from Paris (Gault et al 1990, 1992) (amongst other centres) have shown that although there is a rough correlation between intracranial volume (ICV) and ICP, there are children – particularly those with Apert syndrome – in whom the intracranial volume is actually increased despite their ICP being raised (Fig. 8.3). A more recent study (Stavrou et al 2002) has shown that although for children under 6 months and for those with untreated pan-synostosis (craniostenosis) the ICV is small, after 6 months there is little difference compared to unaffected children (except for those with pan-synostosis) and, once again, children with Apert syndrome have an increased ICV.

There are also regional anatomical differences in ICV to be taken into account. Syndromic craniosynostosis frequently involves the lambdoid sutures and in these children the posterior fossa is likely to be small and the cerebellar tonsils prolapsed through the foramen magnum (the Chiari 1 malformation) (Thompson et al 1997a) (Fig. 8.4). This in turn can predispose to hydrocephalus and in some children cause severe transient occipital headaches associated with coughing, laughing and straining (activities which further raise the ICP) that can only be relieved by a foramen magnum decompression. In children with complex forms of craniosynostosis, the Chiari 1 malformation is seen most frequently in Crouzon and Pfeiffer syndromes. It is a less usual complication of Apert syndrome (Cinalli et al 1995).

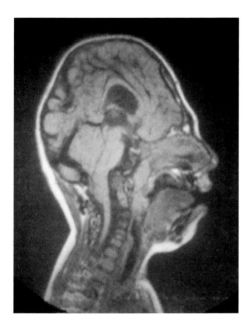

Fig. 8.4 Midline sagittal MR image of a child with Pfeiffer syndrome showing the severe degree of antero-posterior shortening of the whole head, hydrocephalus (enlarged third ventricle) and prolapse of the cerebellar tonsils downwards through the foramen magnum (Chiari 1 malformation).

HYDROCEPHALUS

It is important when discussing hydrocephalus to differentiate between progressive and non-progressive ventricular enlargement. In the Paris study (Renier et al 1982) of 1297 children treated surgically for craniosynostosis (isolated or syndromic), the incidence of ventricular enlargement was estimated overall at 8.1 per cent (just under half of whom received a shunt). It was most common in syndromic cases (12.1 per cent), requiring treatment more often in Crouzon syndrome than in Apert syndrome. It was present in all cases of cloverleaf skull syndrome (Pfeiffer type 2). As already suggested, it was more common in children with the Chiari malformation – and also in those with venous hypertension.

In our experience also, progressive ventriculomegaly sufficient to require some form of CSF diversion is extremely uncommon in single suture synostosis.

Once progressive hydrocephalus has been diagnosed, a ventriculo-peritoneal shunt is usually required, although in those cases in which there is a disproportionate increase in the size of the lateral and third ventricles compared to the fourth ventricle (so that the site of obstruction is likely to be in or around the aqueduct or posterior fossa) it may be possible to relieve the ICP by performing an endoscopic third ventriculostomy (see below).

AIRWAY OBSTRUCTION

Airway obstruction is a complication that occurs frequently in children with the pheno-typically most severe forms of syndromic craniosynostosis (Gonsalez et al 1997, 1998) and, as has already been described, it can be associated not only with transient (physiological)

145

rises in ICP but also with the sustained rises (plateaux) classified by Lundberg as A waves (Figs 8.1 and 8.11). What is this connection? The cerebral veins drain into unvalved and effectively splinted dural sinuses that in turn drain directly via the internal jugular veins into the superior vena cava – a structure that lies within the thoracic cavity. But forced inspiration in the face of upper airway obstruction is more likely to lead to a fall than a rise in intrathoracic pressure, although this will of course rise during obstructed expiration. The explanation is probably multifactorial. There is compression of the easy-to-occlude venous complexes within the neck by the abnormal activity of the accessory muscles of respiration during episodes of airway compromise, and this acts as a resistance in series to the venous obstructions that lie within the skull base (see below) thus augmenting the cranial hypertensive effects of both.

That airway compromise can act as an independent variable, however, in the genesis of chronically raised ICP can be demonstrated by the effect of improving the airway (by introducing continuous positive airway pressure (CPAP) or removing enlarged tonsils and adenoids, for example) on ICP monitoring. With the clearer airway there may be a reduction in both the baseline ICP and in the number and height of A wave plateaux (see 'Case history 2', below), and the appearance of the optic fundi and the VEPs can also be improved (see Chapter 10). All this implies an important causal relationship between airway status and ICP (see section below, 'How does raised ICP cause harm?').

INTRACRANIAL VENOUS HYPERTENSION
Exclusion of cranio-cerebral disproportion, progressive ventricular enlargement and airway obstruction still leaves the majority of children with syndromic craniosynostosis and raised ICP without an aetiological explanation. It is now generally accepted that intracranial venous hypertension is a major contributor (Sainte-Rose et al 1984, Thompson et al 1995b, 1995c, Anderson et al 1997, Taylor et al 2001). This may occur 'passively' as a consequence of an obstructed airway and raised intrathoracic pressure interfering with venous return (as explained above), but it also follows the progressive obstruction to the cranial venous outflows that these children are now known to have. In our own study (Taylor et al 2001) of 24 angiograms in 23 children with known raised ICP, significant anomalies of venous drainage (total non-opacification or >51 per cent stenosis) were observed affecting the jugular-sigmoid complex on one or both sides in 18 cases (Fig. 8.5). Also obvious were venous collaterals that were sometimes prominent enough to be palpated in the retromastoid region (Fig. 8.6). Whether these problems reflect maldevelopment of the venous sinuses as yet another effect of the responsible genetic mutation, or are merely secondary to the bony changes in the skull base, is unknown, although a further study from here (Rich et al 2003) has demonstrated actual narrowing of the jugular foramina in affected children (Fig. 8.7).

Venous hypertension can raise ICP in its own right. It can also contribute to the production of hydrocephalus through its effects upon the absorption of CSF through the arachnoid granulations into the superior sagittal sinus (Sainte-Rose et al 1984). It may also – as has been indicated earlier – be aggravated by airway obstruction.

146

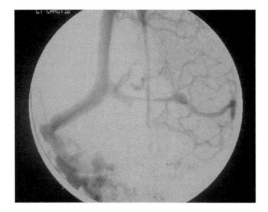

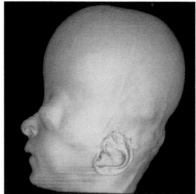

Fig. 8.5 Venous phase of a digital subtraction angiogram showing normal sagittal and right transverse sinuses, narrowing of the lateral half of the left transverse sinus, complete absence of the sigmoid/jugular complex on the left and copious collateral venous channels on the right suggesting obstruction to the sigmoid/jugular complex on that side as well.

Fig. 8.6 'Soft tissue' 3D CT reconstruction of a study of a child with Apert syndrome demonstrating exorbitism due to maxillary hypoplasia and supraorbital ridge recession, prominent scalp veins and extensive venous collaterals giving a lumpy appearance to the retro-mastoid region.

a
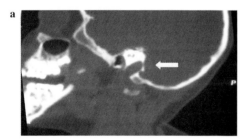

b
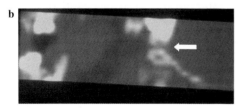

Fig. 8.7 (a) and (b) 'Slices' through the jugular foramina (open arrows) reconstructed from 3D CT datasets of a child with unicoronal synostosis (a – normal) and a child with Crouzon syndrome (b – narrowed). (Note the normal (class I) occlusion of the child in (a) and the abnormal (class III) occlusion in (b).

In summary, therefore, it can be seen that the raised ICP in children with syndromic craniosynostosis is multifactorial, with all four potential contributors acting synergistically with each other in a variety of subtle ways. This complexity of course has important implications when it comes to treatment.

147

What clinical problems are associated with raised ICP in children with craniosynostosis?

The raised ICP of these children has already been likened to that of benign intracranial hypertension (BIH), and, as in that condition, the most frequently reported consequences are ophthalmic (Wall and George 1991).

In a recent examination (Khan et al 2003) of 141 children of this hospital with syndromic craniosynostosis, just under 40 per cent were found to have a visual acuity of Snellen (or equivalent) 6/12 or worse in their *best* eye, while 64.6 per cent had an acuity of 6/12 or worse in at least one eye. Not all this morbidity is due to raised ICP – amblyopia due to previously unrecognised (and/or untreated) astigmatism and various forms of strabismus also play a prominent role. However it does point up the fact that ophthalmological vigilance is vital in these children and that an important component to their visual morbidity is raised ICP (Stavrou et al 2002). It is unusual for such deterioration to progress to complete blindness but this disaster is certainly well described and it is to be hoped that recognition that some degree of visual failure is so common will lead to more children with clinically occult raised ICP being detected before irreversible damage to their eyesight has occurred.

If it is well recognised that raised ICP can affect vision, are there any other clinical functions that are similarly vulnerable? A significant proportion of children with, in particular, syndromic or otherwise complex craniosynostosis may have learning difficulties and delay in other areas of their development, as well as being at risk of developing raised ICP. Are the two connected? The answer at present is that we do not know. There are many other contenders for a role in impeding these children's developmental progress, including chronic hypoxia and sleep deprivation due to airway obstruction, feeding difficulties leading to a failure to thrive, low parental and societal expectations, and hearing loss – not to mention any direct effects upon brain function of the genetic disorder responsible for the syndrome in the first place. If raised ICP is due to hydrocephalus the answer is simple – all aspects of a child's development can be severely affected by raised ICP due to untreated hydrocephalus. But when the rise in ICP is due, say, to chronic venous hypertension, comparison with a condition such as BIH (and perhaps achondroplasia – where intracranial venous pressure is also often raised) would suggest that, the effects on vision aside, raised ICP alone may not be contributing further to the child's disability.

In this context it is instructive to consider the influence of early surgery upon the cognitive development of children with isolated sagittal synostosis and with Apert syndrome.

Children with isolated sagittal synostosis have a higher than 'normal' incidence of delay in their speech and language acquisition – see Chapter 14 (Arnaud et al 1995, Shipster et al 2003). However there is no obvious connection between this and whether or not they have been operated upon, and therefore, while the aetiology of the delay remains unknown, it is not thought to be related to raised ICP.

The situation with Apert syndrome is more complex. In a large Paris study (Renier et al 1996), those children operated upon at less than 1 year of age had a better outcome in terms of their IQ than those operated upon later. But *all* the children in the series were being operated upon once they had been referred to the craniofacial centre, which means that the timing of their surgery reflected also the timing of each child's entry to a specialised service – the moment from which they would, perhaps for the first time, be properly assessed and start receiving treatment for not only raised ICP but also, for example, hearing and respiratory difficulties – potent causes of impaired psychosocial development in these children. An earlier referral also represented earlier interest in the child – this is supported by the fact that those children who had been insitutionalised also fared worse. All this should not be taken as an argument against the possible beneficial effects of early ICP-lowering operations in children with syndromic synostosis – only as a reminder that the situation is complex and it can be difficult to unravel the various aetiological strands when accounting for a child's developmental problems. It is therefore always important to remember how all the various causes of raised ICP in these children are interlinked and, as some of them (airway obstruction, for example) can certainly affect development, there is no excuse for a nihilistic approach when ICP is suspected, even in the presence of apparently normal vision.

How does raised ICP cause harm?
Given the interlinking of the various contributors to the raised ICP that can affect, in particular, children with the syndromic forms of craniosynostosis, it should come as no surprise that it can be difficult to differentiate the 'pure' effects of raised ICP – and analyse how those effects are produced – from those due to each individual contributor (airway obstruction, for example).

One direct effect of raised ICP alone is upon the cerebral perfusion pressure (CPP). CPP is the mean systemic arterial pressure (MAP) minus the mean intracranial pressure and reflects – albeit crudely – the driving force of blood through the brain. In the management of head-injured patients – children and adults – it is now standard practice to concentrate on trying to keep the CPP above at least 50 mmHg (Bruce 1985). In extremes of raised ICP in a hypotensive patient, the ICP can exceed the systemic blood pressure leading to a 'no-flow' situation and brain death. There are, however, physiological mechanisms whose function is to prevent this, the best known of which is the Cushing response in which the brainstem compression seen when the ICP is very high triggers both a rise in blood pressure and a fall in pulse rate. At less agonal levels of ICP, cerebral blood flow (CBF – which is directly related to CPP and inversely related to the cerebro-vascular resistance, CVR) is maintained by a process known as autoregulation. This autoregulatory process triggers cerebral vasodilatation to preserve CBF when MAP falls or ICP rises (Lee and Hoff 2000).

Does this autoregulatory process compensate for the rises in ICP seen particularly during periods of respiratory embarrassment during REM or active sleep in children with syndromic craniosynostosis (Lundberg's A waves)?

We studied (Gonsalez and Hayward 2002) 11 children (10 with syndromic forms of craniosynostosis, 1 with osteopetrosis), monitoring simultaneously both their mean arterial pressure and their ICP. Only two children maintained CPPs above 50 mmHg during their plateaux of raised ICP (some of which lasted for 15 minutes or more) and the lowest

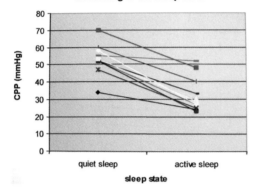

**Mean cerebral perfusion pressure (CPP),
according to the sleep state**

CPP (mmHg)

80
70
60
50
40
30
20
10
0

quiet sleep   active sleep

sleep state

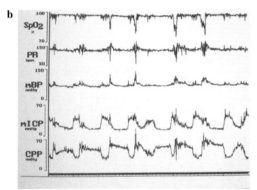

b

SpO2
PR
MBP
MICP
CPP

Fig. 8.8 (a) Mean cerebral perfusion
pressures (CPP) during quiet and active
sleep in a group of 11 children with various
syndromic forms of craniosynostosis.
(b) The overnight record of one of these
children (with Antley–Bixler syndrome),
showing (from above down), peripheral
oxygen saturation, pulse rate, mean arterial
blood pressure, mean ICP and CPP.
Note the dramatic fall in CPP during the
rise of ICP associated with alterations in
oxygen saturation, pulse and BP (the latter
being insufficient to maintain CPP). The
child showed signs of airway compromise
– snoring – during these periods.

CPP recorded was just under 14 mmHg. There were small rises in MAP but these were
insufficient to compensate for the rise in ICP (Fig. 8.8). Clearly this could be a mechanism
whereby raised ICP causes harm, but before jumping to any definite conclusions it is
important to recall again just how little is known about the normal cerebro-vascular
processes in young children and their response to variations in ICP. For example, can an
apparently dangerously low CPP be equated with a significantly reduced CBF (which is
more likely to be the mechanism through which functional damage to the brain might
occur), or can there be dramatic reductions in the child's cerebro-vascular resistance to
provide sufficient compensation – preserving CBF without the need for a matching rise in
MAP? And is it justified to assume that the limits of tolerance for CPP in an apparently well
child (in terms of consciousness) are similar to those accepted for the unconscious child with
traumatic brain injury? It should also be borne in mind that if cerebral vasodilatation is
occurring as the anticipated response to such a fall in CPP then this should in turn lead to
a further rise in ICP. The stage is therefore set for a classic vicious cycle (see Fig. 8.9).

Another question that arises at this point concerns the relative importance of the baseline
ICP versus the pressures reached during the plateaux of Lundberg A waves. Fig. 8.8(b) is
a good example of how extremes of raised ICP spanning almost half the nine and a half hours

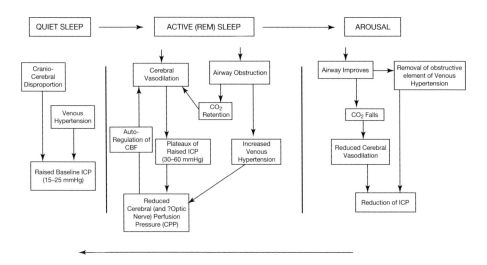

Fig. 8.9 The relationship between raised ICP, venous hypertension and respiratory problems in the production of visual failure in children with syndromic craniosynostosis – a unifying theory.

ICP is moderately raised during quiet sleep due to a combination (in variable proportions) of cranio-cerebral disproportion and venous hypertension. During active (REM) sleep, relaxation of pharyngeal muscle tone around the deformed airway leads to an aggravation of the respiratory compromise, which in turn leads to a rise in retained CO_2 and hypoxia, an increase in ICP and a fall in CPP. The compensatory mechanisms (autoregulation) necessary for the preservation of CBF sufficient to protect cerebral function are stimulated by the hypoxia/rise in CO_2 to produce a state of cerebral vasodilatation, which in turn further increases ICP. This vicious cycle is responsible for the plateau waves of pressure that may peak as high as 50–60 mmHg and last for several minutes until the child changes sleep state or effectively wakes up (arousal). During arousal and in quiet sleep, airway muscle is restored, ventilation becomes more effective, the cycle is broken and ICP falls to its previous levels.

of the study were superimposed upon a normal baseline pressure – a not unusual picture. Indeed in the study by Taylor (Taylor et al 2001) the mean baseline ICP of the 16/23 patients in whom this exceeded 15 mmHg was 20.5 (range 17–30), while the mean height of the plateaux was 37.1 mmHg (range 25–60). Regardless of any as yet unknown effect on CBF of these rather modest changes in baseline pressure, it would seem more likely that it is the plateaux waves that are associated with whatever morbidity can be linked to raised ICP in these children and that their effects are compounded by the respiratory problems with which they are so frequently associated. This hypothesis would also explain why although a small but definite incidence of 'raised' or 'borderline raised' ICP has been reported both by us (Thompson et al 1995d) and by others (Renier et al 1982) in children with single suture synostosis, it has never been generally accepted that this finding can be translated into a source of ophthalmological, neurological or cognitive morbidity – thus leaving the prime indication for surgical intervention the reduction of their cosmetic disability (usually by means of a surgical procedure that will also increase intracranial volume).

Coupled with these difficulties is the fact that we have unequivocal evidence for only one area of clinical morbidity as a consequence of raised ICP – deterioration in vision associated with, first, disc swelling and eventually optic atrophy. Is this due to decreased vascular perfusion? The optic nerves are outgrowths of the central nervous system and it therefore seems reasonable to consider them as vulnerable to alterations in CBF and CPP as the brain itself. However the picture is once again confused because at least one of the other contributors to raised ICP – airway obstruction – can also be associated with disc swelling (see 'Case history 2', in the next section), and venous hypertension can also interfere with perfusion. (Hydrocephalus can of course lead to optic atrophy and blindness in its own right.)

The pathogenesis of this harm is likely to be found in the more restricted ability of the optic nerve (an attenuated length of CNS tissue bathed by CSF within a relatively inelastic dural tube) to autoregulate its blood flow as efficiently as the brain as a whole is likely to be doing under these extreme circumstances. It is, after all, increased venous pressure around the optic nerves in response to raised CSF pressure in other situations of high ICP (a brain tumour, for example) that is probably responsible for the production of papilloedema.

Our present view is that the deleterious effects of raised ICP upon the optic nerves should be considered multifactorial in origin, with all the various processes already described linking with each other in a variety of complex ways.

This linkage may be summarised as follows. In active (or REM) sleep (sleep is a convenient time to study these effects in children) two important events occur – there is a reduction in the tone of the muscles responsible for maintaining an adequate airway in the face of anatomical obstructions, and there is cerebral vasodilatation. The latter initiates a rise in ICP even in 'normal' subjects, while the airway obstruction produces a fall in arterial oxygen saturation and retention of carbon dioxide – the latter a potent cerebral vasodilator. Activation of the accessory muscles of respiration increases any pre-existing venous hypertension and in turn further raises ICP. With the raised ICP comes a significant drop in CPP and, in response to it, more vasodilatation – the brain's autoregulatory reaction to preserve cerebral blood flow – and a further rise in ICP. A vicious cycle now exists – one that will only be broken when the child arouses and corrects both its blood gases and its airway obstruction (by the establishment of normal tone in the muscles responsible for maintaining a patent airway). This sequence is illustrated in Fig. 8.9.

What the raised pressure seen in these children does not do, however, is distort the brain and cause the sort of acute coning syndromes that are associated with expanding mass lesions. The nearest exception to this is the chronic effect of raised pressure upon the contents of a posterior fossa already rendered small in volume because of the effects of the responsible gene mutation, causing the cerebellar tonsils to prolapse through the foramen magnum to produce a Chiari 1 malformation (Thompson et al 1997a). This may in turn cause syringomyelia (extremely rare in our experience) and, less uncommonly, acute headaches associated with the transient rises in ICP that normally accompany coughing, laughing, straining, etc. Such crowding of the posterior fossa may contribute sufficiently to any existing impairment to CSF circulation to cause hydrocephalus, while the rise in ICP caused by hydrocephalus can contribute to tonsillar herniation – a potential vicious cycle (Thompson et al 1997b).

Management of raised ICP

Knowledge of the multiple contributors to raised ICP in children with craniosynostosis allows treatment to be ordered along more logical lines. For some years it has been the practice of many units looking after such children to recommend some form of vault expansion procedure for all children with syndromic craniosynostosis whether or not there is definite evidence for raised ICP. However, it can be appreciated from what has already been explained that such a simplistic approach may not be as universally appropriate as was once thought. An idea of its deficiencies can be appreciated by considering the interplay between cranio-cerebral disproportion, venous hypertension and hydrocephalus in the following case histories.

Case history 1

A baby girl with type 3 Pfeiffer syndrome had normal ventricles on MRI at 6 weeks of age and *no* tonsillar herniation. Her airway was moderately obstructed and palpation of her fontanelle suggested that her ICP was raised. A posterior cranial vault expansion was performed when she was 2 months old but ICP monitoring three months later showed that her ICP was still unequivocally raised. An anterior vault expansion was now performed but, despite this, within eight weeks of the operation her ICP was clinically raised again. Her ventricles had now enlarged significantly and she needed a ventriculo-peritoneal shunt. This relieved her ICP but an MRI one year later showed that her posterior fossa was small and she now had prolapse of her cerebellar tonsils down to the level of C2. She has since had midface surgery to improve her airway (the cosmetic benefits of which she has now grown out of – see comments on relapse in the preceding chapter) and a foramen magnum decompression to treat headaches secondary to her cerebellar impaction.

Case history 2

A boy with Crouzon syndrome and moderate airway obstruction had an anterior and lateral cranial vault expansion performed at the age of 6 months or so when his ophthalmic examination was normal (no papilloedema) but palpation of his anterior fontanelle suggested at least a modest rise in ICP. At the age of two and a half years much of the cosmetic advantage from his frontal advance had been lost, his optic discs were now swollen and there was some increase in latency in his visual evoked potentials (VEPs). His ventricles remained small but his airway obstruction had deteriorated. An adeno-tonsillectomy was performed and a repeat ophthalmic examination two months later showed improvement in both the appearance of his optic discs and his VEPs.

With such complexities in mind, the following general statements about the treatment of raised ICP in craniosynostosis can be made.

1 CRANIO-CEREBRAL DISPROPORTION

As has already been discussed, raised ICP due to this condition alone is not as common as was once believed, but all craniofacial units will still be presented with the occasional child – often with what at first sight appears to be a (phenotypically) less severe case of Crouzon syndrome – who has failing vision and pale optic discs, a small head circumference and accompanying radiographs that show the absence of all vault sutures plus generalised copper-beating. Such a child urgently needs a vault expansion procedure (assuming that hydrocephalus is not an issue) – a procedure that can be applied to the anterior, lateral (biparietal) or posterior parts of the skull (see Chapter 19 for surgical details). Which to choose depends primarily on what surgical procedures are likely to be needed in the future.

2 HYDROCEPHALUS

The treatment of raised ICP due to progressive ventricular dilatation requires some form of CSF diversion. This can be achieved in two ways – by the insertion of a ventriculo-peritoneal shunt (VPS) (Fig. 8.10) or by an endoscopic third ventriculostomy. The latter procedure depends upon the block to the circulation of CSF lying somewhere between the ventricular system and (on the outside of the brain) the tentorium. The condition for which it is most effective in general neurosurgical practice is hydrocephalus due to aqueduct stenosis, but it can be equally useful when the obstruction is in the posterior fossa – due, say, to a tumour there. As has already been explained, in syndromic craniosynostosis, hydrocephalus may be due to a combination of intracranial venous hypertension and impairment of CSF flow through the posterior fossa due to its small size. The former situation (in which the 'block' is at the level of CSF absorption at the arachnoid granulations) is unlikely to be helped by this technique, while the latter (in which the fourth ventricle is significantly smaller than the lateral and third ventricles) may well be (Cinalli et al 1999).

3 AIRWAY OBSTRUCTION

The management of airway obstruction is dealt with in detail in Chapter 9. At this point it is only necessary to point out that, in order of increasing invasiveness, the manoeuvres that may be required include continuous positive airway pressure (CPAP), nasal prongs, removal of tonsils and adenoids, tracheostomy, and advancement of the hypoplastic midface. Choanal stenosis may also require treatment. The potential for the improvement of an obstructed airway to ameliorate the effects of raised ICP has been illustrated in the second case history described above.

4 VENOUS HYPERTENSION

Whatever the fundamental problem responsible for venous hypertension, some method of reducing ICP is required if the threat to the child's vision is to be removed. Although angiographic examinations have demonstrated the likely sites of the venous obstructions in our cases, there exists at present no satisfactory way of reconstructing the anomalous venous

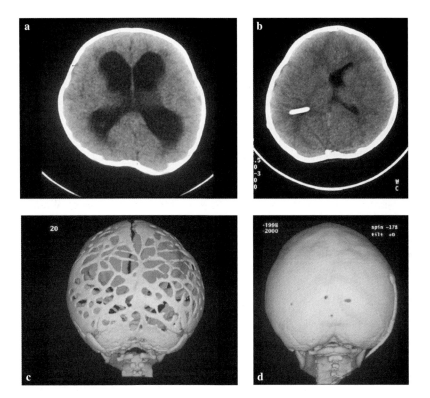

Fig. 8.10 A remarkable degree of 'copper-beating' which resolved after relief of raised intracranial pressure following the insertion of a ventriculo-peritoneal shunt for hydrocephalus. The child has 'non-syndromic' craniosynostosis affecting all vault sutures.
(a) and (b) Axial CT before and after VP shunt insertion.
(c) and (d) 3D CT reconstructions before and after shunt insertion.

anatomy. The literature contains sporadic reports of dural sinus to internal jugular venous shunts (Niwa et al 1988) – and the use of this procedure (and venous decompression) in the raised ICP associated with achondroplasia (Steinbok et al 1989, Lundar et al 1990) – but these tend to be single case histories only. It is for this reason that we do not at present routinely analyse (by digital subtraction angiography or magnetic resonance venography, for example) the venous outflow patterns in children with syndromic forms of craniosyn-ostosis.

Ironically, the treatment of choice for venous hypertension is the same surgical procedure that used to be advocated for what was thought to be the only cause of raised ICP in these children (cranio-cerebral disproportion) – a cranial vault expansion. And highly effective it is, with clinical and ophthalmological examinations as well as repeat ICP monitoring (Fig. 8.11) confirming its success (Liasis et al – personal communication).

The overlap between two quite different causes of raised ICP in even this apparently clear-cut situation can be appreciated from the occasional but well-recognised progression

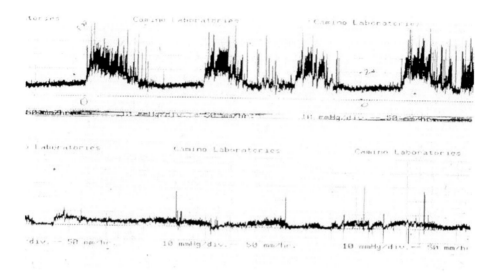

Fig. 8.11 This child with Apert syndrome and raised ICP (top trace) underwent a cranial vault expansion procedure. The ICP monitoring was repeated three months later to confirm the fall in ICP (bottom trace). (Vertical scale – 10 mmHg per line.)

of hydrocephalus following a vault expansion procedure carried out for raised ICP associated with venous hypertension, whether or not there is a state of cranio-cerebral disproportion (Thompson et al 1997b).

SUMMARY OF THE MANAGEMENT OF RAISED ICP

Raised ICP in (predominantly) syndromic craniosynostosis is multifactorial in its aetiology and is a dynamic rather than a 'fixed' complication for these children, with its various causes becoming important at different ages. Its successful treatment therefore needs to take many different factors into account, and it is for this reason that we no longer recommend some form of vault expansion procedure for all our syndromic children when they are first seen, despite the fact that the incidence of raised ICP during their first six years or so may be 50 per cent or even higher. Some of these children may never develop raised ICP, while for those that do, if it is detected and treated early, there should be no ill effects. Also, for some children – as already illustrated – the treatment of choice may not be a vault expansion at all, while for those that do require cranial surgery, the later this is performed, the smaller the risks of relapse.

This raises the question of whether or not a future rise in ICP can be predicted when the present ICP appears to be normal. Some crude predictions can be made on the basis of the syndrome alone – a child with Saethre–Chotzen syndrome, for example, is much less likely to run into raised ICP problems than one with, say, Pfeiffer or Crouzon syndrome. The phenotypic severity of the syndrome and the presence or absence of airway obstruction are also likely to be relevant. There is no evidence available at present to tell us if a particular degree of abnormal venous drainage as assessed by magnetic resonance venography (MRV) in a child with syndromic synostosis and (at present) normal ICP will translate to raised ICP in the years to come. For this reason and because there is at the moment no specific vein-to-vein reconstruction procedure available for these children, we do not routinely investigate them either with digital subtraction angiography or MRV, but clearly this situation will change as further information becomes available.

Monitoring of children with craniosynostosis for raised ICP

In the preceding chapter, which dealt with the general principles of the management of children with craniosynostosis, the vital importance of the initial assessment of, in particular, those with the syndromic or otherwise complex forms was emphasised. One of the purposes of this assessment was to determine whether the child was already suffering from raised ICP, or appeared likely to do so in the future. Early raised ICP obviously requires early treatment, but for those whose pressures are not an immediate cause for concern and for those who have had some form of ICP-lowering intervention, long-term monitoring will be needed.

Again, as has already been explained, the main deleterious effect of raised ICP in these children is deterioration in their vision and, once their fontanelles have closed, it is from their ophthalmic examination that most will be learned about their ICP (headache and other clinical manifestations of raised ICP being unreliable indicators in this context). The three most important components of this ophthalmic surveillance are the child's acuity (when this can be assessed), the appearance of their optic fundi (which ideally should be recorded by 'digital capture' in the ophthalmology clinic at each attendance so that comparisons can be made between one visit and another) and the electro-diagnostic tests – usually the visual evoked potentials (VEPs). (For the details of this monitoring see Chapter 10.)

Children who have had treatment for raised ICP instigated on the basis of ophthalmic concerns are, of course, also monitored closely because, as illustrated by the first case history above, successful treatment of one cause does not guarantee that the problem will not arise again, due either to the same or to a different factor. But how successful is any treatment (depending upon which is the most appropriate) in reversing any ophthalmic abnormalities whose recognition has led to the diagnosis of raised ICP in the first place?

Our experience is that, provided treatment is initiated promptly, it is usually possible to see a marked improvement in both the appearance of the optic fundi and the VEPs when the children are reassessed (see Fig. 10.7, p. 197).

For how long should such monitoring be continued? The answer is that nobody knows for sure – the complexity of the problems surrounding raised ICP in these children having only recently been appreciated. Our own impression is that the period of particular danger lasts from the child's first year until they are 6 or 7 years old, but it will take many more years of experience with what are after all rare cases to tell whether or not this prediction is correct. Certainly a child who has reached this age with no evidence of raised ICP at any time is unlikely to run into trouble, but as most children have ophthalmic problems other than those associated with raised ICP it is likely that they will remain under some form of specialised ophthalmic surveillance for several years to come.

Conclusions

Raised intracranial pressure can complicate all forms of craniosynostosis but the clinical problems it may cause seem to affect predominantly those with syndromic forms – and the area most likely to be involved is vision. All children with a syndromic form of craniosynostosis should be considered at risk of losing vision to a variable degree, and our studies have revealed just how severe and how extensive this ophthalmic morbidity really is.

It seems logical that raised ICP is responsible for any cognitive developmental morbidity, but in this situation it is in competition with other factors such as the primary effects of the genetic mutation itself and often years of hypoxia due to chronic respiratory difficulties, and therefore the case remains to be proven.

We now appreciate that the problem is not just one of 'simple' cranio-cerebral disproportion – a tight brain squeezed within a bony box that because of fused sutures cannot expand to accommodate its growth – but reflects a complex interplay between venous hypertension and respiratory compromise due to upper airway obstruction which affects also the pathogenesis (when present) of hydrocephalus.

We know too that raised ICP is not a 'one-off' phenomenon that the child either has or does not have. The situation is a changing, dynamic one, with the possibility that a child with Crouzon syndrome (say) seen aged 1 year with normal ICP is still capable of developing raised ICP and then losing vision a year or two later.

The keys to reducing the morbidity due to raised ICP complicating syndromic forms of craniosynostosis are: awareness of the frequency of the problem; an understanding of its complexity; a commitment to regular ophthalmological monitoring, with invasive ICP monitoring reserved for cases where the diagnosis is in doubt; and finally the expertise with which to act (not necessarily with some form of vault expansion operation) once the diagnosis has been made.

REFERENCES

Anderson PJ, Harkness WJ, Taylor W, Jones BM, Hayward RD (1997) Anomalous venous drainage in a case of non-syndromic craniosynostosis. *Childs Nerv Syst* 13(2): 97–100.

Arnaud E, Renier D, Marchac D (1995) Prognosis for mental function in scaphocephaly. *J Neurosurg* 83(3): 476–479.

Bruce D (1985) Cerebrovascular dynamics. In: James HE, Anas NG, Perkin RM, editors. *Brain Insults in Infants and Children*, Orlando: Grune and Stratton, pp 52–57.

Cinalli G, Renier D, Sebag G, Sainte-Rose C, Arnaud E, Pierre-Kahn A (1995) Chronic tonsillar herniation in Crouzon's and Apert's syndromes: the role of premature synostosis of the lambdoid suture. *J Neurosurg* 83(4): 575–582.

Cinalli G, Sainte-Rose C, Chumas P, Zerah M, Brunelle F, Lot G, Pierre-Kahn A, Renier D (1999) Failure of third ventriculostomy in the treatment of aqueductal stenosis in children 2. *J Neurosurg* 90(3): 448–454.

Eide PK, Helseth E, Due-Tonnesson B, Lundar T (2002) Assessment of continuous intracranial pressure recordings in childhood craniosynostosis. *Pediatr Neurosurg* 37(6): 310–320.

Fok H, Jones BM, Gault DG, Andar U, Hayward R (1992) Relationship between intracranial pressure and intracranial volume in craniosynostosis. *Br J Plast Surg* 45(5): 394–397.

Gault DT, Renier D, Marchac D, Ackland FM, Jones BM (1990) Intracranial volume in children with craniosynostosis. *J Craniofac Surg* 1(1): 1–3.

Gault DT, Renier D, Marchac D, Jones BM (1992) Intracranial pressure and intracranial volume in children with craniosynostosis. *Plast Reconstr Surg* 90(3): 377–381.

Gonsalez S, Hayward R (2002) Cerebral perfusion pressures in children with syndromic craniosynostosis. (Personal communication.)

Gonsalez S, Hayward R, Jones B, Lane R (1997) Upper airway obstruction and raised intracranial pressure in children with craniosynostosis. *Eur Respir J* 10(2): 367–375.

Gonsalez SL, Thompson D, Hayward R, Lane R (1998) Breathing patterns in children with craniofacial dysostosis and hindbrain herniation. *Eur Respir J* 11(4): 866–872.

Hayward R, Nischal K, Thompson D, Dunaway D, Jones BMJ (2001) What is the natural history of raised intracranial pressure in syndromic craniosynostosis? In: Lauritzen CGK, editor. *Craniofacial Surgery 9*. Bologna: Monduzzi Editire, pp 29–32.

Khan SH, Nischal KK, Dean F, Hayward RD, Walker J (2003) Visual morbidity in craniosynostoses – a review of 141 cases. *Br J Ophthalmol* 87(8): 999–1003.

Lee KL, Hoff JT (2000) Raised intracranial pressure and its effect on brain function. In: Crockard A, Hayward R, Hoff JT, editors. *Neurosurgery: The Scientific Basis of Clinical Practice*, 3rd edn, vol. 1. Oxford: Blackwell Science, pp 393–409.

Lundar T, Bakke SJ, Nornes H (1990) Hydrocephalus in an achondroplastic child treated by venous decompression at the jugular foramen. *J Neurosurg* 73: 138–140.

Lundberg N (1960) Continuous recording and control of ventricular fluid pressure in neurosurgical practice. *Acta Psychiatr Scand* 36(suppl): 1–193.

Minns RA (1991) *Problems of Intracranial Pressure in Childhood*. London: Mac Keith Press.

Mursch K, Brockmann K, Lang JK, Markakis E, Behnke-Mursch J (1998) Visually evoked potentials in 52 children requiring operative repair of craniosynostosis 1. *Pediatr Neurosurg* 29(6): 320–323.

Nischal K (2002) Can raised intracranial pressure exist antenatally in children with complex craniosynostosis? (Personal communication.)

Niwa J, Ohtaki M, Morimoto S, Nakagawa T, Hashi K (1988) Reconstruction of the venous outflow using a vein graft in dural arteriovenous malformation associated with sinus occlusion. *No Shinkei Geka* 16(11): 1273–1280.

Pople IK, Quinn MW, Bayston R, Hayward RD (1991) The Doppler pulsatility index as a screening test for blocked ventriculo-peritoneal shunts. *Eur J Pediatr Surg* 1(suppl 1): 27–29.

Renier D (1989) Intracranial pressure in craniosynostosis: pre- and postoperative recordings – correlation with functional results. In: Persing JA, Edgerton MT, Jane J, editors. *Scientific Foundations and Surgical Treatment of Craniosynostosis*, Baltimore: Williams & Wilkins, pp 263–269.

Renier D, Sainte-Rose C, Marchac D, Hirsch JF (1982) Intracranial pressure in craniostenosis. *J Neurosurg* 57(3): 370–377.

Renier D, Arnaud E, Cinalli G, Sebag G, Zerah M, Marchac D (1996) Prognosis for mental function in Apert's syndrome. *J Neurosurg* 85(1): 66–72.

Rich P, Cox TCS, Hayward R (2003) The jugular foramen in complex and syndromic craniosynostosis and its relationship to raised intracranial pressure. *Am J Neurorad* 24: 45–51.

Sainte-Rose C, LaCombe J, Pierre-Kahn A, Renier D, Hirsch JF (1984) Intracranial venous sinus hypertension: cause or consequence of hydrocephalus in infants? *J Neurosurg* 60(4): 727–736.

Samuel M, Marchbanks RJ, Burge DM (1998) Tympanic membrane displacement test in regular assessment in eight children with shunted hydrocephalus. *J Neurosurg* 88: 983–995.

Shipster C, Hearst D, Somerville A, Stackhouse J, Hayward R, Wade A (2003) Speech, language and cognitive development in children with isolated sagittal synostosis. *Dev Med Child Neurol* 45: 34–43.

Siddiqi SN, Posnick JC, Buncic R, Humphreys RP, Hoffman HJ, Drake JM, Rutka JT (1995) The detection and management of intracranial hypertension after initial suture release and decompression for craniofacial dysostosis syndromes 1. *Neurosurgery* 36(4): 703–708.

Stavrou P, Sgouros S, Willshaw HE, Goldin JH, Hockley AD, Wake MJ (2002) Visual failure caused by raised intracranial pressure in craniosynostosis. *Childs Nerv Syst* 13(2): 64–67.

Steinbok P, Hall J, Flodmark O (1989) Hydrocephalus in achondroplasia: the possible role of intracranial venous hypertension 1. *J Neurosurg* 71(1): 42–48.

Taylor WJ, Hayward RD, Lasjaunias P, Britto JA, Thompson DN, Jones BM, Evans RD (2001) Enigma of raised intracranial pressure in patients with complex craniosynostosis: the role of abnormal intracranial venous drainage. *J Neurosurg* 94(3): 377–385.

Thompson DN, Harkness W, Jones B, Gonsalez S, Andar U, Hayward R (1995a) Subdural intracranial pressure monitoring in craniosynostosis: its role in surgical management. *Childs Nerv Syst* 11(5): 269–275.

Thompson DN, Hayward RD, Harkness WJ, Bingham RM, Jones BM (1995b) Lessons from a case of kleeblattschadel. Case report. *J Neurosurg* 82(6): 1071–1074.

Thompson D, Hayward R, Jones B (1995c) Anomalous intracranial venous drainage: implications for cranial exposure in the craniofacial patient. *Plast Reconstr Surg* 95(6): 1126.

Thompson DN, Malcolm GP, Jones BM, Harkness WJ, Hayward RD (1995d) Intracranial pressure in single-suture craniosynostosis. *Pediatr Neurosurg* 22(5): 235–240.

Thompson DN, Harkness W, Jones BM, Hayward RD (1997a) Aetiology of herniation of the hindbrain in craniosynostosis. An investigation incorporating intracranial pressure monitoring and magnetic resonance imaging. *Pediatr Neurosurg* 26(6): 288–295.

Thompson DN, Jones BM, Harkness W, Gonsalez S, Hayward RD (1997b) Consequences of cranial vault expansion surgery for craniosynostosis. *Pediatr Neurosurg* 26(6): 296–303.

Tuite GF, Chong WK, Evanson J, Narita A, Taylor D, Harkness WF, Jones BM, Hayward RD (1996a) The effectiveness of papilledema as an indicator of raised intracranial pressure in children with craniosynostosis. *Neurosurgery* 38(2): 272–278.

Tuite GF, Evanson J, Chong WK, Thompson DN, Harkness WF, Jones BM, Hayward RD (1996b) The beaten copper cranium: a correlation between intracranial pressure, cranial radiographs, and computed tomographic scans in children with craniosynostosis. *Neurosurgery* 39(4): 691–699.

Wall M, George D (1991) Idiopathic intracranial hypertension. A prospective study of 50 patients 1. *Brain* 114(pt 1A): 155–180.

Welch K (1980) The intracranial pressure in infants. *J Neurosurg* 52(5): 693–699.

Whittle IR, Johnston IH, Besser M (1984) Intracranial pressure changes in craniosynostosis. *Surg Neurol* 21(367): 372.

9
AIRWAY MANAGEMENT IN SYNDROMIC CRANIOSYNOSTOSIS

Susanna Leighton and Roderick Lane

Introduction

Airway obstruction in children is an important problem that may cause significant morbidity and even mortality. It may present in the neonatal period if it is entirely due to a congenital abnormality (either anatomical or functional), or it may present in the older child as growth and physiological changes occur (such as adenotonsillar hypertrophy) that alter structure or function.

Children with syndromic craniosynostosis, because of abnormal midfacial growth affecting the structure and function of the pharynx, have a high risk of airway obstruction at the pharyngeal level. This typically presents as stertorous breathing, which may only be present at night and is then termed sleep disordered breathing (SDB). If severe, it may be associated with subtle daytime symptoms such as cognitive and behavioural problems that are not recognised, or are attributed to the underlying disorder in these children. It is also associated with failure to thrive. There is a complex relationship between SDB and intracranial hypertension; the latter may be multifactorial in these children. There is a risk, too, of significant cardiorespiratory morbidity and even sudden death if severe cases of SDB are unrecognised and untreated (Wilkinson et al 1981).

Because of the abnormal anatomy of the pharyngeal airway and high risk of SDB, it is important that children with syndromic craniosynostosis have an airway assessment as part of their initial clinical evaluation and regularly thereafter. Parents' reports of airway and other symptoms in SDB tend to be unreliable, so objective assessment by respiratory sleep study is also mandatory.

We have established a management protocol in these children in which we hope to treat and prevent symptoms and complications of airway obstruction while minimising the morbidity of interventions. The ultimate aim is to optimise the outcome for the patient both functionally and cosmetically by the time adulthood is reached.

Sleep and breathing

The concept that sleep profoundly affects breathing has only become clear in the last 30 years (see review by Phillipson 1978). While studies of the effects of sleep on breathing date back to the nineteenth century, it was not until the 1940s that Magnussen (1944) showed in healthy adults that ventilation was diminished during sleep and alveolar carbon dioxide tension (P_ACO_2) was increased. In the subsequent decade crucial work by Aserinsky and

Kleitman (1953) and Dement and Kleitman (1957) showed that sleep was not a uniform state but that it could be divided into different periods based on the pattern of neural (electroencephalogram (EEG)) and muscular (electromyogram (EMG)) activity, and in particular the pattern of involuntary eye movements (electro-oculogram (EOG)). They were able broadly to divide sleep into periods of sleep accompanied by rapid eye movements (REM) and periods without these characteristic signs (non-REM). These different sleep states had important implications for the control of breathing, which had quite different characteristics in the two states. Bulow (1963) subsequently published a more comprehensive description of the effects of sleep on breathing when he made comparisons of respiration between periods of quiet wakefulness and periods of non-REM sleep. Differences in breathing patterns during REM when compared with non-REM sleep were subsequently described by a number of investigators (Aserinsky 1965, Schmidt-Nowara and Snyder 1983, Gould et al 1988, Pack 1995).

In general, breathing patterns in non-REM sleep are regular with little variation in tidal volume or respiratory rate. The overall level of ventilation is approximately 15 per cent lower than during quiet wakefulness, and this results in a small alteration in blood gases with the partial pressure of carbon dioxide in the arterial blood (P_aCO_2) rising by between 3 and 7 mmHg, and the partial pressure of oxygen in the arterial blood (P_aO_2) falling by between 4 and 9 mmHg, with arterial oxygen saturation (S_aO_2) falling by approximately 1–2 per cent from awake levels. The decrease in ventilation appears to be the result of a decrease in the level of central ventilatory drive coupled with a failure to compensate for the sleep-related increase in upper airway resistance that results from the decline in upper airway muscle tone associated with sleep.

During REM sleep there are further important changes in respiration. REM sleep breathing patterns are characterised by irregularities in both tidal volume and respiratory rate and, in adults, breathing may be interrupted by central apnoeas lasting up to 30 seconds. The overall level of ventilation is difficult to assess but is probably either similar to, or slightly less than, that seen in non-REM sleep. Blood gases are likely to be similarly affected as by non-REM sleep but have more variable levels as a result of the variability of minute ventilation.

Sleep apnoeas are recognisable interruptions of breathing and are classified as central, obstructive or mixed depending on their underlying cause. Central apnoeas are characterised by a cessation of airflow at the nose and mouth with no apparent respiratory effort (Fig. 9.1) and are the consequence of a cessation in the phasic central neural drive to breathe. In contrast, obstructive apnoeas are seen when there is a cessation of airflow at the nose and mouth but continued, or even increased, respiratory effort (Fig. 9.2). The respiratory efforts during an obstructive apnoea are rendered ineffective by the loss of upper airway patency due to collapse. It is also possible to have partial airway obstruction when the airway patency is reduced; this is characterised by increased respiratory effort but diminished airflow in response to the increased upper airway resistance. Mixed apnoeas are described when elements of both central and obstructive apnoeas are seen in association, without interruption by any effective respiration. The length of apnoea considered abnormal varies with age. Premature infants, for example, may exhibit central apnoeas of up to 20 seconds'

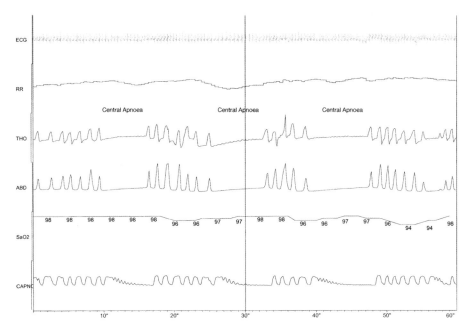

Fig. 9.1 Central sleep apnoea. This 1-minute segment was recorded in a 5-month-old infant. A series of central sleep apnoeas lasting approximately 15–20 seconds is evident. During the apnoeas there is an absence of respiratory effort with no discernible movements on the thoracic (THO) or abdominal (ABD) channels. An absence of airflow can be deduced from the pattern of the expired PCO_2 trace (CAPNO) with a decline to almost zero during the apnoeic episodes. The high frequency oscillations seen on the PCO_2 trace (CAPNO) during the apnoeas are caused by small 'puffs' of CO_2 being expelled from the airway as a consequence of the heart beating within the thorax; these confirm that the airway is open and exclude the possibility of an obstructive cause for the apnoea.

duration before they are considered abnormal, whereas older infants and children may exhibit shorter periods of obstructive apnoea, which can be clinically significant. A measure of the significance of an apnoea may be judged by its association with significant hypoxia, hypercapnia or bradycardia.

Central apnoea and hypopnoea

Central apnoeas are characterised by a cessation in airflow at the nose and mouth with no discernible respiratory effort. They are considered clinically significant if they are associated with significant changes in blood gases (S_aO_2 <92 per cent, end-tidal partial pressure of carbon dioxide ($P_{et}CO_2$) >55 mmHg) and/or significant bradycardia. Central apnoeas are frequently associated with arousals (EEG, autonomic or movement) which cause sleep fragmentation and poor sleep quality; this may have detrimental effects on daytime behaviour and growth.

Craniofacial patients may be considered as a risk group for central respiratory control problems for two reasons. First, the abnormal anatomy of the cranial base may lead to a

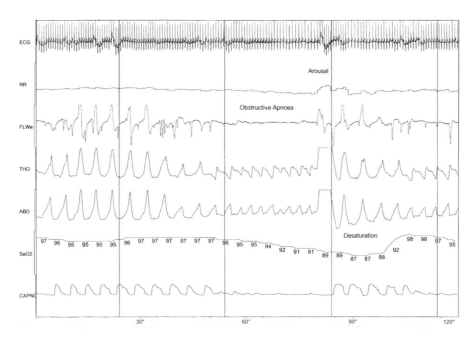

Fig. 9.2 Obstructive sleep apnoea. This 2-minute segment was recorded in a 5-year-old child with Crouzon syndrome. An obstructive apnoea lasting for approximately 30 seconds is indicated, with absence of airflow (FLWe) despite continued thoracic (THO) and abdominal (ABD) respiratory efforts. There is significant oxygen desaturation (SaO_2) with a dip of 10 per cent from a baseline of 97 per cent to a nadir of 87 per cent. The expired PCO_2 trace (CAPNO) diminishes to near zero during the apnoeic episode. Heart rate (RR) shows a mild fall during the latter part of the apnoea. The apnoeic episode is terminated by an arousal with a sharp rise in heart rate (RR) and a resumption of effective respiration and recovery of oxygen saturation (SaO_2).

mechanical distortion of the brainstem wherein lie the respiratory control centres. Second, the intracranial hypertension, which is often seen in these patients, may cause anomalies of respiratory control due to increased pressure exerted on the brainstem structures. In extreme cases the brainstem may herniate through the foramen magnum of the skull base; this may be visualised on MRI.

The first description of chronic hindbrain herniation in a patient with syndromic craniosynostosis was in an infant with Pfeiffer syndrome (Saldino et al 1972); it has subsequently been described in patients with cloverleaf skull malformation, Crouzon and Apert syndromes (Vanes 1988, Francis et al 1992, Cinalli et al 1994, Thompson et al 1994). The caudal displacement of the cerebellar tissue through the foramen magnum and into the cervical canal may be associated with anatomical changes in the brainstem, with lesions of the cerebellum and compression of the medulla. From a respiratory point of view, herniation of the hindbrain may affect brainstem neurological structures including ponto-medullary respiratory centres, and the cranial nerve nuclei and roots of the nerves innervating upper airway musculature. Malfunction of these structures may lead to feeding difficulties, stridor, breath-holding spells, upper airway obstruction and central sleep apnoea or hypoventilation.

Patients with Arnold–Chiari malformation are susceptible to acute cord compression syndromes, particularly under circumstances where there may be acute changes in intracranial pressure (e.g. obstructive sleep apnoea with swings in P_aCO_2). If the brainstem becomes compressed, these individuals may develop central alveolar hypoventilation and/or frank central apnoeas. Under these circumstances they may require mechanical ventilation intermittently or all the time.

In a study in our sleep laboratory (Gonsalez et al 1998), a group of 13 children with syndromic craniosynostosis and hindbrain herniation (confirmed on MRI) underwent overnight cardiorespiratory sleep studies without sedation. Clinically significant central apnoeas with falls in S_aO_2 to less than 90 per cent were found in only two cases. In contrast, ten of the patients showed a degree of upper airway obstruction, ranging in severity from mild to severe. A further two patients had previously undergone tracheostomy to alleviate severe obstructive sleep apnoea. We concluded that in a selected group of children with syndromic craniosynostosis and hindbrain herniation, the predominant sleep-related breathing problem was obstructive apnoea and that, despite expectations, central apnoeas and mixed apnoeas were only infrequently seen in the minority of patients.

Brainstem compression may also be associated with an increased risk of airway obstruction. Patients with Arnold–Chiari malformation are at risk of developing bilateral vocal fold paralysis (Graham 1963, Fitzsimmonds 1965, Snow and Rodgers 1965); this is most frequent in infants, commonly presenting with airway symptoms between 1 and 12 months of age. Affected infants develop progressive inspiratory stridor, which may become worse during sleep. This may progress to constant stridor with CO_2 retention and respiratory failure. Normal respiratory control involves a co-ordinated dilatation of the upper airway musculature in order to maintain upper airway patency during the imposition of negative intra-luminal pressures during inspiration. During expiration, the vocal folds occupy their normal relaxed partially open position; during inspiration, the folds are normally abducted, opening the airway lumen. Vocal fold abduction is controlled by the recurrent laryngeal branch of the Vagus nerve (C.X). Malfunction can be brought on as a result of traction on the nerve roots, or by compression or stretching of the medulla itself (Papasozomenos and Roessmann 1981).

Obstructive apnoeas and hypopnoeas
A patent upper airway is a prerequisite for successful respiration. The upper airway is a collapsible muscular tube that includes the nasopharynx, oropharynx and laryngopharynx. Its patency is determined by its diameter and the tonic activity of the pharyngeal dilators and their phasic contraction in response to the negative upper airway pressure generated during inspiration. During sleep, reduced tone of these dilators and diminished reflex dilatation lead to physiological airway narrowing, especially during REM sleep. This physiological narrowing can result in SDB, especially if the craniofacial morphology is abnormal, resulting in an airway of less than average diameter at any point. Craniofacial abnormalities such as the syndromic craniosynostoses, Treacher–Collins syndrome (Sher et al 1989) and Pierre–Robin sequence (Sher 1992) all predispose to SDB. It is also common in achondroplasia (Waters et al 1993), the mucopolysaccharidoses (Semenza and Pyeritz

1988) and syndromic obesity (Prader–Willi syndrome) (Hertz et al 1993). If the tone of the upper airway musculature is abnormal, either hypotonic or hypertonic, this may also increase the risk of SDB (Trang et al 1993). Children with Down syndrome have both narrow airways and reduced muscular tone and thus have a high risk of SDB (Marcus et al 1991).

Nasal obstruction can contribute to SDB. The likely mechanism is that high nasal resistance to airflow necessitates the generation of high negative intrathoracic pressures. Opening the mouth to augment the airway causes the tongue to move posteriorly, thus narrowing the airway and further contributing to the conditions necessary for collapse. Large tonsils and adenoids are associated with SDB (Brouillette et al 1982, Frank et al 1983) but there is no strong evidence of a correlation between their size and the severity of airway obstruction (Croft et al 1990); it is rather their size relative to the size of the airway that is important.

In the syndromic craniosynostoses, although the membranous bones of the facial skeleton fail to grow normally, the cartilaginous components are unaffected. Thus the facial dysplasia is severe with the maxilla grossly hypoplastic in all dimensions and the nose and mandible relatively prominent. There is foreshortening of both the anterior and the posterior cranial base and the maxilla is retrognathic in relation to the former. This results in a reduction in pharyngeal depth, height and width. There is also a reduction in the height and width of the posterior choanae leading to choanal stenosis which is often misdiagnosed clinically as choanal atresia in these patients (Sculerati et al 1998).

A long velum and a mandibular body short in length contribute to the pharyngeal crowding in three dimensions. The tongue is displaced posteriorly by the mandibular hypoplasia and obstruction may occur at tongue base level (Kakitsuba et al 1994). The palate is typically narrow and high-arched. In Apert and Crouzon syndromes there are lateral palatal swellings due to soft tissue deposits of mucopolysaccharides lying along the lateral arches of the alveolus (Solomon et al 1973); these are separated by a narrow median groove which may be misdiagnosed as a cleft palate. The swellings often become more prominent with maturity.

In our series, children with Pfeiffer syndrome (32 per cent) were more likely to need airway support for symptoms or complications of SDB than those with Crouzon syndrome (27 per cent) or Apert syndrome (19 per cent) (unpublished data). A proportion of children with Apert syndrome may have a cleft palate and this is associated with a reduced need for airway intervention. Those with Antley–Bixler and Saethre–Chotzen syndromes do not appear to have more airway problems in childhood than the general population.

Obstructive apnoeas are defined as periods of cessation of airflow measured at the nose and mouth, but during which respiratory efforts continue and, more often than not, increase (crescendo). The apnoeic period is associated with detrimental changes in blood gases (falling S_aO_2, rising P_aCO_2), and possibly reflex bradycardia (Table 9.1). During the apnoea there is a progressive increase in the drive to breathe, leading to increasing respiratory efforts against the closed airway, and progressively greater negative intrathoracic pressures, resulting in respiratory-related dips in blood pressure (pulsus paradoxus). The apnoea is terminated by an arousal that is probably triggered by the increasing levels of afferent input from the respiratory chemoreceptors, and by increased activity from mechanoreceptors

TABLE 9.1
Components of the obstructive/arousal cycle leading to sleep
fragmentation with associated nocturnal and daytime consequences

Apnoea/hypopnoea	Arousal (terminates apnoea/ hypopnoea)	Consequences
• No airflow (oro-nasal)/$\downarrow$ flow (<50%)	• Effective airflow resumes	• Fragmented sleep
• Upper airway collapse/partial collapse	• Airway patency restored	• Excess of light sleep
• $\uparrow$ respiratory effort (crescendo)/ (sustained)	• $\downarrow$ respiratory effort	• Loss of deep sleep
• $\uparrow$ −ve intrathoracic pressure swings	• Normalised intrathoracic pressure swings	• Unrefreshing sleep
• $\downarrow S_aO_2$, $\uparrow P_aCO_2$	• $\uparrow S_aO_2$, $\downarrow P_aCO_2$	• Poor sleep quality
• $\uparrow$ pulsus paradoxus	• $\uparrow$ sympathetic activity	• $\downarrow$ growth/failure to thrive (FTT)
• $\uparrow$ metabolic rate	• $\uparrow$ BP (surge)	• $\uparrow$ behavioural problems

within the lung, airway and chest wall. Arousal serves to increase the level of drive to the musculature supporting the upper airway, causing airway dilatation and allowing effective respiration to resume. Arousal is also associated with a reflex increase in heart rate and a surge in blood pressure as a consequence of a sudden increase in sympathetic drive. The patient typically takes three or four large effective breaths, sufficient to restore blood gases, before returning to a deeper sleep state, at which point airway tone is again lost and the obstructive cycle begins again.

There is no universally accepted definition of obstructive sleep apnoea. In adults the definition proposed by Guilleminault et al (1976b) is widely accepted. They defined sleep apnoea as 30 or more apnoeic episodes, of greater than ten seconds' duration each, occurring within an eight-hour sleep period. However, clinically, patients with significant symptoms (daytime hypersomnolence, impaired daytime function) will commonly have apnoeic episodes lasting considerably longer than ten seconds, associated with significant oxygen desaturation, and several hundred episodes per night. In children, the criteria for diagnosis of obstructive sleep apnoea based on duration and frequency of apnoeic events are even more poorly established.

There is a clinical spectrum of SDB in children, ranging from primary snoring, through upper airway resistance syndrome (UARS) and obstructive hypoventilation syndrome (OHS), to obstructive sleep apnoea syndrome (OSAS), as severity increases. Primary snoring is noise generated by turbulent airflow in the pharynx; there is no associated apnoea, hypopnoea, hypoxaemia or sleep fragmentation due to arousals. In children it is most commonly due to physiological adenotonsillar hypertrophy. Peak incidence is in the 3- to 6-year age group when it affects up to 10 per cent of normal children (Ali et al 1993), resolving with maturity. In upper airway resistance syndrome, snoring is associated with partial upper airway obstruction during sleep and increased inspiratory effort (Guilleminault et al 1982). There is sleep fragmentation and there may be daytime symptoms but there are no gas exchange abnormalities. In obstructive hypoventilation syndrome there is continuous partial upper airway obstruction during sleep, with at least 50 per cent reduction in

TABLE 9.2
**Criteria for scoring the severity of upper airway obstruction during sleep based
on clinical observations and sleep study findings (from Gonsalez et al 1997)**

Severity	Clinical observations	Sleep study findings

Mild	Slightly increased respiratory efforts
	Usually mouth breathing
	± slight intercostal or suprasternal
	  inspiratory recession
	± snoring
	Without restless sleep
		Ribcage and abdominal signals in-phase, or
		  slightly out-of-phase
		Baseline S_aO_2 within normal limits (>92%)
		± few brief drops in S_aO_2 (never <90%)

Moderate	Moderately increased respiratory efforts
	Usually mouth breathing
	± slight intercostal or suprasternal inspiratory
	  recession
	± snoring and snorting
	With disrupted, restless sleep
		Ribcage and abdominal signals out-of-phase
		Baseline S_aO_2 within normal limits (>92%)
		More frequent, repeated periods of desaturation
		  to the mid-80s %

Severe	Markedly increased respiratory efforts
	Mouth breathing
	Marked intercostal or suprasternal inspiratory
	  recession
	± nasal flare
	Loud snoring and snorting
	Disrupted, restless sleep
		Ribcage and abdominal signals out-of-phase
		Prolonged periods of paradoxical breathing
		Prolonged periods of arterial oxygen
		  desaturation

airflow, causing mild oxygen desaturation (Rosen et al 1992); there may also be a degree of hypercapnia. Again there is sleep fragmentation and its ensuing problems. Obstructive sleep apnoea syndrome is characterised by episodic complete upper airway obstruction during sleep with increased respiratory effort, paradoxical respiratory movements and sleep fragmentation with reduced arterial oxygen saturation with or without hypercapnia (Guilleminault et al 1976b). It is thought to affect 2–3 per cent of normal children and, like primary snoring, peaks in the 3- to 6-year age group (Goldstein et al 1994). A diagnosis of SDB in a child may therefore be more difficult than in an adult and cannot necessarily be based solely on 'objective' sleep study indices. In our practice we use a combination of sleep study findings and direct clinical observations of the sleeping child in order to grade the degree of nocturnal airway obstruction (Table 9.2).

Obstruction (partial or complete) is generally considered significant if associated with hypoxaemia (falls in S_aO_2 to less than 90 per cent) and hypercapnia (P_aCO_2 >45 mmHg), and/or when sleep-related breathing difficulties and sleep fragmentation or deprivation result in clinically significant effects such as failure to thrive, cor pulmonale or behavioural problems. A history of disordered sleep patterns is often the first indication of obstructive sleep apnoea in a child. More detailed questioning of the parents, possibly with the use of a sleep diary to record nocturnal events of the period of, say, a week, may reveal other signs and symptoms of sleep apnoea (Table 9.3). Sleep laboratory recordings can then be used to establish the presence and severity of sleep breathing disturbances and their effects on overall sleep quality.

TABLE 9.3
**Paediatric sleep questionnaire for children with obstructive
sleep apnoea syndrome (OSAS) (from Chervin et al 2000)**

Surname:_____   Forename:_____

Hospital No:_____   DOB:_____

Date:_____

While sleeping does your child . . .

. . . snore more than half the time? . . . . .Y / N   [A2]

. . . always snore? . . . . .Y / N   [A3]

. . . snore loudly? . . . . .Y / N   [A4]

. . . have 'heavy' or 'loud' breathing? . . . . .Y / N   [A5]

. . . have trouble breathing, or struggle to breathe? . . . . .Y / N   [A6]

Have you ever . . .

. . . seen your child stop breathing during the night? . . . . .Y / N   [A7]

Does your child . . .

. . . tend to breathe through the mouth during the day? . . . . .Y / N   [A24]

. . . have a dry mouth on waking up in the morning? . . . . .Y / N   [A25]

. . . occasionally wet the bed? . . . . .Y / N   [A32]

Does your child . . .

. . . wake up feeling *un*refreshed in the morning? . . . . .Y / N   [B1]

. . . have a problem with sleepiness during the day? . . . . .Y / N   [B2]

Has a teacher or other supervisor commented that your child appears sleepy during the day? . .Y / N   [B4]

Is it hard to wake your child up in the morning? . . . . .Y / N   [B6]

Does your child wake up with headaches in the morning? .Y / N   [B7]

Did your child stop growing at a normal rate at any time since birth? . . . . .Y / N   [B9]

Is your child overweight? . . . . .Y / N   [B22]

This child often . . .

. . . does not seem to listen when spoken to directly. . . . . .Y / N   [C3]

. . . has difficulty organising tasks and activities. . . . . .Y / N   [C5]

. . . is easily distracted by extraneous stimuli. . . . . .Y / N   [C8]

. . . fidgets with hands or feet or squirms in seat. . . . . .Y / N   [C10]

. . . is 'on the go' or often acts as if 'driven by a motor'. . . . . .Y / N   [C14]

. . . interrupts or intrudes on others (e.g. butts into conversations or games). . . . . .Y / N   [C18]

Score Y = 1, N (or No Response) = 0

Snore Score	(A2+A3+A4+A5)	= _____
Sleepiness Score	(B1+B2+B4+B6)	= _____
Behavioural Score	(C3+C5+C8+C10+C14+C18)	= _____
Other Score=	(A6+A7+A24+A25+A32+B7+B9+B22)	= _____
Total Score		= _____
Mean Score	(Total Score / 22 * 100%)	= _____ *

*(Cutoff Mean Score > 0.33)

A recent study in our own practice (van Someren et al 2000) confirmed that in our hands the use of a structured questionnaire for the parents, together with a formal sleep study, formed the best basis for the diagnosis of SDB. The use of questionnaire and clinical history in the absence of a formal sleep study was found to give an accurate assessment of the severity of sleep breathing problems in only 42 per cent of cases. In 17 per cent of cases the clinician underestimated the severity of SDB when subsequently assessed by sleep study, while in 16 per cent of cases the clinician overestimated the severity. In 10 per cent of cases the clinical impression was markedly different (more than two grades in Table 9.2) from the sleep study assessment.

Clinical features of obstructive sleep apnoea syndrome (OSAS)
Nocturnal symptoms and signs of OSAS usually include heavy snoring, restlessness and sweating. There may be a history of nightmares or night terrors. Intermittent apnoeas and increased respiratory effort are often noted. Children may adopt unusual sleeping positions to optimise the airway, typically with a hyperextended neck and mouth-open posture, or prone with the knees tucked under the chest and the head turned to the side. There is an association with enuresis (Weider and Hauri 1985).

Daytime symptoms and signs include nasal obstruction, mouth breathing and hyponasal speech. In addition, the complex cumulative physiological effects of repeated upper airway obstruction during sleep may have adverse effects on cardiac function, somatic growth and neuro-behavioural function (Guilleminault et al 1976a) including daytime hyperactivity, aggression, social withdrawal and hypersomnolence (Brouillette et al 1982, Frank et al 1983, Brouillette et al 1984, Mandel and Reynolds 1985, Potsic et al 1986), reduced attentional capacity, memory and cognitive function with developmental delay (Guilleminault et al 1981, Brouillette et al 1982), and in older children problems with academic performance (Weissbluth et al 1983). These symptoms are thought to be due to arousals disrupting the functions of the sleeping brain. However, while there is much anecdotal evidence there are relatively few data from well-controlled studies at present.

The ability to remain at a task and to attend to external stimuli plays an important role in learning, and social and academic development. Recent studies have provided the first limited data on the detrimental effects of SDB on attention capacity in children (Owens-Stively et al 1997, Blunden et al 2000). They suggest that children with sleep-related breathing disorders are less reflective, more impulsive and show poorer sustained and selective attention. Importantly, two further studies have suggested that these effects are reversible with successful treatment of the upper airway obstruction during sleep (Guilleminault et al 1982, Ali et al 1996).

Two studies using standard psychometric tests have shown significantly reduced memory performance in children with sleep-related breathing disorders (Rhodes et al 1995, Blunden et al 2000). Children with moderate/severe OSAS were shown to perform in the intellectually deficient ranges compared to controls who produced scores within the average range, while those with mild SDB tended to fall in the low normal range. These results suggest a dose-dependent effect of SDB on memory capacity.

Only three published studies have looked at intelligence (IQ) in school-aged children with sleep-related breathing disorders. Two studies (Rhodes et al 1995, Blunden et al 2000) found significantly reduced IQ scores, while the third (Ali et al 1996) did not. Further studies are needed to clarify this relationship.

It can be shown that children with SDB show diminished academic performance (Stradling et al 1990, Guilleminault et al 1996). Conversely, it has been shown that poor academic achievers include a high preponderance of children with SDB (Weissbluth et al 1983, Gozal 1998, Gozal and Pope 2001). Importantly, it has also been demonstrated that treatment of these children with sleep-related breathing problems by tonsillectomy or adenotonsillectomy has been followed by an improvement in academic performance (Guilleminault et al 1982, Gozal 1998).

Questionnaires of parents and teachers suggest that behavioural problems are common in children with sleep-related breathing disorders. Children have been found to show increased levels of internalised problematic behaviours (shy, withdrawn, anxious) (Guilleminault et al 1981, Brouillette et al 1984) and externalised behaviours (impulsivity, hyperactivity, aggression) (Stradling et al 1990, Ali et al 1993, 1996, Guilleminault et al 1996). Inattention-hyperactivity is frequently found, with a reported prevalence rate of 20–42 per cent (Guilleminault et al 1981, Weissbluth et al 1983, Stradling et al 1990). Conversely, children with inattention-hyperactivity show a high prevalence of sleep-disordered breathing (Weissbluth et al 1983, Chervin et al 1997). Treatment of nocturnal breathing problems has been shown to improve daytime behaviour (Guilleminault et al 1982, Chervin et al 1997).

Unlike adults with OSAS, excessive daytime sleepiness (EDS) is not usually a feature in children (Carroll and Loughlin 1992); this is thought to be due to the fact that arousals in children are usually movement arousals rather than EEG or behavioural arousals as they are in adults. The diagnosis of EDS in children is difficult as tiredness may manifest as hyperactivity (Chervin et al 1997). However, daytime sleepiness is reported in some children (Brouillette et al 1984, Ali et al 1993, Guilleminault et al 1996, Blunden et al 2000).

Intracranial hypertension (>15 mmHg) is frequent in children with syndromic craniosynostosis. Its aetiology is multifactorial but OSAS may be an important cause (Gonsalez et al 1997). It may be asymptomatic, or children may notice headache or failing vision. Like SDB, it can also have an effect on behaviour.

There may be poor growth and failure to thrive (Brouillette et al 1982, Everett et al 1987, Carroll and Loughlin 1992) due both to the increased energy expenditure necessary to breathe during sleep and to reduced growth hormone secretion owing to sleep fragmentation (Lind and Lundell 1982, Goldstein et al 1987). Successful treatment, however, results in catch-up growth. Unlike adults, obesity (Carroll 1996) and systemic hypertension (D'Andrea et al 1993) are uncommon features in children.

Cardiorespiratory complications occur as a consequence of recurrent severe hypoxia, hypercarbia and acidosis. They include dysrhythmias, pulmonary hypertension and cor pulmonale (Menashe et al 1965, Levy et al 1967, Guilleminault et al 1976b, Brouillette et al 1982). These are reversible within 48 hours of treatment of OSAS (Sofer et al 1988). Acute cardiorespiratory failure may be triggered by an upper respiratory tract infection and result in sudden death (Wilkinson et al 1981). Such complications are rare now with recognition of OSAS and earlier diagnosis and treatment. The long-term cardiorespiratory effects of mild SDB are unknown; there may be an increased risk of systemic hypertension in later life (Baharav et al 1994).

Diagnosis

The diagnosis of SDB in children is based on the history from the parents, clinical findings on examination and the results of investigations. The criterion standard investigation for the diagnosis of OSAS is polysomnography (PSG). Other investigations advocated include radiology, cephalometry (in which standardised measurements of distances and angles from identifiable bony landmarks are taken), fluoroscopy, endoscopy, computerised tomography and magnetic resonance imaging. They may provide information about the level of obstruction but their indications are not standardised and their value is unclear. Furthermore, investigations in the awake child may not provide information relevant to the status of the airway during sleep and, paradoxically, sedation may not mimic normal sleep either. Pulse oximetry, if it confirms a pattern of cyclic desaturation, can be helpful but there is a high false negative rate for OSAS and it cannot diagnose UARS or OHS (Brouillette et al 2000). The reference technique for the diagnosis of UARS is oesophageal manometry which shows wide swings in pressure in this condition; pulse transit time has been shown to correlate with these pressure changes and can be used as a clinical measure (Pitson et al 1995).

It has been shown that clinical histories from parents tend to overestimate the significance of mild airway symptoms and underestimate the severity of serious problems (Goldstein et al 1994, Carroll et al 1995), perhaps because of chronicity. We have also found this in our own series. In syndromic children, respiratory problems may be overshadowed by other, apparently more severe, problems such as cosmesis or developmental delay and be discounted by the parents. Furthermore, expectations of children with multiple problems may be low, and symptoms such as developmental delay may be attributed to the syndrome itself rather than other potentially remediable causes such as SDB, hearing impairment or visual problems.

Clinical examination will confirm the abnormal craniofacial morphology. Patency of the nasal airways, status of the palate, and size of the tonsils and adenoids should be assessed as well as the general condition of the child and any signs of chronic respiratory distress. If there is a suspicion of cardiorespiratory complications, an electrocardiogram and a chest radiograph should be examined for evidence of right ventricular hypertrophy. Measurement of height and weight and comparison with standardised growth charts may confirm failure to thrive, especially if the child is monitored over a period of time. Feeding difficulties are common in the syndromic craniosynostoses and failure to thrive may be attributed to this cause alone, but SDB is also an important cause and should be considered.

Respiratory sleep studies are not usually carried out before adenotonsillectomy for normal children with symptoms and signs of OSAS or UARS but are recommended by the American Thoracic Society (1996) for a number of more complex situations including children with craniofacial anomalies. It has been estimated that as many as 85 per cent of children with syndromic craniosynostosis who have not had corrective surgery have some degree of upper airway obstruction during sleep, and in 61 per cent it is clinically significant (moderate to severe) (Gonsalez et al 1997). Formal sleep studies should therefore be routine to evaluate regularly the function of the airway for this group of children.

Respiratory sleep studies

There is general agreement that sleep-related breathing disorders need to be documented objectively but there remains controversy over the type of investigation needed, what to look for, and what degree of abnormality constitutes a problem worth treating.

Historically, sleep studies developed in research laboratories looking at classical sleep patterns using electrophysiological measures (EEG, EOG, EMG) to document sleep architecture and to identify the effects of problems, such as insomnia and depression. The primary interest was in classifying the nature and patterns of sleep. Sleep was classified based upon a system that was later to become standardised by a consensus committee (Rechtschaffen and Kales 1968). It was broken down into epochs of 20 or 30 seconds for analysis purposes. Each epoch was classified as wake, non-REM (stages I–IV), or REM; numerous indices were then generated to quantify the amount and the distribution of each of these sleep states in order statistically to describe the overall sleep architecture. Monitoring of sleep-related breathing problems arrived at a later date and the measurement of respiratory variables was added to the neurophysiological montage. The tendency was for breathing patterns and anomalies to be analysed within the same rigid framework as the neurophysiological signals, generating a wealth of indices of respiratory disturbance.

The rigid, epoch-based approach to the analysis of respiratory sleep studies still holds sway in many sleep laboratories today, particularly in the USA. However, other centres, often with more limited resources, have adopted a rather more pragmatic approach to respiratory sleep studies. The most essential element of a respiratory, as opposed to a neurophysiological, sleep study is to identify the nature and the severity of any respiratory anomalies, and to establish the degree of sleep fragmentation or disruption that results from these respiratory problems. To this end, measurements are made that describe the pattern and effectiveness of breathing, on the one hand, and evaluate the degree of sleep disruption, on the other. These studies aim to document the nature and extent of sleep-related breathing anomalies and to discern whether any sleep disruption is the consequence of the respiratory anomalies or the result of another, non-respiratory, cause. As previously described, respiratory anomalies can be broadly divided into two types; central events are characterised by a diminution or absence of respiratory effort, whereas obstructive events manifest as a diminution or absence of respiratory airflow as a consequence of upper airway collapse and despite a continuation of respiratory effort. Sleep disruption may result from respiratory events. Arousals (an acute transition to a lighter stage of sleep or even wakefulness) occur in response to the stimuli of increased respiratory effort, diminished P_aO_2, or elevated P_aCO_2 (Gleeson et al 1990, Gleeson and Zwillich 1992).

Traditional polysomnography typically includes documentation of:

* gross sleep architecture and arousals derived from neurophysiological recordings (EEG, EOG, EMG);

- respiratory patterns discerned from recordings of oro-nasal airflow (apnoea, hypopnoea), and from ribcage and abdominal movements (respiratory effort);
- ECG to give information about heart rate changes (increased heart rate with arousal, reflex bradycardia with hypoxia) and dysrhythmias (possibly stimulated by hypoxia);
- upper airway obstruction, as evidenced by snoring, monitored by direct sound recordings or from characteristic patterns on the oro-nasal flow tracing;
- changes in arterial blood gases (arterial oxygen saturation (S_aO_2) and non-invasive arterial PCO_2) which give measures of the adequacy of ventilation;
- posture, which may be important as upper airway obstruction may be exacerbated in certain positions;
- leg movements, documented from EMG recordings from an anterior leg muscle. Periodic leg movements are an example of a non-respiratory cause of sleep fragmentation.

Originally these multi-channel recordings were made on paper running at a speed of 10–15 mm/s, which gave 20–30 s/page and thus determined the epoch length for subsequent analysis. Analysis was by hand and required the sleep state for each epoch to be determined, and any respiratory or cardiac events to be identified, classified and annotated (Fig. 9.3). Even today, when recordings are made digitally and stored on computer, the analysis of a sleep study epoch by epoch can take many hours by a skilled individual.

The analysis of respiratory events is, in itself, time-consuming and requires not inconsiderable skill and experience.

RESPIRATORY AIRFLOW

The measurement of oro-nasal airflow and the deduction of apnoea or hypopnoea is notoriously difficult, particularly as the signal generated by the measuring devices (usually a thermistor) is not related to true flow rates in a linear fashion, and is prone to artifact if the measuring device is displaced by even a small amount. Alternative methods of recording flow, such as continuous CO_2 sampling from the nostrils, are also imperfect, although they can give useful additional information about changes in alveolar and arterial PCO_2 levels.

RESPIRATORY EFFORT

The most reliable and accurate measurement of respiratory effort is the measurement of intra-oesophageal pressure (P_{oes}) using a catheter passed via the nose with its tip located in the lower third of the oesophagus. However, this clearly invasive procedure is poorly tolerated by patients (particularly children), is technically demanding and time-consuming to set up, and may, in itself, lead to sleep disruption.

Recently, teams in Oxford (Pitson et al 1995) and Grenoble (Smith et al 1999) have worked to establish alternatives to P_{oes} to measure respiratory effort. The phenomenon of changes in arterial blood pressure associated with inspiratory efforts (pulsus paradoxus) has been recognised for some time. Each inspiratory effort generates a small fall in intrathoracic pressure; as the heart is located within the thoracic cavity, it is subject to these pressure changes with the net result that the small respiratory pressure swings are superimposed on

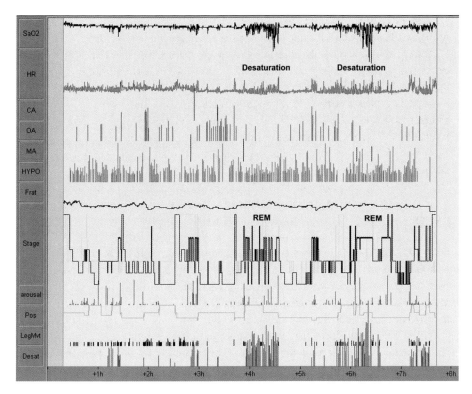

Fig. 9.3 10-year-old child with moderate-severe obstructive sleep apnoea. This 8-hour graphical summary shows: arterial oxygen saturation (SaO_2 per cent), heart rate (HR, bpm), central apnoea (CA), obstructive apnoea (OA), mixed apnoea (MA), hypopnoea (HYPO) duration, respiratory rate from the flow signal (Frat, breath/min), sleep stage hypnogram (wake, REM, Stage 1, 2, 3, 4, reading downwards), arousals, body position (Pos), leg movements (LegMvt), and magnitude of oxygen desaturations (Desat). Sleep was described as restless with frequent movements and arousals. Frequent and prolonged obstructive apnoeas (OA) and hypopnoeas (HYPO) are seen, particularly during rapid eye movement (REM) sleep periods with oxygen desaturation (SaO_2), and cardiac variability (HR). The degree of oxygen desaturation (Desat) becomes progressively worse with each successive REM period. Sleep quality is poor with a high degree of sleep fragmentation (arousal) and a high number of sleep state changes (Stage).

the arterial blood pressure trace (Lea et al 1990). With partial or total obstruction of the upper airway there is a marked increase in magnitude of the respiratory efforts, with increasingly negative intrathoracic pressure swings which are reflected in the pulsus paradoxus pattern seen on the arterial pressure trace (Fig. 9.4).

Clearly, continuous measurements of arterial blood pressure during sleep are impractical. However, the measurement of pulse transit time (PTT) has been validated in recent years as an alternative, surrogate measure of blood pressure. Pulse transit time is a measure of the time taken for an arterial pulse waveform to travel between two points on the arterial system. Commercially available systems now allow the measurement of the time interval between ventricular contraction (detected from the ECG 'R' wave) and the arrival of the

175

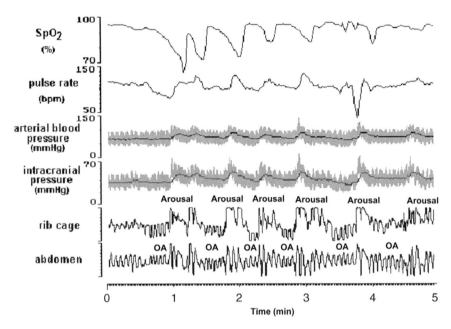

Fig. 9.4 A 5-minute segment recorded in an 18-month-old infant with Crouzon syndrome and severe obstructive sleep apnoea. The trace shows repeated obstructive apnoeas (OA) interspersed by acute arousals from sleep. The breathing pattern shows periods of paradoxical respiratory movements (ribcage vs. abdomen) during apnoeic episodes (OA) interspersed by episodes of 3–4 effective breaths during periods of arousal. Severe dips in arterial oxygen saturation (SaO$_2$) result from each obstructive episode with dips to below 70 per cent. Arousals are seen between each obstructive episode indicated by acute rises in pulse rate. Recordings of arterial blood pressure (brachial arterial line) and intracranial pressure (indwelling subdural pressure transducer) show characteristic respiratory oscillations (pulsus paradoxus) during obstructive episodes with acute rises in pressure during arousal episodes.

pulse waveform at the periphery (detected from the plethysmographic waveform of the pulse oximeter, located on the finger in adults, or toe in infants and young children). The time taken for the waveform to cover this distance is primarily dependent on the tension in the arterial wall and thus inversely related to arterial blood pressure (Fig. 9.5).

Analysis of the breath-to-breath changes in the PTT trace allows the degree of respiratory effort to be quantified, while an abrupt fall in PTT is indicative of an autonomic arousal and is a measure of sleep disruption. We have validated the use of PTT as a measure of severity of obstruction in a group of children with OSAS ranging from mild to severe (Table 9.2) (Massa et al 2000).

RESPIRATORY PATTERNS

Ribcage and abdominal movements give an important indication of respiratory patterns and their interrelationship can give information about the degree of respiratory effort and the nature of the apnoea or hypopnoea. There are a number of devices that allow the measurement of ribcage and abdominal movements: inductance plethysmography uses two

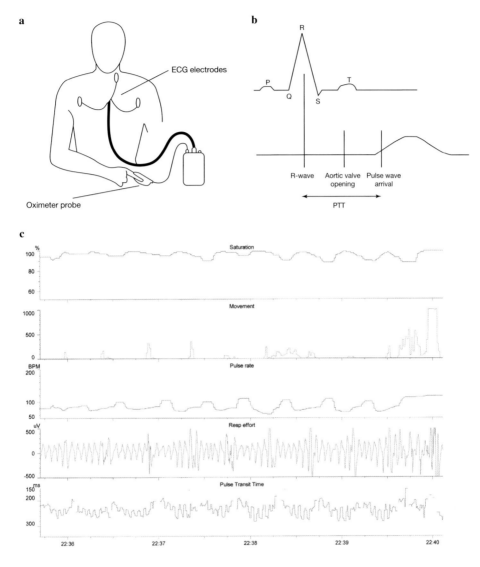

Fig. 9.5 The use of pulse transit time (PTT) as a measure of inspiratory effort and arousal in a patient with obstructive sleep apnoea. PTT is measured as the time lag between ECG 'R'-wave (ventricular contraction) and onset of the pulse wave form detected at the finger by the pulse oximeter ((a) and (b)). The primary determinant of PTT is arterial pressure, with an inverse relationship between mean arterial pressure and PTT. By deriving PTT during a sleep study one is able to derive a non-invasive indicator of blood pressure changes. In the patient with obstructive sleep apnoea the magnitude of the breath-by-breath troughs in PTT is an indication of inspiratory effort (pulsus paradoxus), while the non-breathing-related peaks are markers of arousal. The sleep recording shows a 4-minute segment of a study on a patient with moderate obstructive sleep apnoea. Arousals are indicated by: gross body movements, acute rises in pulse rate, increased respiratory efforts and a peak of pulse transit time. Obstructive apnoeas (OA) are characterised by diminished respiratory excursions, arterial oxygen desaturation and increasing levels of inspiratory effort shown by the progressively deeper dips in the PTT waveform.

elasticated belts that encircle each compartment (ribcage at the level of the axilla, abdomen beneath the lower ribs and above the umbilicus) and give a signal that is proportional to volume. Strain gauges similarly placed offer an alternative that gives information about the expansion and contraction of the two compartments but the changes seen are not directly related to volume and thus only semi-quantitative.

The interplay between the ribcage and abdominal signals can be used to indicate the level of respiratory effort. During unloaded breathing the two compartments expand and contract in synchrony (Fig. 9.6(a)). With increased upper airway resistance and increased inspiratory effort the two signals become progressively more asynchronous (Fig. 9.6(b)), with the abdominal expansion tending to lead the ribcage. In extreme circumstances, such as total upper airway occlusion, the ribcage and abdomen show a characteristic pattern of paradoxical motion (Fig. 9.6(c)). It is important to remember, however, that in infants and young children the ribcage is not fully developed and remains very compliant (non-rigid), and paradoxical movement with the ribcage being drawn in during inspiratory efforts may be seen when work of breathing is increased but without total upper airway obstruction.

The complexity and subtleties of the changes seen in the respiratory patterns make analysis complex and require interpretation by a skilled individual. As yet, automated, computerised systems have failed to offer an alternative to manual scoring of the respiratory patterns.

ARTERIAL BLOOD GAS TENSIONS
While the pattern of breathing is important, an assessment of the overall effect of respiratory anomalies is best judged from how well, or otherwise, arterial blood gases are maintained. With modern sleep systems, non-invasive measurements of both arterial oxygenation

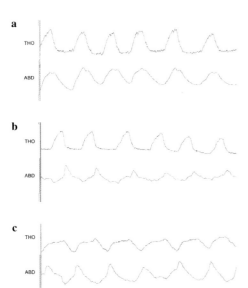

Fig. 9.6 The relationship between thoracic (THO) and abdominal (ABD) movements. Each trace shows a period of approximately 20 seconds of breathing. In (a), thoracic and abdominal movements are in-phase with synchronous movements of the two compartments. (b) shows an example of partial asynchrony, with the inspiratory peaks of the two traces no longer fully aligned. Partial asynchrony is often a sign of increased work of breathing and may be associated with increased inspiratory effort associated with increased upper airway resistance. (c) shows an example of respiratory paradox with the two compartments working in opposition. Paradoxical movements may be seen during episodes of upper airway obstruction; however, they should be interpreted with caution in young children whose chest walls are easily deformable.

and PCO_2 levels are possible. The development of pulse oximetry with the ability to make continuous, non-invasive measurements of arterial oxygen saturation (S_aO_2) has probably been the single most important contribution to respiratory sleep medicine.

To what extent S_aO_2 measurements can substitute for measurements of actual respiratory events is not clear. While numerous attempts have been made to look at the relationship between the number and frequency of hypoxic dips and measures of apnoea/hypopnoea, it is difficult to reach any firm conclusions as there are too many variables to consider (differences between oximeters, different definitions of hypoxic events (≥ 3 per cent, ≥ 4 per cent, >4 per cent dips), correlated to differently defined apnoeas and hypopnoeas (duration and percentage decrease in airflow). While it emerges that there is generally a good relationship between hypoxic dip events and respiratory events, there are circumstances when S_aO_2 becomes a poor index of the severity of obstruction. It is recognised that there is a wide variation between individuals in the magnitude of the stimulus needed to cause arousal. So while many patients obstruct for a period sufficient to cause oxygen desaturation and generate an event identifiable from oximetry, a significant number of individuals arouse more easily and therefore rescue their airway before any significant change in S_aO_2 (Gleeson et al 1990, Gleeson and Zwillich 1992) (Fig. 9.7).

The use of oximetry alone, therefore, is liable to miss patients with significant upper airway obstruction, but who readily arouse. These individuals may have all the symptoms of OSAS, including fragmented sleep and daytime consequences, but will not be picked up from these limited sleep studies. In a study comparing the analysis of oximetry alone with full polysomnography, Brouillette et al (2000) showed that an S_aO_2 study which showed significant periods of hypoxaemia during sleep was clinically significant; however, the absence of hypoxaemia cannot be used to exclude OSAS. Many symptomatic children do not desaturate even though they may demonstrate hypercapnia, partial upper airway obstruction and marked sleep disturbance on PSG.

SNORING

Snoring is an important marker of upper airway narrowing; however, it is important to remember that during periods of total upper airway obstruction snoring is absent; therefore treat with caution the parent who enthusiastically reports that their child has now stopped snoring during sleep. The extent and nature of snoring can be assessed from a direct audio recording or from a graphical channel on the PSG.

ECG

The ECG and heart rate analysis can be used to give an approximate indication of wakefulness, non-REM (quiet) sleep, and REM (active) sleep in the absence of neurophysiological recordings. Acute heart rate increases can be used as an index of arousal, while bradycardia associated with apnoea is clinically important in infants. The ECG may also be examined for dysrhythmias that may be sleep-state-related or associated with hypoxia. In reality, the usual single lead ECG may be inadequate for serious diagnostic purposes and any suspicion of ECG anomalies is better investigated using conventional ECG Holter monitoring.

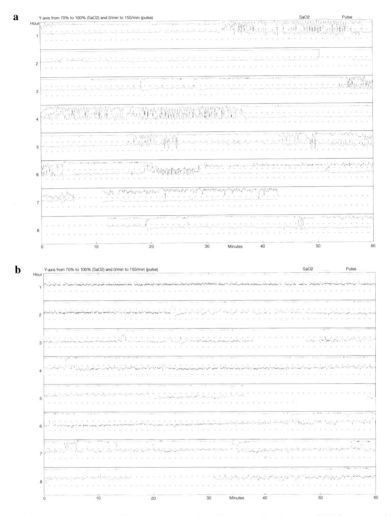

Fig. 9.7 8-hour records of arterial oxygen saturation (SaO$_2$) and pulse rate (PR) in two patients with obstructive sleep apnoea, but with contrasting patterns of response. Each panel shows a sequence of eight 1-hour strips, with each strip depicting SaO$_2$ (ranging between 70 per cent and 100 per cent), and pulse rate (ranging between 0 and 150 beats/min). The SaO$_2$ trace is the uppermost trace in each strip.

The first patient shows a 'typical' pattern of obstructive sleep apnoea. SaO$_2$ and PR tend to be stable during periods of quiet sleep (e.g. first 30 mins of hour 1, most of hours 2 and 3, etc.), but become unstable during periods of active or rapid eye movement (REM) sleep, with frequent dips in SaO$_2$ (oxygen desaturation) and acute PR rises (arousals) (e.g. latter half of hour 1, first half of hour 4, etc.). This patient had a mean SaO$_2$ = 96 per cent, with an average of 16 dips in SaO$_2$ greater than 4 per cent per hour, with dips to a mean nadir of 89 per cent. Pulse rate shows frequent acute rises (arousals) with a mean rate of 30 arousals per hour.

The second patient also has obstructive sleep apnoea, but is a 'non-dipper'. Arterial oxygen saturation (SaO$_2$) remains stable throughout sleep at a mean level of 98 per cent with no significant dips. Nevertheless, sleep is fragmented with an average of 47 arousals (acute PR rises) per hour, and inspiratory effort (estimated from pulse transit time) is significantly elevated at a level suggestive of severely increased upper airway resistance (partial obstruction).

180

International recommendations

The American Thoracic Society (ATS) has published two official statements on cardiorespiratory sleep studies in children (ATS 1996, 1999). To date, there are no published recommendations specific to the UK. In relation to craniofacial patients, sleep studies are recommended in the following circumstances:

- To differentiate benign/primary snoring (i.e. snoring not associated with apnoea or hypoventilation) from pathological snoring (associated with partial or complete airway collapse, dipping S_aO_2 and sleep disruption).
- To investigate disturbed sleep patterns, excessive daytime sleepiness, cor pulmonale, failure to thrive, and unexplained polycythaemia, especially in the presence of snoring.
- To investigate a child with observed snoring and clinically significant airway obstruction (apnoea, retractions, paradox), either observed or on video record, in order to confirm the diagnosis of OSAS or to optimise treatment.
- To determine if the level of OSAS is severe enough to warrant surgery, or if it is anticipated that the child may need intensive postoperative care following adenotonsillar or pharyngeal surgery. There is an increased surgical risk in children less than 2 years old, in those with a respiratory disturbance index (RDI) >10 events/hr, and in those with craniofacial anomalies, particularly midfacial hypoplasia, retrognathia and micrognathia (Schafer 1982, Shprintzen 1988, McColley et al 1992, Rosen et al 1994).
- Follow-up sleep studies are recommended in children previously diagnosed with OSAS in whom symptoms persist following therapy. A sleep study should be delayed at least four weeks following any surgery to allow postoperative oedema to resolve.
- Follow-up and review of OSAS patients treated with continuous positive airway pressure (CPAP) or a nasopharyngeal airway.

Children with mild/moderate OSAS with complete resolution of snoring and disturbed sleep patterns after therapy do not require follow-up sleep studies. However, for children with severe OSAS, or those under a year of age, follow-up sleep studies are suggested to assure resolution of clinically significant abnormalities (Suen et al 1995). Irrespective of whether a sleep study is ordered, the parents and primary carers should be taught the signs and symptoms of a recurrence of OSAS. The child should be followed up with routine clinical assessments to ensure early detection of the recurrence of OSAS.

SIMPLER ALTERNATIVES TO FULL POLYSOMNOGRAPHY

Historically, respiratory sleep studies grew out of neurophysiological sleep studies. While still controversial, there is increasing support for the idea of simplified sleep studies for the assessment of respiratory problems. The idea is attractive from practical and financial points of view and because of the time involved. Furthermore, in the paediatric field the idea of simpler, less invasive studies is in itself attractive. The question really is how simple can a study be for it to retain the sensitivity and specificity of the criterion standard polysomnogram. In the real world, a balance has to be struck between that which is ideal and that which is feasible, practical and clinically acceptable. Clinically, a test needs to identify correctly individuals whose disease severity warrants treatment, and can then be used to follow up these patients post-therapy to confirm the effectiveness of therapy. In reality, there is little agreement between sleep centres as to what constitutes the ideal 'limited' sleep study. However, most would agree that the aims of any 'limited' sleep study should allow the assessment of:

- **respiratory effort** (ribcage and abdominal movements, snoring, or, possibly, a high quality video recording);
- **respiratory efficacy** (e.g. S_aO_2 and/or end-tidal PCO_2);
- **sleep fragmentation** (EEG, or acute heart rate rises, acute blood pressure rises, or gross body movement from leg EMG, pressure sensitive mattress or high quality video recording).

At Great Ormond Street Hospital, our approach is to use three levels of respiratory sleep study:

1 Limited cardiorespiratory studies with video/sound recording (Visilab, Stowood Scientific Instruments, Oxford, UK)
The majority of patients are studied with a system that records a limited number of cardiorespiratory signals (with minimal patient contact to accommodate children), with a high quality video and sound recording using an infra-red video camera allowing a picture to be recorded in an apparently dark room. The signals recorded include:

- arterial oxygen saturation (S_aO_2)   pulse oximeter
- pulse rate (PR)   pulse oximeter
- respiratory pattern   strain gauge (mid-thoracic)
- heart rate (HR) and dysrhythmias   electrocardiogram (ECG)
- movement (arousals)   infra-red video recording
- sound (snoring)   video recording
- respiratory effort and arousals   PTT – derived from ECG and oximeter

The system has been validated in children in a collaborative study between Great Ormond Street Hospital and the Royal Free Hospital (van Someren et al 2000). The system was found to be robust in a paediatric clinical setting and the results valid when compared to full cardiorespiratory sleep studies in the same patients. The biggest shortcoming of the system was in the computerised automated scoring of arousals (movement) from the video record, where the individual reporting the sleep study needed to be aware that many of the automatically scored arousals were actually movements from the parent or nurse caring for the patient. Nevertheless, these artifactual movements could be eliminated by reference to the appropriate period in the real-time video recording (Fig. 9.7(a)).

2 Oximetry alone (Biox 3800, Ohmeda, UK or Pulsox 3i, Minolta, Japan)
The recording of oximetry alone is simple to perform and generates records of:

- arterial oxygen saturation (S_aO_2)   pulse oximeter
- pulse rate (PR)   pulse oximeter

Most modern pulse oximeters are able to store the S_aO_2 and PR data in an internal memory for periods of 12 hours or more. These data can subsequently be downloaded to a computer for analysis using appropriate software. It should be noted that 'spot' recordings of S_aO_2 taken during the night are unreliable as a means of identifying the severity of obstruction, with apparently normal values of S_aO_2 reported in cases where there is in fact serious obstruction. In our practice, oximetry-only sleep studies are only performed in patients in whom a more comprehensive sleep study has been previously performed and in whom we have a clear picture of the nature and severity of their condition. Follow-up studies to monitor progress or response to treatment may be possible using oximetry alone.

3 Multi-channel cardiorespiratory monitoring (+/- video/sound)
(Alice 4, Respironics, USA)
Our third level of study uses a computerised full polysomnography system, although we generally do not use any of the electrophysiological channels (EEG, EOG, EMG) unless there is a suspicion that there is a relationship between neurological events (e.g. epilepsy) and respiratory events (e.g. apnoea). The choice to use the cardiorespiratory channels only is largely for practical reasons, as to set up, calibrate and supervise full polysomnography requires experienced, technically able staff to attend the overnight monitoring. Furthermore, these complex studies are not really feasible in the normal ward environment and are better suited to a dedicated sleep laboratory. The full polysomnography system is, however, ideal for making comprehensive recordings during sleep of a full cardiorespiratory montage including:

- arterial oxygen saturation (S_aO_2)   pulse oximeter
- pulse rate (PR)   pulse oximeter
- end-tidal PCO_2 ($P_{et}CO_2$)   side stream infra-red PCO_2 analyser sampling via nasal cannulae
- respiratory pattern   ribcage (RC) and abdominal (ABD) strain gauges
- heart rate (HR) and dysrhythmias   electrocardiogram (ECG)
- oro-nasal airflow   thermistors or intra-nasal pressure
- snoring   throat microphone
- body position   position sensor on chest
- arm and leg movements   accelerometers attached to wrist and ankle
- movement (arousals)   infra-red video recording
- sound (snoring)   video recording.

The computerised analysis system allows subsequent interactive analysis of respiratory and cardiac events. The video and sound recording is a useful adjunct to these studies, and although the present video system is analogue, recent technical developments mean that future polysomnography systems will include digital video and sound that are recorded synchronously on to the polysomnography system, allowing greater convenience and accuracy to the operator scoring the sleep study, as they will be able to view the video record in one window synchronised with the cardiorespiratory traces in another window.

These more detailed studies are generally performed in children less than 18 months of age, in whom central respiratory problems are likely to be seen, and in older children where central problems may be anticipated (e.g. raised intracranial pressure, brainstem herniation, etc.), or in patients with chronic hypoventilation in whom neuromuscular or skeletal abnormalities may be manifesting in poor ventilation that worsens during sleep.

INTERPRETATION

The interpretation of a sleep study involves the integration of the patterns seen in the sleep study recording with the information available from the patient's sleep history and physical examination. Clearly, OSAS is not an 'all-or-nothing' condition, but is best thought of as a continuum ranging from normality through different degrees of severity. We use a system of classification that categorises the patient based upon clinical observations of the sleeping child, and the sleep study results. Using these two measures we classify an individual as normal, mild OSA, moderate OSA or severe OSA (Table 9.2).

While the use of rigid indices of severity of OSA (e.g. apnoea/hypopnoea index, or S_aO_2 dip/hr) with arbitrary cut-offs between normality and disease – e.g. normal <1 obstructive apnoea/hr (ATS 1996), or ≤3 S_aO_2 dip/hr (Stradling et al 1990) – may be appropriate in describing patient groups in research studies, they are probably over-simplistic when dealing with individual patients. While age-related normative data exist for numerous respiratory variables (Brouillette 1992, ATS 1996, 1999), interpretation of clinical sleep studies requires a more flexible, intuitive approach. Those analysing, interpreting and reporting the sleep studies thus need considerable experience and a good knowledge of the individual patient.

Treatment

Treatment of symptomatic SDB in children depends on the cause and severity, the age of the patient, family and social circumstances and patient compliance with treatment. Intervention may be mandatory in severe cases where there is a risk of cardiopulmonary complications, but is also considered for snoring children with normal sleep studies or mild abnormality when significant daytime symptoms, that may be the result of nocturnal upper airway obstruction, are present. Clearly the risks and complications of any planned intervention must be weighed in every individual against the risks of leaving their condition untreated.

In adults, weight reduction and pharmacotherapy are therapeutic options but this is not the case in children. Treatment is directed towards relieving the obstruction or bypassing it. Theoretically, options available include nasal prong airways, adenotonsillectomy,

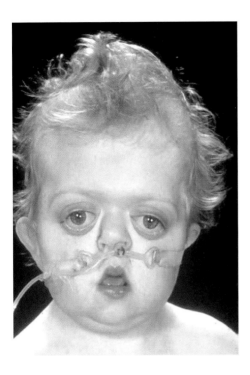

Fig. 9.8 This child with Pfeiffer syndrome has had her airway obstruction treated with a nasopharyngeal airway.

uvulopharyngopalatoplasty (UPPP), splitting of the soft palate with or without resection of the posterior palate margin, nasal continuous positive airway pressure (nasal-CPAP), tracheostomy and Le Fort III osteotomy and maxillary advancement or monobloc advancement, to increase the diameter of the pharynx. After surgical correction of the obstructed airway, close postoperative monitoring in the first 24 to 48 hours is essential as the correction of the blood oxygen and carbon dioxide levels may affect respiratory control centres, resulting in respiratory arrest.

A nasopharyngeal airway (Fig. 9.8) can be useful in the first few months of life, when the infant is an obligate nasal breather, if there is significant choanal stenosis. It requires regular suction to remain patent, and regular changing. It is associated with feeding difficulties, especially nasal regurgitation of milk and is seldom tolerated in the older child. Occasionally, however, it may be useful on a temporary basis after cleft palate repair until postoperative oedema has settled or, on a long-term basis, to bypass obstruction at tongue base level, particularly if only inserted at night, thus avoiding daytime cosmetic and feeding issues (unpublished data). The ideal position of the airway is with the tip lying just above the epiglottis. There is a positive correlation between the length of the tube and the crown/heel length, which can be used to guide the clinician, but optimal position must still be confirmed by clinical assessment (Fig. 9.9) (Heaf et al 1982).

Adenotonsillectomy is the standard treatment for childhood SDB generally (Lim and McKean 2003) and although the pathophysiology of SDB in children with syndromic craniosynostosis is multifactorial, adenotonsillectomy may be beneficial if there is

Fig. 9.9 A lateral radiograph is a convenient method for assessing the length of a nasopharyngeal airway.

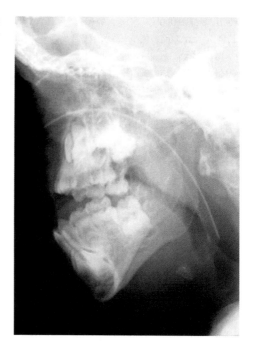

adenotonsillar hypertrophy or even if there is not; even a small increase in pharyngeal airway diameter may alter the airflow dynamics and raise the critical closing pressure. In affected children SDB may persist after adenotonsillectomy but may be less severe (unpublished data); factors predicting which children may benefit from adenotonsillectomy have not been established.

UPPP is not widely used to treat childhood OSAS although it has been successful in children with neuromuscular disorders (Kosko and Derkay 1995). Palate splitting with or without resection of the posterior palate margin is not routinely employed either although it has been reported in syndromic craniosynostosis (Moore 1993). It carries the potential for increasing the problem of middle ear effusion and for later speech disorders and velopharyngeal incompetence, especially after maxillary advancement – although theoretically these could be corrected by later closure of the pseudocleft, with or without pharyngoplasty.

Nasal-CPAP is very beneficial for patients who have not received sufficient benefit from adenotonsillectomy or who are not suitable candidates for surgery (Gonsalez et al 1996). Positive pressure is used to stent the collapsing airway. The level of pressure required to eliminate obstructive apnoeas, and correct nocturnal ventilation and oxygenation, is determined in the paediatric sleep laboratory and must then be serially evaluated and adjusted as the child grows. Complications from nasal-CPAP include irritation over the nasal bridge from the mask, nasal congestion and non-compliance. Compliance has improved with advances in equipment and mask design and can be further improved by intensive behavioural intervention. At our institution we have had 45 patients with syndromic craniosynostosis established successfully on nasal-CPAP for airway management

(Massa et al 2002). The time taken to acclimatise has varied from one night to two months. The advantages of nasal-CPAP are that it is non-invasive and that it only has to be applied during sleep. It may be ineffective if the adenoids are obstructive or there is significant choanal stenosis resulting in insufficient airway patency to allow the pressure to act as a splint. Adenoidectomy should be considered prior to a trial of nasal-CPAP; the possibility of cleft palate or a submucous cleft with bifid uvula should be remembered in Apert syndrome; either is a contraindication to adenoidectomy because of the risk of precipitating velopharyngeal incompetence.

Tracheostomy is an effective method of bypassing multilevel obstruction and always relieves obstructive sleep apnoea syndrome. It has been advocated as the first step in the management of all patients with severe craniofacial anomalies and breathing problems, regardless of planned subsequent treatment (Lauritzen et al 1986). However long-term paediatric tracheostomy carries significant risks in terms of morbidity and mortality. The tube is subject to obstruction and requires constant vigilance with regular suction and tube changes. There are adverse effects on feeding, speech and language development, education and socialisation. Children with syndromic craniosynostosis may already have significant handicaps in these areas. We therefore endeavour to avoid long-term tracheostomy in this group of patients. However, it is sometimes unavoidable; 10 of 147 children with a diagnosis of Apert, Crouzon or Pfeiffer syndrome underwent tracheostomy in our series (unpublished data); this compares favourably with other series in which rates as high as 48 per cent have been reported (Sculerati et al 1998). Temporary tracheostomy may rarely be indicated in older children for intra-operative and postoperative airway management if intubation is difficult. It is, however, mandatory if interdental wiring is being undertaken or halo distraction is performed in children on nasal-CPAP.

Surgical correction of the midface by Le Fort III osteotomies and maxillary advancement or monobloc advancement may improve airway calibre but the benefit for SDB is unpredictable and may not be maintained (Jarund and Lauritzen 1996). Conventional techniques using bone grafts and titanium plates were associated with increased risks for revision surgery, often necessary in adolescence for children who have had early surgery, as growth is disordered and there tends to be relapse. However, modern techniques using distraction osteogenesis may be equally or more effective in correcting deformity without increasing the risks of later surgery, and the results for airway improvement are encouraging (Dunaway 2002, personal communication). The most successful results for facial form and occlusion are achieved only after facial growth is completed so we reserve early craniofacial surgery for children with at least two functional problems rather than those with airway problems alone.

Summary
Our philosophy of management is to perform sleep studies on every child who presents with syndromic craniosynostosis and to interpret the results in conjunction with the history and clinical findings. If there is evidence of symptomatic SDB and adenotonsillar hypertrophy, adenotonsillectomy is the first step in airway management, unless adenoidectomy is contraindicated because of cleft palate, in which case tonsillectomy and possibly partial

adenoidectomy may be undertaken. The airway is then re-evaluated. If moderate to severe OSAS persists, the next step is a trial of nasal-CPAP. Only if this is unsuccessful would tracheostomy or maxillary advancement be considered, and the decision as to which should be undertaken is taken by the multidisciplinary craniofacial team as a whole, taking into consideration other functional problems and in discussion with the parents.

REFERENCES

Ali NJ, Pitson DJ, Stradling JR (1993) Snoring, sleep disturbance, and behaviour in 4–5 years olds. *Arch Dis Child* 68: 360–366.
Ali NJ, Pitson D, Stradling JR (1996) Sleep disordered breathing: effects of adenotonsillectomy on behaviour and psychological functioning. *Eur J Pediatr* 155: 56–62.
Aserinsky E (1965) Periodic respiratory pattern occurring in conjunction with eye movements during sleep. *Science* 150: 763–766.
Aserinsky E, Kleitman N (1953) Regularly occurring periods of eye motility, and consequent phenomena, during sleep. *Science* 118: 273–274.
ATS (American Thoracic Society) (1996) Standards and indications for cardiopulmonary sleep studies in children. ATS Statement. *Am J Respir Crit Care Med* 153: 866–878.
ATS (American Thoracic Society) (1999) Cardiorespiratory sleep studies in children. Establishment of normative data and polysomnographic predictors of morbidity. *Am J Respir Crit Care Med* 160: 1381–1387.
Baharav A, Kotagal S, Rubin BK, Gibbons V, Pratt J, Karim J, Akselrod S (1994) Obstructive sleep apnea and the autonomic cardiovascular control: an investigation by power spectrum analysis of heart rate variability. *Am J Respir Crit Care Med* 149: A558. (Abstract.)
Blunden SL, Lushington K, Kennedy D, Martin J, Dawson D (2000) Behaviour and neurocognitive function in children aged 5–10 years who snore compared to controls. *J Clin Neuropsychol* 22: 554–568.
Brouillette RT (1992) Assessing cardiopulmonary function during sleep in infants and children. In: Beckerman RC, Brouillette RT, Hunt CE, editors. *Respiratory Control Disorders in Infants and Children.* Baltimore: Williams and Wilkins, pp 125–141.
Brouillette R, Fernbach SK, Hunt CE (1982) Obstructive sleep apnea in infants and children. *J Pediatr* 100: 31–40.
Brouillette R, Hanson D, David R, Klemka L, Szatkowski A, Fernbach S, Hunt C (1984) A diagnostic approach to suspected obstructive sleep apnea in children. *J Pediatr* 105: 10–14.
Brouillette RT, Morielli A, Leimanis A, Waters KA, Luciano R, Ducharme FM (2000) Nocturnal pulse oximetry as an abbreviated testing modality for pediatric obstructive sleep apnea. *Pediatrics* 105: 405–412.
Bulow K (1963) Respiration and wakefulness in man. *Acta Physiol Scand* 59(suppl 209): 1–110.
Carroll JL (1996) Sleep-related upper-airway obstruction in children and adolescents. *Child Adolesc Psychiatr Clin North Am* 5: 617–647.
Carroll JL, Loughlin GM (1992) Diagnostic criteria for obstructive sleep apnea syndrome in children. *Pediatr Pulmonol* 14: 71–74.
Carroll JL, McColley SA, Marcus CL, Curtis S, Loughlin GM (1995) Inability of clinical history to distinguish primary snoring from obstructive sleep apnea syndrome in children. *Chest* 108: 610–618.
Chervin RD, Dillon JE, Bassetti C, Ganoczy DA, Pituch KJ (1997) Symptoms of sleep disorders, inattention and hyperactivity in children. *Sleep* 20: 1185–1192.
Chervin RD, Hedger K, Dillon JE, Pituch KJ (2000) Pediatric sleep questionnaire (PSQ): validity and reliability for sleep-disordered breathing, snoring, sleepiness, and behavioural problems. *Sleep Med* 1: 21–32.
Cinalli G, Renier D, Marchac D, Sainte-Rose C, Arnaud E, Pierre-Khan A (1994) Chiari malformation in craniofacial premature synostosis. *Childs Nerv Syst* 10: 411. (Abstract.)
Croft CB, Brockbank MJ, Wright A, Swanston AR (1990) Obstructive sleep apnoea in children undergoing routine tonsillectomy and adenoidectomy. *Clin Otolaryngol* 15: 307–314.
D'Andrea LA, Rosen CL, Haddad GG (1993) Severe hypoxemia in children with upper airway obstruction during sleep does not lead to significant changes in heart rate. *Pediatr Pulmonol* 16: 362–369.
Dement WC, Kleitman N (1957) Cyclic variations in EEG during sleep and their relation to eye movements, body motility, and dreaming. *Electroencephalogr Clin Neurophysiol* 9: 673–690.

Everett A, Knock W, Saulsbury F (1987) Failure to thrive due to obstructive sleep apnea. *Clin Pediatr* 26: 90–92.

Fitzsimmonds JS (1965) Laryngeal stridor and respiratory obstruction associated with meningomyelocele. *Arch Dis Child* 40: 687–688.

Francis PM, Beales S, Rekate HL, Pittman HW, Manwaring K, Reiff J (1992) Chronic tonsillar herniation and Crouzon's syndrome. *Pediatr Neurosurg* 18: 202–206.

Frank Y, Kravath RE, Pollak CP, Weitzman ED (1983) Obstructive sleep apnea and its therapy: clinical and polysomnographic manifestations. *Pediatrics* 71: 737–742.

Gleeson K, Zwillich CW (1992) Adenosine stimulation, ventilation, and arousal from sleep. *Am Rev Respir Dis* 145: 453–457.

Gleeson K, Zwillich CW, White DB (1990) The influence of increasing ventilatory effort on arousal from sleep. *Am Rev Respir Dis* 142: 295–300.

Goldstein SJ, Wu RHK, Thorpy MJ, Shprintzen J, Marion RE, Saenger P (1987) Reversibility of deficient sleep entrained growth hormone secretion in a boy with achondroplasia and obstructive sleep apnea. *Acta Endocrinol* 116: 95–101.

Goldstein NA, Sculerati N, Walsleben JA, Bhatia N, Friedman DM, Rapoport DM (1994) Clinical diagnosis of pediatric obstructive sleep apnea validated by polysomnography. *Otolaryngol Head Neck Surg* 111: 611–617.

Gonsalez S, Thompson D, Hayward R, Lane R (1996) Treatment of obstructive sleep apnoea using nasal CPAP in children with craniofacial dysostoses. *Childs Nerv Syst* 12: 713–719.

Gonsalez S, Hayward R, Jones B, Lane R (1997) Upper airway obstruction and raised intracranial pressure in children with craniosynostosis. *Eur Respir J* 10(2): 367–375.

Gonsalez S, Thompson D, Hayward R, Lane R (1998) Breathing patterns in children with craniofacial dysostosis and hindbrain herniation. *Eur Respir J* 11: 866–872.

Gould GA, Gugger M, Molloy J, Tsara V, Shapiro CM, Douglas NJ (1988) Breathing pattern and eye movement density during REM sleep in humans. *Am J Respir Dis* 138: 874–877.

Gozal D (1998) Sleep disordered breathing and school performance in children. *Pediatrics* 102: 616–620.

Gozal D, Pope DW (2001) Snoring during early childhood and academic performance at age thirteen to fourteen years. *Pediatrics* 107: 1394–1399.

Graham MD (1963) Bilateral vocal cord paralysis associated with meningomyelocele and the Arnold–Chiari malformation. *Laryngoscope* 73: 85–92.

Guilleminault C, Eldridge F, Simmons F, Dement WC (1976a) Sleep apnea in eight children. *Pediatrics* 58: 23–31.

Guilleminault C, Tilkian A, Dement W (1976b) The sleep apnea syndromes. *Ann Rev Med* 27: 465–484.

Guilleminault C, Korobkin R, Winkle R (1981) A review of 50 children with obstructive sleep apnea syndrome. *Lung* 159: 275–287.

Guilleminault C, Winkle R, Korobkin R, Simmons B (1982) Children and nocturnal snoring: evaluation of the effects of sleep-related respiratory resistive load and day time functioning. *Eur J Pediatr* 139: 165–171.

Guilleminault C, Pelayo R, Leger D, Clerk A, Bocian RCZ (1996) Recognition of sleep disordered breathing in children. *Pediatrics* 98: 871–882.

Heaf DP, Helms PJ, Dinwiddie R, Matthew DJ (1982) Nasopharyngeal airways in Pierre Robin syndrome. *J Pediatr* 100: 698–703.

Hertz G, Cataletto M, Feinsilver SH, Angulo M (1993) Sleep and breathing patterns in patients with Prader Willi syndrome: effects of age and gender. *Sleep* 16: 366–371.

Jarund M, Lauritzen C (1996) Craniofacial dysostosis: airway obstruction and craniofacial surgery. *Scand J Plast Reconstr Surg Hand Surg* 30: 275–279.

Kakitsuba N, Sadaoka T, Motoyama S, Fujiwara Y, Kanai R, Hayashi I, Takahashi H (1994) Sleep apnea and sleep-related breathing disorders in patients with craniofacial synostosis. *Acta Otolaryngol Suppl* 517: 6–10.

Kosko JR, Derkay CS (1995) Uvulopalatopharyngoplasty: treatment of obstructive sleep apnea in neurologically impaired pediatric patients. *Int J Pediatr Otorhinolaryngol* 32: 241–246.

Lauritzen C, Lilja J, Jarlstedt J (1986) Airway obstruction and sleep apnea in children with craniofacial anomalies. *Plast Reconstr Surg* 77: 1–6.

Lea S, Ali NJ, Goldman M, Loa L, Fleetman J, Stradling JR (1990) Systolic blood pressure swings reflect inspiratory effort during simulated obstructive sleep apnoea. In: Horne J, editor. *Sleep '90*. Bochum: Pontenagel Press, pp 178–181.

189

Levy AM, Tabakin BS, Hanon JS, Narkewicz RM (1967) Hypertrophied adenoids causing pulmonary hypertension and severe congestive heart failure. *N Engl J Med* 277: 506–511.

Lim J, McKean M (2003) Adenotonsillectomy for obstructive sleep apnoea in children (Cochrane review). In: *The Cochrane Library*, Issue 1, Oxford: Update Software.

Lind M, Lundell B (1982) Tonsillar hyperplasia in children. *Arch Otolaryngol Head Neck Surg* 108: 650–654.

McColley SA, Carroll JL, April MM, Naclerio RN, Loughlin GM (1992) Respiratory compromise after adenotonsillectomy in children with obstructive sleep apnea syndrome. *Arch Otolaryngol Head Neck Surg* 118: 940–943.

Magnussen G (1944) *Studies on the Respiration during Sleep*. London: Lewis.

Mandel EM, Reynolds CF (1985) Sleep disorders associated with upper airway obstruction in children. *Int J Pediatr Otorhinolaryngol* 9: 173–182.

Marcus CL, Keens TG, Bautista DB, Von Pechmann WS, Davidson-Ward SL (1991) Obstructive sleep apnea in children with Down syndrome. *Pediatrics* 88: 132–139.

Massa F, Wallis C, Laverty A, Lane R (2000) Relationship of pulse transit time (PTT) to severity of sleep breathing disorders (SBD) in children. *Eur Respir J* 16: 272S.

Massa F, Gonsalez S, Laverty A, Wallis C, Lane R (2002) The use of nasal continuous airway pressure to treat obstructive sleep apnoea. *Arch Dis Child* 87: 438–443.

Menashe VD, Farrehi F, Miller M (1965) Hypoventilation and cor pulmonale due to chronic upper airway obstruction. *J Pediatr* 67: 198–203.

Moore MH (1993) Upper airway obstruction in the syndromal craniosynostoses. *Br J Plast Surg* 46: 355–362.

Owens-Stively J, McGuinn M, Berkelhammer L, Marcotte A, Nobile C, Spirito A (1997) Neuropsychological and behavioural correlates of obstructive sleep apnea in children. *Sleep Res* 26(suppl): 452. (Abstract.)

Pack AI (1995) Changes in respiratory motor activity during rapid eye movement sleep. In: Dempsey JA, Pack AI, editors. *Regulation of Breathing*. New York: Marcel Dekker, pp 983–1002.

Papasozomenos S, Roessmann U (1981) Respiratory distress and Arnold–Chiari malformation. *Neurology* 31: 97–100.

Phillipson EA (1978) Control of breathing during sleep. *Am Rev Respir Dis* 118: 909–939.

Pitson DJ, Sandell A, van der Hout R, Stradling JR (1995) Use of pulse transit time as a measure of inspiratory effort in patients with obstructive sleep apnoea. *Eur Respir J* 8:1669–1674.

Potsic WP, Pasquariello PS, Corsobaranak C, Marsh RR, Miller LM (1986) Relief of upper airway obstruction by adenotonsillectomy. *Otolaryngol Head Neck Surg* 94: 476–480.

Rechtschaffen A, Kales A (1968) *A Manual of Standardised Terminology, Techniques and Scoring System for Sleep Stages in Human Subjects*. Washington DC: National Institutes of Health. Publication no. 204.

Rhodes SK, Shimoda KC, Waid LR, O'Neil PM, Oexmann MJ, Collop NA, Willi SM (1995) Neurocognitive deficits in morbidly obese children with obstructive sleep apnea. *J Pediatr* 127: 741–744.

Rosen CL, D'Andrea L, Haddad GG (1992) Adult criteria for obstructive sleep apnea do not identify children with serious obstruction. *Am Rev Respir Dis* 146: 1231–1234.

Rosen GM, Muckle RP, Mahowald MW, Goding GS, Ullevig C (1994) Postoperative respiratory compromise in children with obstructive sleep apnea syndrome: can it be anticipated? *Pediatrics* 93: 784–788.

Saldino RM, Steinbach HL, Epstein CJ (1972) Familial acrocephalosyndactyly (Pfeiffer syndrome). *Am J Roentgenol Radium Ther Nucl Med* 116: 609–622.

Schafer ME (1982) Upper airway obstruction and sleep disorders in children with craniofacial anomalies. *Clin Plast Surg* 9: 555–567.

Schmidt-Nowara W, Snyder MJ (1983) A quantitative analysis of the relationship between REM and breathing in normal man. *Sleep Res* 12: 75–82.

Sculerati N, Gottlieb MD, Zimbler MS, Chibbaro PD, McCarthy JG (1998) Airway management in children with major craniofacial anomalies. *Laryngoscope* 108: 1806–1812.

Semenza GL, Pyeritz RE (1988) Respiratory complications of mucopolysaccharide storage disorders. *Medicine* 67: 209–219.

Sher AE (1992) Mechanisms of airway obstruction in Robin sequence: implications for treatment. *Cleft Palate Craniofac J* 29: 224–231.

Sher AE, Shprintzen RJ, Thorpy MJ (1989) Endoscopic observations of obstructive sleep apnea in children with anomalous upper airways: predictive and therapeutic value. *Int J Pediatr Otorhinolaryngol* 17: 1–11.

Shprintzen RJ (1988) Pharyngeal flap surgery and the pediatric upper airway. *Int Anesthesiol Clin* 26: 79–88.

Smith RP, Argod J, Pepin J-L, Levy PA (1999) Pulse transit time: an appraisal of potential clinical applications. *Thorax* 54: 452–458.

Snow JB, Rodgers KA (1965) Bilateral abductor paralysis of the vocal cords secondary to Arnold–Chiari malformation and its management. *Laryngoscope* 75: 316–321.

Sofer S, Weinhouse E, Tal A, Wanderman KL, Margulis G, Leiberman A, Gueron M (1988) Cor pulmonale due to adenoidal or tonsillar hypertrophy or both in children: non invasive diagnosis and follow-up. *Chest* 93: 119–122.

Solomon LM, Medenica M, Pruzansky S, Kreiborg S (1973) Apert syndrome and palatal mucopolysaccharides. *Teratology* 8: 287–291.

Stradling JR, Thomas G, Warley ARH, Williams P, Freeland A (1990) Effect of adenotonsillectomy on nocturnal hypoxaemia, sleep disturbance and symptoms in snoring children. *Lancet* 335: 249–253.

Suen JS, Arnold JE, Brooks LJ (1995) Adenotonsillectomy for the treatment of obstructive sleep apnea in children. *Arch Otolaryngol Head Neck Surg* 121: 525–530.

Thompson D, Gonsalez S, Lane R, Jones B, Harkness W, Hayward R (1994) Chronic tonsillar herniation in craniosynostosis – causes and effects. *Childs Nerv Syst* 10: 411. (Abstract.)

Trang TTH, Desguerre I, Goldman M, Delaperche MF, Gaultier CI (1993) Sleep-related breathing pattern in young children with neuromuscular disorders. *Am Rev Respir Dis* 147: A760. (Abstract.)

Vanes JL (1988) Arnold–Chiari malformation in an infant with Kleeblattschädel: an acquired malformation? *Neurosurgery* 23: 360–362.

Van Someren V, Burmeister M, Alusi G, Lane R (2000) Are sleep studies worth doing? *Arch Dis Child* 83: 76–81.

Waters KA, Everett F, Sillence D, Fagan E, Sullivan CE (1993) Breathing abnormalities in sleep in achondroplasia. *Arch Dis Child* 69: 191–196.

Weider DJ, Hauri PJ (1985) Nocturnal enuresis in children with upper airway obstruction. *Int J Pediatr Otorhinolaryngol* 9: 173–182.

Weissbluth M, Davis AT, Poncher J, Reiff J (1983) Signs of airway obstruction during sleep and behavioural, developmental and academic problems. *Dev Behav Pediatr* 4: 119–121.

Wilkinson AR, McCormick MS, Freeland AP, Pickering D (1981) Electrocardiographic signs of pulmonary hypertension in children who snore. *BMJ* 282: 1579–1581.

10
OCULAR ASPECTS OF CRANIOSYNOSTOSIS

Ken K. Nischal

Introduction

Craniofacial disorders may comprise various entities such as clefting anomalies, tumours, e.g. fibrous dysplasia, orbito-facio-cranial trauma and the craniosynostoses. Each may have significant ocular involvement but the focus of this chapter is the craniosynostoses.

Craniosynostosis is the premature closure of one or more cranial sutures and this may be associated with systemic features or an isolated finding (Fries and Katowitz 1990). When a suture closes prematurely, growth of the skull continues parallel to the suture but is arrested or retarded perpendicular to it (see Fig. 10.1). Premature closure of the coronal sutures results in a relative recession of the frontal process (see Fig. 10.2) which may affect the action of the extraocular muscles (see later).

As previously discussed, mutations in FGFR2 (fibroblast growth factor receptor type 2) have been shown to cause Crouzon, Jackson–Weiss, Apert and Pfeiffer syndromes (Jabs et al 1994, Reardon et al 1994, Wilkie et al 1995). Fibroblast growth factor is involved in a variety of activities including mitogenesis, angiogenesis and wound healing. FGFR is a membrane-spanning tyrosine kinase receptor (De Moerlooze and Dickson 1997). FGFR2 mutations shown to be responsible for the syndromic craniosynostoses mentioned are thought to cause a gain-of-function effect rather than a loss-of-function effect (Galvin et al 1996), which may explain then the increased closure rate of the sutures concerned. Other FGFR types have also been implicated including FGFR1 (Pfeiffer syndrome) (Muenke et al 1994) and FGFR3 (Crouzon syndrome with acanthosis nigricans, and certain cases of non-syndromic unicoronal synostosis – Muenke's syndrome) (Meyers et al 1995, Reardon et al 1997). FGFR3 has also been implicated in some cases of achondroplasia. Crouzon, Apert and Pfeiffer syndromes all share features such as midfacial hypoplasia of varying degrees with shallow orbits, craniosynostoses, but differ from the systemic features involved (as discussed earlier). Patients with Saethre–Chotzen syndrome display mild syndactyly with webbing between the fingers and often show ptosis. Some cases of Saethre–Chotzen syndrome have been shown to be due to mutations in the TWIST gene (Howard et al 1997), a transcription factor gene, which controls myogenesis. Craniofrontonasal dysplasia is an X-linked dominant condition, in which females only are affected. There is often marked hypertelorism, craniosynostoses and a very mild cleft of the tip of the nose.

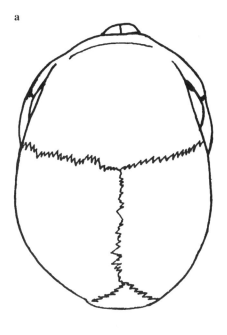
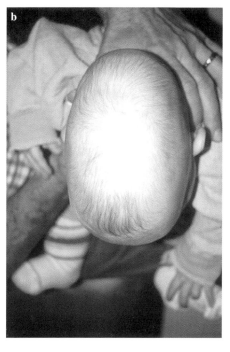

Fig. 10.1 (a) Superior view of the skull showing the sagittal suture, coronal sutures and lambdoid sutures. (b) A patient with sagittal synostosis; the anterior–posterior diameter is increased while the bi-parietal diameter is decreased. This is due to the fact that the growth parallel to the suture that closes early is increased while the growth perpendicular to it is decreased.

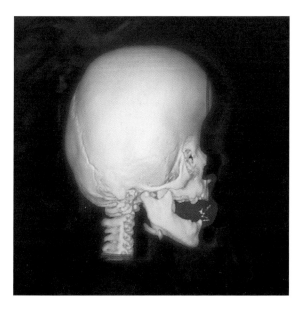

Fig. 10.2 3D CT of a child with bi-coronal synostosis. This has resulted this time in a decreased anterior–posterior diameter and an increased bi-parietal diameter; the decreased anterior–posterior diameter means that the frontal process is relatively recessed as shown.

The role of the ophthalmologist

The ocular aspects of the craniosynostoses may be considered in terms of detection and prevention of visual loss, ocular motility problems, binocular vision, lacrimal duct problems and miscellaneous ocular problems.

VISUAL LOSS

The most important role for the ophthalmologist is the detection of visual loss. This may be due to optic neuropathy, amblyopia and corneal scarring secondary to exposure keratopathy (Hertle et al 1991). Amblyopia is a loss in vision due to abnormal visual stimuli or input, which develops up to the age of approximately 8 years. Countering any detected cause for the amblyopia (e.g. giving spectacle correction if needed) and then patching the better eye can reverse it. This latter is called occlusion therapy. It stimulates normal visual development in the affected eye. Amblyopia may be due to a difference in refractive error of the two eyes (anisometropic amblyopia), moderate to severe refractive error of both eyes (ametropic amblyopia), abnormal shape of the cornea leading to astigmatism (meridional amblyopia), deprivation of light stimulus (deprivation amblyopia) or ocular misalignment (strabismic amblyopia).

In a retrospective review (Khan et al 2003) of 141 cases of syndromic craniosynostoses (Apert, Crouzon, Pfeiffer and Saethre–Chotzen) we found 40.3 per cent of patients had 1 dioptre or more of astigmatism in at least one eye with mean age at last examination of 68.1 months (SD 53.8). Age-matched normals range from 2.3 to 30 per cent at 2–3 years

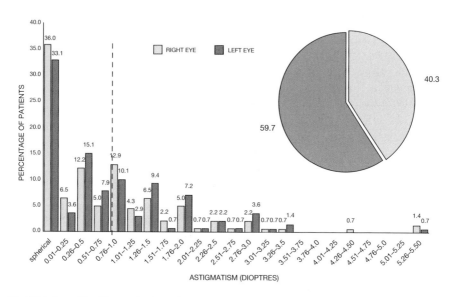

Fig. 10.3 Overall incidence of astigmatism. Pie chart insert shows that 40.3 per cent of patients have one dioptre or more of astigmatism.

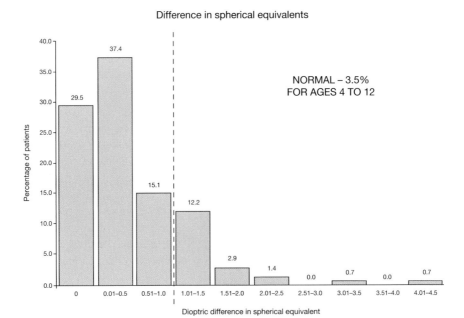

Fig. 10.4 Difference in spherical equivalent refraction between the two eyes by varying amounts; 18 per cent of patients were found to have one dioptre or more of difference between the two eyes (anisometropia). Normal age-match controls would have an incidence of 3.5 per cent of one dioptre or more of anisometropia.

old (Favian 1966, Gwiazda et al 1984) and 6 to 18 per cent at 8 years of age (Hirsch 1963, Dobson et al 1984). This is important because astigmatism is strongly amblyogenic if untreated with appropriate spectacle correction (see Fig. 10.3).

We also found anisometropia of 1 dioptre or more in 18 per cent of patients (age-matched normals 3.5 per cent (Gupta and Gupta 2000)), which again indicates an increased risk of amblyogenic visual loss if untreated (see Fig. 10.4).

Refractive error is common then in craniosynostoses and astigmatism may be significant. The astigmatism may be secondary to corneal scarring, ptosis, and the abnormal shape of the orbits, which in itself is secondary to the synostoses.

Accurate refraction is very important and customised spectacles are essential if the child is to accept the refractive error correction. The problem, especially with the syndromic synostoses, is that several factors have made the examination of these children very difficult; midfacial hypoplasia often leads to crowded upper airways making breathing difficult and laboured, while exposure keratopathy makes these children photophobic and intensely upset during examination with any type of light-emitting instrument. It is essential to consider examination under anaesthetic in children who have had inadequate assessment in the clinic. Co-operation between the ophthalmologist and craniofacial surgeons allows reduction of general anaesthetics by co-ordinated scheduling. At Great Ormond Street Hospital for Children our clinical co-ordination nurse facilitates this.

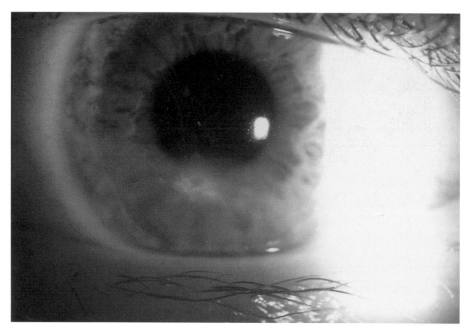

Fig. 10.5 Corneal scarring secondary to exposure keratopathy in child with Apert syndrome.

Exposure keratopathy, commonly seen in craniosynostotic patients (Fries and Katowitz 1990) (see Fig. 10.5), is due to proptosis from shallow orbits secondary to midfacial hypoplasia and a short skull base. These children often sleep with their eyes slightly open and this results in desiccation of the cornea with breakdown of the corneal epithelium. If it is prolonged, inflammatory responses result in invasion of the cornea with blood vessels, fibrovascular membrane formation and permanent scarring. The result is deprivation of stimulus and/or astigmatism. Lubrication especially at night is very important, but sometimes this is not enough and traditionally tarsorraphy has been advocated in such cases. Although tarsorraphy still has a role in these difficult cases it is limited since the main problem is midface hypoplasia and midfacial distraction creates more orbital volume (Polley et al 1995). In severe cases where there is often subluxation of the globe with severe exposure keratopathy midfacial distraction is an option that should be considered. In cases of massive chemosis postoperatively a blanket decision to perform tarsorraphies may not be rational. If the orbit is tight, the globe cannot be retropulsed easily, and then large tarsorraphies will increase the intraorbital pressure and therefore the intraocular pressure. Under these circumstances the optic nerve is at greater risk of damage. Proptosis and chemosis are the body's coping mechanism with too much orbital tissue – a large tarsorraphy negates this mechanism. Small lateral tarsorraphies are sometimes useful to provide some protection in cases of recurrent chemosis or corneal breakdown in children who will not allow sufficient application of lubricating eye ointment (see Fig. 10.6).

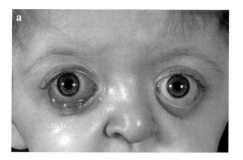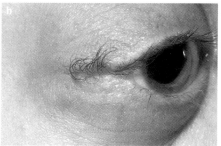

Fig. 10.6 (a) Chemosis of the right conjunctiva due to exposure because of proptosis. (b) Small lateral tarsorrhaphy to deal with the type of exposure shown in (a).

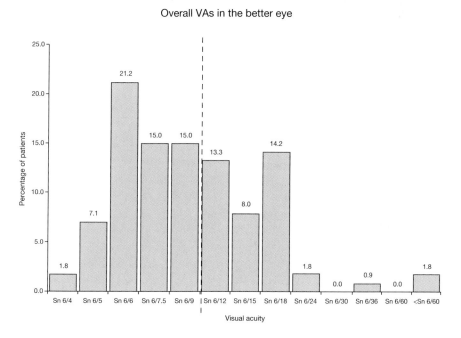

Overall VAs in the better eye

Fig. 10.7 Visual outcome in terms of Snellen equivalent. Just under 40 per cent of patients had 20/40 or worse vision (dotted line) in their better eye.

The visual outcome results in our study (Khan et al 2003) showed 39.8 per cent of patients had visual acuity of *20/40 or worse* in their better eye (see Fig. 10.7). The cause of the visual loss may be due to amblyopia, optic neuropathy or both.

Visual loss due to optic neuropathy has been described in children with syndromic craniosynostoses (Fries and Katowitz 1990, Hertle et al 1991). Traditionally the ophthalmologist has been asked to check these children's fundi for evidence of papilloedema, which

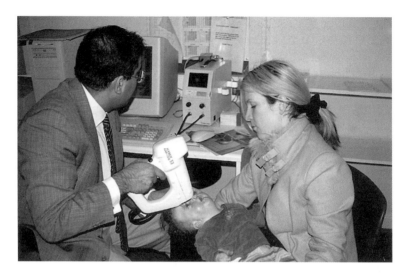

Fig. 10.8 Using the Nidek digital hand-held camera to take optic disc recordings in a child with Pfeiffer syndrome.

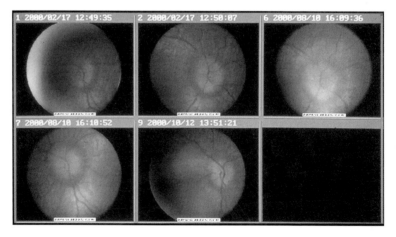

Fig. 10.9 Digitally captured images of the same patient on different visits, using the Nidek camera. The two pictures at the bottom show clear evidence of a decrease in optic nerve swelling with time, whereas the two pictures on the top right show no decrease in swelling of the optic disc on that side with time.

is not always easy. Several factors have made the examination of these children very difficult; as already mentioned, midfacial hypoplasia often leads to crowded upper airways making breathing difficult and laboured, while exposure keratopathy makes these children photophobic and intensely upset during examination with a bright indirect ophthalmoscope. We use digital photography (Nidek) which uses infra-red to image the optic disc through a dilated pupil; when an adequate image is obtained a momentary flash allows colour images to be stored on hard disk (see Fig. 10.8). This allows serial images to be stored at follow-up visits allowing objective comparisons (see Fig. 10.9).

Unfortunately there is good evidence that the optic disc appearance is not a reliable indicator of raised intracranial pressure or optic neuropathy (Tuite et al 1996). Mursch et al (1998) have shown that 25 per cent of 52 patients with craniosynostoses displayed abnormal flash visual evoked potentials (VEP) responses with normal-looking optic discs. We have found that 66 per cent of 184 patients with both syndromic and non-syndromic craniosynostoses (111 syndromic and 73 non-syndromic) had abnormal pattern reversal VEPs in terms of amplitude, latency, morphology, or any combination of these, compared to age-matched normals (Thompson et al 2002). It is our practice now to record baseline VEPs in all patients attending the craniofacial clinic for the first time. This then allows for the use of follow-up VEPs to look for deterioration.

In some cases continued deterioration of the pattern VEP in the presence of stable visual acuity has prompted craniofacial intervention which has resulted in an improvement in the amplitude and latency of the pattern VEP, especially at the smaller check sizes (see Fig. 10.10).

The cause of optic neuropathy is controversial. Certainly the phenomenon of cranio-cerebral disproportion is well described in the literature but it is clear that raised intracranial pressure may be present in the absence of reduced intracranial volume (Fok et al 1992). Evidence in the ophthalmic literature suggests that in elderly patients sleep apnoea syndrome may account for both papilloedema and anterior ischemic optic neuropathy (Purvin et al 2000, Mojon et al 2002) resulting in visual loss.

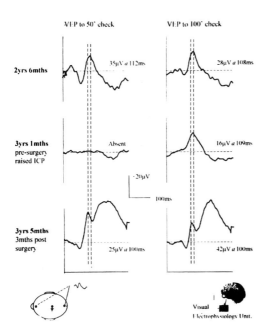

Fig. 10.10 Pattern reversal visual evoked potentials recording before and after bi-parietal expansion. It can be seen that for 50-minute checks the response becomes attenuated but after craniofacial intervention the amplitude has increased significantly. This is true for both 50-minute and 100-minute checks. (Courtesy of Dorothy Thompson and Alki Liasis.)

Patients with syndromic craniosynostosis often have breathing difficulties and sleep apnoea has been well described in this group of children, with raised intracranial pressure being postulated as a consequence of hypercapnia (Gonzalez et al 1997). However, is it possible that sleep apnoea could cause hypoxic damage? The craniofacial unit at Great Ormond Street Hospital for Children has shown that in complex syndromic craniosynostoses there is decreased flow in the sigmoid-jugular sinus complex with a consequent florid collateral circulation through the stylomastoid emissary venous complex (Taylor et al 2001). This results in venous hypertension, raised intracranial pressure and also excessive collateral vasculature. Whether these events result in disordered autoregulation is unknown, but if they did, it would lead to hypoxia during sleep apnoeic episodes. Add to this that some patients with craniosynostoses may also suffer from hydrocephalus and the causes of optic neuropathy are complex (see Fig. 10.11).

In summary, optic disc swelling may result from cranio-cerebral disproportion, hydrocephalus, intracranial venous hypertension, hypercapnia from obstructive sleep apnoea or a combination of any of these factors, while sleep apnoea may also cause hypoxic damage to an already compromised (from chronic swelling) optic nerve.

There is still the issue of continued visual loss in the absence of swollen optic discs. Evidence from the literature (Lepore 1992, Huff et al 1996, Wang et al 1998) suggests that idiopathic intracranial hypertension may occur without papilledema, and some authors have postulated that this may be due to optic nerve sheath anomalies or lamina cribrosa changes

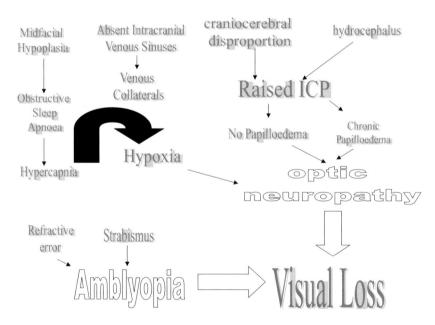

Fig. 10.11 Scheme showing potential causes of optic neuropathy in patients with syndromic craniosynostosis (K.K. Nischal and R. Hayward).

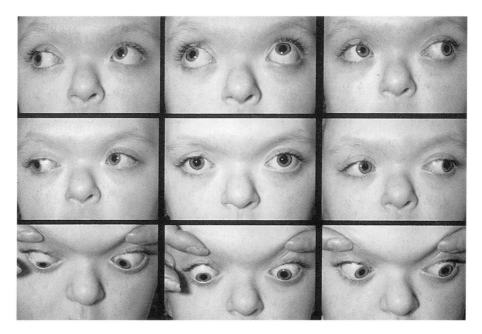

Fig. 10.12 Child with Apert syndrome. Figure shows nine positions of gaze. When the child looks up, the deviation between the two eyes increases, but when she looks down it decreases: this is called a V pattern.

due to increased collagen or decreased elasticity (Lepore 1992). Whether this is so in cases of syndromic craniosynostoses is as yet unknown but it may well be a possibility.

In summary, visual loss may be due to amblyopia, exposure keratopathy, optic neuropathy or any combination of these. The ophthalmologist must be aware of all three factors in order to intervene or direct intervention to prevent irreversible visual loss.

OCULAR MOTILITY AND BINOCULAR VISION

Strabismus (ocular misalignment) has been well described in both syndromic and non-syndromic craniosynostoses (Diamond and Whitaker 1984, Miller 1984, Morax 1984b, Carruthers 1988, Fries and Katowitz 1990, Roarty et al 1994).

Horizontal strabismus in primary position of gaze has been well described. If the angle of deviation changes with up- or downgaze then the horizontal strabismus is said to have a pattern – e.g. if a child is divergent (exotropia) in primary position of gaze and then the deviation *increases* on upgaze but *decreases* on downgaze, he or she is said to have a 'V' pattern exotropia; if the deviation had *decreased* in upgaze and *increased* in downgaze it would be termed an 'A' pattern exodeviation (see Fig. 10.12).

The V pattern exotropia is recognised as perhaps the commonest category seen in craniosynostotic patients (Ortiz Monasterio et al 1976, Morax et al 1983) (see Fig. 10.6). However, we found 38 per cent of patients with syndromic craniosynostoses (Apert, Pfeiffer, Crouzon and Saethre–Chotzen) presented with an exotropia in primary position, 32 per cent

201

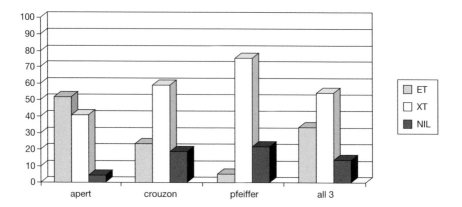

Fig. 10.13 Incidents of horizontal strabismus in those patients who had horizontal strabismus in primary position of gaze. It can be seen that exotropia appears to be the commonest type of horizontal strabismus except in cases of Apert syndrome.

Fig. 10.14 Alphabet patterns: the overwhelming majority of patients with a pattern deviation to their horizontal strabismus had a V pattern deviation.

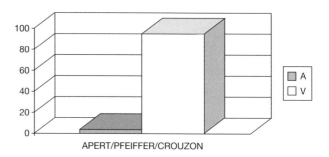

with esotropia (convergent), and 24 per cent were straight in the primary position (Khan et al 2003). By syndrome, Saethre–Chotzen and Apert presented with more esotropia than exotropia, while the reverse was true for Crouzon and Pfeiffer. This finding may be explained by the fact that some of our patients had already had craniofacial procedures by the time they attended our clinic and the tendency to esotropia post-craniofacial surgery is well established (Morax 1984a). Forty-four per cent of patients in our study were noted to have an alphabet pattern, of which 95 per cent showed a 'V' pattern as opposed to an 'A' (see Figs 10.13 and 10.14).

Binocular vision develops if the eyes are appropriately aligned. Stereopsis is a measure of binocularity which is commonly used by the ophthalmologist and his or her colleagues, namely orthoptists who are specialists in eye movement disorders. Stereopsis in patients with craniosynostoses is difficult to assess because a child may have a constant deviation in the primary position of gaze but have stereopsis and binocularity in another field of gaze where the eyes are aligned. This is an unusual situation but one that may be seen commonly in the craniosynostoses. Equally some cases may have stereopsis in the primary position but have an ocular deviation and no binocularity in any other field of gaze. Although it is safe to suggest that good stereopsis is rare in the syndromic craniosynostoses (Nelson et al 1981) the tendency to esotropia post-craniofacial surgery only leads to symptoms in those cases where stereovision is present preoperatively but has not been tested for. We reported diplopia postoperatively (Walker et al 2001) in three cases of hypertelorism correction (one with craniofrontonasal dysplasia, one with midline encephalocoeles and one with a clefting syndrome).

The type of craniofacial surgery may affect subsequent strabismus surgery; two cases of syndromic craniosynostoses who had never previously had strabismus surgery were found to have massive subconjunctival fibrosis at their first strabismus surgery (Rattigan and Nischal 2003). Both patients had undergone frontal advancement procedures previously which presumably had allowed blood to track into the subtenon space (i.e. subconjunctival). Vertical deviations in primary position of gaze are also well described in the craniosynostoses (Snir et al 1982, Pinchoff and Sandall 1985, Dufier et al 1986, Pollard 1988) and are attributed to overaction of the inferior oblique muscle due to a relative recession of the frontal process in cases of coronal synostosis, creating a mechanical disadvantage for the superior oblique muscle with subsequent overaction of the ipsilateral inferior oblique (see Fig. 10.15). While this holds true for non-syndromic uni- and bi-coronal synostoses, it is less likely to be the whole answer in the syndromic synostoses where midfacial

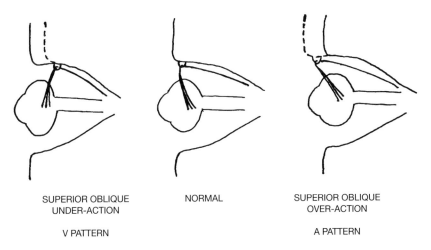

SUPERIOR OBLIQUE
UNDER-ACTION

NORMAL

SUPERIOR OBLIQUE
OVER-ACTION

V PATTERN

A PATTERN

Fig. 10.15 (see also Figure 10.2) The figure in the middle shows the normal relationship of the superior oblique tendon to the insertion to the superior oblique posterior to the equator of the eyeball. In cases of relative recession of the frontal process (left), the vector force of contraction of the muscle is changed because the angle between the tendon and the insertion of the muscle has changed. This leads to a mechanical disadvantage which leads to the antagonist muscle (the inferior oblique muscle) overacting, and can explain the V pattern that is often seen in these children. The figure on the right shows what happens when the frontal process is relatively advanced (for example in congenital or early childhood hydrocephalus), in which case the superior oblique is given an added advantage and an A pattern ensues.

203

hypoplasia also results in recession of the maxilla and floor of the orbit resulting in a mechanical disadvantage of the inferior oblique. Other mechanisms for vertical deviations in primary position of gaze include absent or anomalous superior rectus muscles (Weinstock and Hardesty 1965, Morax 1982, Snir et al 1982, Pollard 1988). In fact more than one rectus muscle may be absent or anomalous. The surgical correction of hypotropia due to anomalous or absent superior rectus muscles can be difficult but we have found a Foster-type modification of the Knapp procedure to be useful in such cases (Rattigan and Nischal 2003). Orbital imaging is important in all cases of suspected absent muscles but not always possible.

Not only can the extraocular muscles be absent, anomalous in position and in size, but they can also be structurally abnormal (Margolis et al 1977). Clinically this can be appreciated per-operatively when rectus muscles can feel gristly and inelastic.

Cheng et al (1993) described a dynamic anomaly of eye movements seen in some patients with syndromic craniosynostoses of cosmetic concern to some patients. This is an upshoot in adduction with a coincident downshoot of the abducting eye on lateroversions (see Fig. 10.16). Reports of pure inferior oblique weakening having little or no effect on the upshots in adduction (Coats et al 2000) confirmed the need for an additional explanation of the anomalous eye movements. Cheng suggested that these eye movements could be

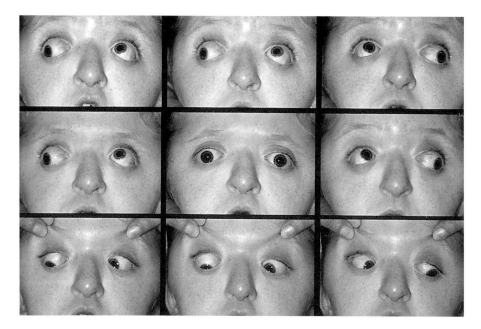

Fig. 10.16 Nine positions of gaze of another child with Apert syndrome. When the child looks to the left the right eye shoots up while the left eye shoots down. Similarly, when the child looks to the right the left eye shoots up and the right eye shoots down. These are the anomalous horizontal eye movements described in the text. In this particular case it can also be seen that in elevation the right eye does not elevate very well. This should raise the suspicion of absent or anomalous superior rectus muscle which has been described in this syndrome.

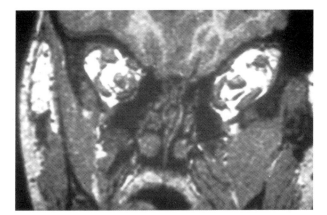

Fig. 10.17 Coronal MRI of a child with craniofrontonasal dysplasia showing that the extra-ocular muscles are exocyclorotated. This means that the superior rectus muscle is displaced laterally, the inferior rectus displaced medially, the medial rectus displaced superiorly, and the lateral rectus displaced inferiorly.

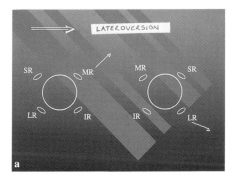 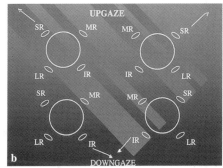

Fig. 10.18 (a) Schematic showing the effect of the vector forces on contraction of the displaced muscles when the child or patient looks to the left. The medial rectus now has a vector force superiorly as well as in adduction and the lateral rectus has a vector force inferiorly as well as abduction.
(b) Vector force on contraction of the displaced muscles, explaining the V pattern that is often seen in children with craniosynostosis.

explained by the fact that many of these patients have exocyclorotated orbits and extraocular muscles, resulting in an upwardly displaced medial rectus, downwardly displaced lateral rectus, laterally displaced superior rectus and medially displaced inferior rectus (see Fig. 10.17).

The resultant vector forces of the displaced muscles on contraction explained the abnormal eye movements on lateroversions as well as the 'V' pattern horizontal strabismus described earlier (see Fig. 10.18). We have found a downward displacement of the medial rectus and upward displacement of the lateral rectus together with anteriorisation of the inferior oblique to be an effective procedure to treat these anomalous horizontal eye movements (see Fig. 10.19). Not all patients with craniosynostosis have exocyclorotated orbits or extraocular muscles but many do. Orbital imaging is the criterion standard of diagnosing exocyclorotated extraocular muscles but this is not always possible to perform especially without general anaesthesia.

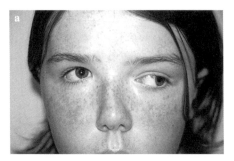 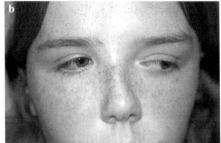

Fig. 10.19 (a) A child with non-syndromic craniosynostosis looking to the left preoperatively. (b) Looking to the left postoperatively. This girl had surgery to move the displaced muscles (medial rectus and lateral rectus on the right side) into a more normal position, and the inferior oblique muscle on that side has been extirpated. It was not possible to anteriorise it because she had already had three operations on that inferior oblique previously at other centres.

Fig. 10.20 Marked exocyclorotation of the fundus in a child with syndromic craniosynostosis.

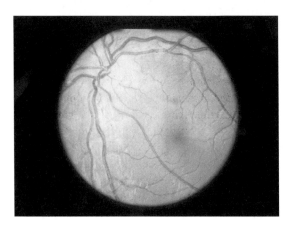

   Clinical clues to possible exocyclorotation of the orbit and muscles include marked exocyclorotation of the fundus (see Fig. 10.20) and the presence of these anomalous eye movements (upshoot in adduction with coincident downshoot in abduction) on lateroversions.

   When assessing the vertical deviation in primary position it is worth remembering that orbital dystopia is common in cases of unicoronal synostosis. We found 19 of 22 cases of unicoronal synostosis to have orbital dystopia (i.e. a vertical disparity between the level of the two orbits – see Fig. 10.21) (Dickinson et al 2001). It is noteworthy that some patients will develop diplopia or confusion after orbital dystopia correction, though in my experience these patients do not have detectable stereovision preoperatively. This suggests that they may have some form of crude binocularity. In all such cases it is worth considering the timing of craniofacial surgery for correction of the orbital dystopia. As stated earlier the visual system is plastic until the age of about 8 years; any change in the sensory input well before this age is unlikely to result in visual problems due to disruption of any (amount or type of) binocularity.

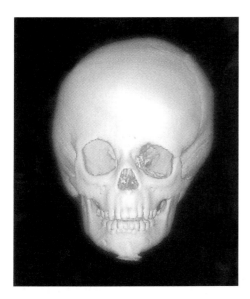

Fig. 10.21 3D CT of a child with right unicoronal synostosis in whom orbital dystopia is present radiologically.

Although at first sight the child with craniosynostoses may appear to have complex eye movements, their management is just like that of any other child with strabismus.

A family history is important because often the parent may be similarly affected (e.g. Crouzon syndrome, Saethre–Chotzen syndrome). Visual function assessment should include VEP in addition to acuity and colour vision measurement. A drop in vision may be due not only to amblyopia and/or refractive error but also to optic neuropathy even in the absence of a swollen optic disc. The presence of stereovision should be checked, especially if the child is about to undergo hypertelorism correction where postoperative diplopia might be distressing to the child and parents if not forewarned.

Any strabismus surgery should be delayed until after craniofacial surgery and the type of craniofacial surgery performed prior to any strabismus surgery noted. Certain types of craniofacial surgery may result in subconjunctival fibrosis, which lengthens the time needed before strabismus surgery can be performed. Only after orbital imaging (if possible) should any surgery be undertaken. The absence of rectus muscles should also be considered and a surgical plan with alternatives prepared prior to operation. Anomalous eye movements on lateroversions can be difficult to treat, but transposing the horizontal recti to a more normal position together with anteriorisation of the inferior oblique is an option.

LACRIMAL DUCT PROBLEMS

Problems with tear overflow are commonly seen in children with craniofacial disorders. The two main groups that are affected are the children with midline clefts and those with Saethre–Chotzen syndrome. Simple probing of the nasolacrimal duct should be attempted but is often unhelpful either because of absence of the puncta or because of a bony abnormality within the nasolacrimal duct itself. If it is the former then a conjunctivo-dacrocystorhinostomy (CJDCR) may be needed, and if it is the latter a dacrocystogram

(DCG) is needed to localise the bony abnormality. Open dacrocystorhinostomy (DCR) may then be performed or endonasal DCR, usually with the assistance of the ENT surgeon.

MISCELLANEOUS OCULAR PROBLEMS

Ptosis repair can be problematic especially in children with Saethre–Chotzen syndrome. The difficulty is that these children often have very poor levator palpebrae superioris function and need a brow suspension from a very early stage. They develop abnormal head postures (usually chin up) to be able to see straight ahead and this has an adverse affect on their motor development. Autologous fascia lata is the material of choice but often cannot be performed before the age of 4 years. It is not acceptable to wait to this age if there is evidence of amblyopia which is not being successfully treated with patching and spectacle correction or if there is evidence of motor development delay. Under such circumstances artificial materials such as mersilene mesh or prolene may be used. Very occasionally if there is moderate levator function and a healthy corneal surface, a levator resection may be performed.

Lid colobomas may be seen in Treacher–Collins syndrome, Goldenhar syndrome and other clefting syndromes. Lubrication of the globe is essential in these circumstances until definitive lid reconstruction can be performed.

Very rarely glaucoma may be present in the craniosynostoses (Lowry and MacLean 1977) and the examining physician should be wary of a child with 'beautiful big eyes' as these may well be due to buphthalmos in cases of congenital or infantile glaucoma.

REFERENCES

Carruthers JDA (1988) Strabismus in craniofacial dysostosis. *Graefe's Arch Clin Exp Ophthalmol* 226: 230–234.

Cheng H, Burdon MA, Shun-Sin GA, Czypionka S (1993) Dissociated eye movements in craniosynostosis: a hypothesis revived. *Br J Ophthalmol* 77: 563–568.

Coats DK, Paysse EA, Stager DR (2000) Surgical management of V-pattern strabismus and oblique dysfunction in craniofacial dysostosis. *J AAPOS* 4(6): 338–342.

De Moerlooze L, Dickson C (1997) Skeletal disorders associated with FGFR mutations. *Curr Opin Genet Dev* 7: 378–385.

Diamond GR, Whitaker L (1984) Ocular motility in craniofacial reconstruction. *Plast Reconstr Surg* 73: 31–35.

Dickinson K, Neill-Dwyer J, Chong K, Nischal KK (2001) Presence of orbital dystopia in unicoronal synostosis. In: Claes Lauritzen, editor. *Craniofacial Surgery IX, Proceedings of the IX International Congress of the International Society of Craniofacial Surgery*. Bologna: Monduzzi Editore, pp 15–18.

Dobson V, Fulton AB, Sebris SL (1984) Cycloplegic refraction of infants and young children: the axis of astigmatism. *Invest Ophthalmol Vis Sci* 25: 83–87.

Dufier JL, Vinuriel MC, Renier D, Marchac D (1986) Les complications ophtalmolgiques des cranio-facistenoses. *J Fr Ophtalmol* 9: 273–278.

Favian G (1966) Ophthalmological examination of 1200 children up to age 2. *Acta Ophthalmol* 44: 473–479.

Fok H, Jones BM, Gault DG et al (1992) Relationship between intracranial pressure and intracranial volume in craniosynostosis. *Br J Plast Surg* 45(5): 394–397.

Fries PD, Katowitz JA (1990) Congenital craniofacial anomalies of ophthalmic importance. *Surv Ophthalmol* 35: 87–119.

Galvin BD, Hart KC, Meyer AN et al (1996) Constitutive receptor activation by Crouzon syndrome mutations in FGFR2 and FGFR2/neu chimeras. *Proc Natl Acad Sci USA* 93: 7894–7899.

Gonzalez S, Hayward R, Jones B et al (1997) Upper airway obstruction and raised intracranial pressure in children with craniosynostosis. *Eur Respir J* 10(2): 367–375.

Gupta M, Gupta Y (2000) A survey on refractive error and strabismus among schoolchildren in a school at Aligarh. *Indian J Public Health* 44(3): 90–93.

Gwiazda J, Scheiman M, Mohindra I et al (1984) Astigmatism in children: changes in axis and amount from birth to six years. *Invest Ophthalmol Vis Sci* 25: 88–92.

Hertle RW, Quinn GE, Minguini N, Katowitz JA (1991) Visual loss in patients with craniofacial synostosis. *J Paediatr Ophthalmol Strab* 28: 344–349.

Hirsch MJ (1963) Changes in astigmatism during the first eight years in school – an interim report from the Ojai Longitudinal Study. *Am J Optom Arch Am Acad Optom* 40: 127–132.

Howard TD, Paznekas WA, Green ED et al (1997) Mutation in TWIST, a basic helix-loop-helix transcription factor in Saethre–Chotzen syndrome. *Nat Genet* 15(1): 36–41.

Huff AL, Hupp SL, Rothrock JF (1996) Chronic daily headache with migrainous features due to papilloedema-negative idiopathic intracranial hypertension. *Cephalgia* 16(6): 451–452.

Jabs EW, Scott AF, Meyers G et al (1994) Jackson–Weiss and Crouzon syndromes are allelic with mutations in FGFR2. *Nat Genet* 8: 275–279.

Khan S, Nischal KK, Dean F, Hayward R, Walker J (2003) Visual morbidity in craniosynostoses – review of 141 cases. *Br J Ophthalmol* 87(8): 999–1003.

Lepore FE (1992) Unilateral and highly asymmetric papilledema in pseudotumor cerebri. *Neurology* 42 (3 pt 1): 676–678.

Lowry RB, MacLean JR (1977) Syndrome of mental retardation, cleft palate, eventration of diaphragm, congenital heart defect, glaucoma, growth failure and craniosynostosis. *Birth Defects Orig Artic Ser* 13(3B): 203–228.

Margolis S, Pachter BR, Breinin GM (1977) Structural alterations of extraocular muscle associated with Apert's syndrome. *Br J Ophthalmol* 61: 683–689.

Meyers GA, Orlow SJ, Munro IR et al (1995) FGFR3 transmembrane mutation in Crouzon syndrome with acanthosis nigricans. *Nat Genet* 11: 462–464.

Miller MT (1984) Ocular abnormalities in craniofacial malformations. *Int Ophthalmol Clin* 24: 143–163.

Mojon D, Hedges TR III, Ehrenberg B et al (2002) Association between sleep apnea syndrome and nonarteritic anterior ischemic optic neuropathy. *Arch Ophthalmol* 120(5): 601–605.

Morax S (1982) Absence du muscle droit superieur dans le syndrome d'Apert. *J Fr Ophtalmol* 5: 323–326.

Morax S (1984a) Change in eye position after cranio-facial surgery. *J Maxillofac Surg* 12: 47–55.

Morax S (1984b) Oculo-motor disorders in craniofacial malformations. *J Maxillofac Surg* 12: 1–10.

Morax S, Pascal D, Barraco P (1983) Signification du syndrome 'V' avec double 'Up shoot'. *J Fr Ophtalmol* 6: 295–310.

Muenke M, Schell U, Hehr A et al (1994) A common mutation in the FGFR1 gene in Pfeiffer syndrome. *Nat Genet* 8: 269–274.

Mursch K, Brockmann K, Lang JK, Markakis E, Behnke-Mursch J (1998) Visually evoked potentials in 52 children requiring operative repair of craniosynostosis. *Pediatr Neurosurg* 29(6): 320–323.

Nelson LB, Ingoglia S, Breinin GM (1981) Sensorimotor disturbances in Craniostenosis. *J Pediatr Ophthalmol Strab* 18(5): 32–40.

Ortiz Monasterio F, Fuente del Campo A, Limon-Brown E (1976) Mechanism and correction of V syndrome in craniofacial dysostosis. In: *Symposium on Plastic Surgery in the Orbital Region*. St Louis: Mosby, pp 246–254.

Pinchoff BS, Sandall G (1985) Congenital absence of the superior oblique tendon in craniofacial dysostosis. *Ophthalmic Surg* 16: 375–377.

Pollard ZF (1988) Bilateral superior oblique muscle palsy associated with Apert's syndrome. *Am J Ophthalmol* 106: 337–340.

Polley JW, Figueroa AA, Charbel FT, Berkowitz R, Reisberg D, Cohen M (1995) Monobloc craniomaxillofacial distraction osteogenesis in a newborn with severe craniofacial synostosis: a preliminary report. *J Craniofac Surg* 6(5): 421–423.

Purvin VA, Kawasaki A, Yee RD (2000) Papilledema and obstructive sleep apnea syndrome. *Arch Ophthalmol* 118(12): 1626–1630.

Rattigan S, Nischal KK (2003) Foster modification of Knapp procedure for anomalous superior rectus muscles in syndromic craniosynostoses. *J AAPOS* 7(4): 279–282.

Reardon W, Winter RM, Rutland P et al (1994) Mutations in the fibroblast growth factor receptor 2 gene (FGFR2) cause Crouzon syndrome. *Nat Genet* 8: 98–103.

Reardon W, Wilkes D, Rutland P et al (1997) Craniosynostosis associated with FGFR3 pro250arg mutation results in a range of clinical presentations including unisutural sporadic craniosynostosis. *J Med Genet* 34: 632–636.

Roarty JD, Pron GE, Siegel-Bartelt J, Posnick JC, Buncic JR (1994) Ocular manifestations of frontonasal dysplasia. *Plast Reconstr Surg* 93: 25–30.

Snir M, Gilad E, Ben-sira I (1982) An unusual extraocular muscle anomaly in a patient with Crouzon's disease. *Br J Ophthalmol* 66: 253–257.

Taylor WJ, Hayward RD, Lasjaunias P et al (2001) Enigma of raised intracranial pressure in patients with complex craniosynostosis: the role of intracranial venous drainage. *J Neurosurg* 94(3): 377–385.

Thompson DA, Nischal KK, Liasis A, Hardy S, Hagan R, Hayward R (2002) The prevalence of visual dysfunction in craniosynostosis. Presented at ISCEV, July 2002, Loeven, Belgium.

Tuite GF, Chong WK, Evanson J, Narita A, Taylor D, Harkness WF, Jones BM, Hayward RD (1996) The effectiveness of papilledema as an indicator of raised intracranial pressure in children with craniosynostosis. *Neurosurgery* 38(2): 272–278.

Walker J, Jones BM, Nischal KK (2001) Diplopia post craniofacial reconstruction for hypertelorism. In: Claes Lauritzen, editor. *Craniofacial Surgery IX, Proceedings of the IX International Congress of the International Society of Craniofacial Surgery*. Bologna: Monduzzi Editore, pp 215–216.

Wang SJ, Silberstein SD, Patterson S et al (1998) Idiopathic intracranial hypertension without papilledema: a case control study in a headache center. *Neurology* 51(1): 245–249

Weinstock FR, Hardesty HH (1965) Absence of superior rectus in craniofacial dysostosis. *Arch Ophthalmol* 74: 152–153.

Wilkie AM, Slaney SF, Oldridge M et al (1995) Apert syndrome results from localised mutations of FGFR2 and is allelic with Crouzon syndrome. *Nat Genet* 9: 165–172.

11

THE DENTAL AND ORTHODONTIC MANAGEMENT OF CRANIOSYNOSTOSIS

Robert D. Evans and Rachel Bradford

Introduction

Craniosynostosis, in the syndromic and to a lesser extent in the non-syndromic forms, affects the growth and development of the facial skeleton, which in turn affects the relationship between the jaws and therefore the teeth (occlusion). Although tooth development does not appear to be affected, the eruption of the dentition is frequently delayed. In addition, the maxilla in the syndromic forms is hypoplastic, to a varying degree, and results in insufficient space for the teeth – this is referred to as dental crowding. Complex craniofacial surgery frequently alters the relationship between the jaws and therefore the teeth. The stage/timing of tooth development and eruption and/or the position of unerupted teeth in the maxilla affects timing of surgery.

Tooth development/eruption and establishment of the occlusion

For a concise overview of this subject read chapters 3, 4 and 5 in *Orthodontics and Occlusal Management* (Shaw 1993).

The development of the teeth (odontogenesis) is a highly co-ordinated and complex process which relies upon cell-to-cell interactions that result in the initiation and generation of the tooth (Cobourne 1999). All teeth develop from a structure called the dental lamina which forms *in utero* between 4 and 6 weeks of age. The early tooth buds develop into tooth germs and consist of the enamel organ (which produces the enamel), dental papilla (which produces the dentine/pulp) and the dental sac (which produces the cementum). The buds for the permanent teeth develop on the lingual aspect of the deciduous teeth. This results in the development of 20 deciduous and 32 permanent teeth (Tables 11.1(a) and 11.1(b)).

The eruption of the deciduous dentition starts with the lower incisors (age 6–8 months) and ends at approximately 28 months with the eruption of the second molars. The permanent dentition starts to erupt between the ages of 6 and 7 years of age with the eruption of the first permanent molars and lower central incisors. Over the next 4–5 years the remainder of the permanent dentition erupts so that by the age of 13, with the exception of the third molars, all the permanent teeth should be present (Tables 11.2(a) and 11.2(b)). Many theories have been put forward to explain tooth eruption – when considering all the evidence we still do not know precisely how tooth eruption is controlled. However, the eruptive

TABLE 11.1(a)
Development of deciduous teeth

Teeth	Calcification starts (weeks in utero)	Crown completed (months)	Root completed (years)
Central incisor	14	2	1.5
Lateral incisor	16	2.5	2
Canine	17	9	3
First molar	15	6	2.5
Second molar	18	10	3

Source: Shaw (1993).

TABLE 11.1(b)
Development of permanent teeth

Teeth	Calcification starts	Crown completed (years)	Root completed (years)
Maxilla			
Central incisor	3 months	3.5	9
Lateral incisor	11 months	4.5	10
Canine	4 months	4.5	14
First premolar	1.5 years	6.5	12
Second premolar	2 years	7.0	13
First molar	At birth	3.5	9
Second molar	3 years	7.0	15
Third molar	8 years	13.0	20
Mandible			
Central incisor	3 months	3.0	8
Lateral incisor	3 months	3.5	9
Canine	4 months	4.5	13
First premolar	1.5 years	5.5	12
Second premolar	2.3 years	7.0	13
First molar	At birth	3.5	9
Second molar	3 years	7.0	14
Third molar	9 years	13.0	20

Source: Shaw (1993).

process for children with craniosynostosis, based on clinical experience, is essentially normal, i.e. teeth erupt.

The establishment of the relationships between the teeth within and between the arches is a highly complex process involving a number of factors:

- Skeletal – the relationship between the maxilla and mandible in all three planes of space (horizontal, vertical and transverse).
- Dental – size of teeth in relationship to the size of the jaws.
- Soft tissues – the effect of the circumoral soft tissues, e.g. lips, tongue, etc.
- Habits, e.g. thumb or finger sucking.

TABLE 11.2(a)
Eruption of the deciduous dentition (months)

Teeth	Girls Mean	SD	Boys Mean	SD
Maxilla				
Central incisor	9.8	1.59	9.6	1.85
Lateral incisor	11.1	2.37	10.4	2.40
Canine	19.5	3.17	18.7	3.15
First molar	15.6	1.89	15.5	2.08
Second molar	7.9	3.75	27.7	4.31
Mandible				
Central incisor	7.9	2.13	7.5	2.10
Lateral incisor	13.4	3.13	13.0	3.12
Canine	20.3	3.26	19.1	3.19
First molar	15.9	1.73	15.6	3.22
Second molar	26.2	3.44	26.3	3.82

Source: Hagg and Tarranger (1986).

TABLE 11.2(b)
Eruption of the permanent dentition (years)

Teeth	Girls Mean	SD	Boys Mean	SD
Maxilla				
Central incisor	7.2	0.75	6.8	0.57
Lateral incisor	8.3	0.86	7.9	0.37
Canine	11.6	1.17	10.8	1.30
First premolar	10.8	1.20	10.3	1.25
Second premolar	11.5	1.20	11.0	1.61
First molar	6.5	0.67	6.3	0.60
Second molar	12.4	1.07	12.0	1.15
Mandible				
Central incisor	6.3	0.59	6.0	0.57
Lateral incisor	7.5	0.81	7.0	0.74
Canine	10.7	1.03	9.5	1.04
First premolar	11.1	1.22	10.3	1.34
Second premolar	11.8	1.28	11.2	1.43
First molar	6.4	0.72	6.1	0.66
Second molar	12.0	1.11	11.6	1.24

Source: Hagg and Tarranger (1986).

The description of the relationships between the maxillary and mandibular teeth can be done in a number of ways. One of the more commonly used methods is based on the antero-posterior incisor relationship. In a class I incisor relationship (Fig. 11.1(a)) the lower incisor edges occlude with or lie immediately below the cingulum plateaux (middle of the palatal surfaces) of the upper central incisors. This is the type of occlusion regarded as ideal and a desirable outcome. In a class II incisor relationship the lower incisor edges lie posterior to the cingulum plateaux of the upper central incisors. Class II is subdivided

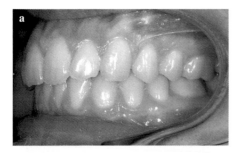

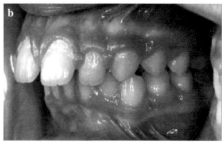

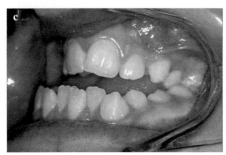

Fig. 11.1 (a) Class I incisor and molar relationship. (b) Class II incisor relationship. (c) Class III incisor relationship.

into two divisions: division 1 – the overjet (horizontal distance between the lower incisors and the incisal edges of the upper incisors) is increased and the upper incisors are either proclined or at a normal angulation (Fig. 11.1(b)); and division 2 – the upper central incisors are retroclined or upright and the overjet is usually minimal but can be increased. Conversely, if the lower incisor edges lie anterior to the cingulum plateaux of the upper incisors, a class III incisor relationship exists (Fig. 11.1(c)). The overjet will be reduced or reversed.

Development/eruption of the teeth in craniosynostosis

Monitoring the development/eruption of both the deciduous and permanent dentition is carried out by an orthodontist working as part of the interdisciplinary team.

Non-syndromic

For children with non-syndromic craniosynostosis this process usually occurs without any specific problems with the teeth (both deciduous and permanent) erupting at the normal milestones. Very occasionally there may be a marked delay in the eruption of the deciduous teeth – no direct intervention is needed. Both parents and orthodontist need to be patient!

Syndromic

The dental development and oral manifestations in Apert syndrome are well described and include: delayed eruption, ectopic eruption and shovel-shaped incisors. A mean developmental dental delay of 0.96 years with a trend to increase with age has been reported (Kaloust

214

et al 1997). Kreiborg and Cohen (1992) reported delayed eruption of primary and secondary teeth. Erupting teeth remained buried in thickened/fibrous gingival tissues for extended periods of time. The precise reason for the delay in eruption is not clear. The eruptive process does not appear to be adversely affected by the underlying causes of the craniosynostosis. A more likely explanation is a mechanical interference caused by the fibrous oral mucosa and lack of space in the developing dental arch (particularly the maxillary dental arch) caused by the maxillary deficiency.

Kreiborg and Cohen (1992) found that a third of their patients had shovel-shaped incisors. This trait is only found in about 1–3.5 per cent of Caucasians (Gorlin 1990). A reduced mesio-distal diameter of maxillary second and third molars was also observed in some cases – this might be explained by the extremely restricted space in the tuberosity region.

The dental findings in Crouzon, Pfeiffer and Saethre–Chotzen syndromes have received much less attention than those in Apert syndrome. Goho (1998) in a single case report of Saethre–Chotzen syndrome noted multiple dental anomalies including teeth with broad, bulbous crowns, thin, narrow tapering roots and diffuse pulp stones in the pulp chambers of all posterior teeth. Alvarez et al (1993) in a report of a child with Pfeiffer syndrome (type 3) described the presence of multiple natal teeth which included mandibular incisors and maxillary first molars.

From a practical point of view the delayed eruption of teeth is not a particular problem. However, the reduced maxillary size leads, all too frequently, to problems with impaction or ectopic eruption. The first permanent molars, which normally erupt at age 6 years, can occasionally become impacted on the distal surface of the second deciduous molars. Very occasionally this can also affect the mandibular first permanent molars. If this problem does not resolve spontaneously it may be necessary to extract the second deciduous

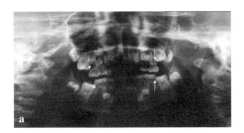 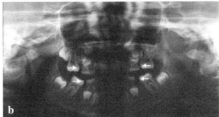

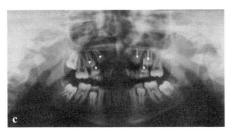

Fig. 11.2 DPT radiographs of a child with Crouzon syndrome showing the effect of the extraction of all four second deciduous molars (arrowed) on the eruption of the previously impacted first permanent molars. The lower second premolars are developmentally absent. The upper arch is very crowded with insufficient space for the canine, first and second premolars (arrowed in (c)).

Fig. 11.3 The maxillary arch of a patient with Apert syndrome showing severe dental crowding.

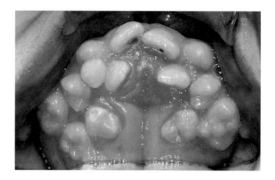

molar(s) to facilitate the eruption of the first permanent molar(s) (Fig. 11.2). The second and third permanent maxillary molars may develop occlusally and buccally to ectopic first molars, with severe delay of eruption or retention of molars.

In the maxillary anterior region, the lateral incisors are frequently blocked out completely and are positioned palatally because of lack of space. The maxillary molar and incisor regions should therefore be monitored radiographically from the age of 5–6 years. With premature loss of the second deciduous molars in the maxilla, the first permanent molars will drift mesially with subsequent loss of space for the second premolars, which will then erupt palatally (Kreiborg and Cohen 1992) (Fig. 11.3).

General dental care

GENERAL MANAGEMENT
During the early years the primary focus of the dental team is maintaining good general dental health, i.e. no caries, gingivitis or periodontal problems, all of which are completely preventable.

All children with craniosynostosis (syndromic and non-syndromic) are reviewed by an orthodontist as part of their initial craniofacial assessment (see Chapter 17). Advice is given about general dental care, i.e. diet, oral hygiene and the use of fluoride supplements, and parents are encouraged to seek general dental care locally, i.e. with the family general dental practitioner (dentist).

The vast majority of children with non-syndromic craniosynostosis do not need any specialist paediatric dental care because they do not present with any specific dental problems, i.e. the teeth develop and generally erupt at the normal milestones. This applies to both the deciduous and permanent dentition.

For children presenting with the more complex 'syndromic' forms of craniosynostosis, general dental care can either be provided by the family dentist or, more commonly, in the case of the Great Ormond Street Hospital for Children, by hospital-based paediatric dental staff. This is because access to local dental care is frequently difficult for families to arrange and it is easier and more efficient to schedule dental 'checks' and treatment as part of the staged management protocols.

THE EVIDENCE

Mustafa et al (2001) undertook a prospective study to compare levels of dental caries, bacterial dental plaque, gingivitis, enamel defects and caries-related microflora, in a group of 57 children with craniosynostosis and their matched controls. The dental health of a group of children with craniosynostosis (from Great Ormond Street Hospital for Children) was generally better than that of the matched controls. This was not expected but appears to reflect the cumulative effect of continuous/independent dental health education from birth. Some of the children experienced difficulty with tooth brushing and this indicates a need for increased help with oral hygiene techniques including the use of modified toothbrush handles or an electric toothbrush, which are easier to hold and use.

Craniofacial morphology and occlusal abnormalities

FACIAL ASYMMETRY

The aetiology of the majority of facial asymmetries is suborbital. In contrast, early fusion of either of the coronal sutures (unicoronal synostosis) can be associated with a mild to moderate facial asymmetry which may be described as a facial scoliosis. Although not documented, most of the asymmetry resolves following fronto-orbital surgery. However, there is a group of patients for whom the asymmetry remains and reflects the degree of the original deformity. The underlying skeletal asymmetry causes an occlusal/dental asymmetry. In the less affected cases the underlying asymmetry can be accepted and any orthodontic treatment carried out will 'camouflage' the underlying skeletal problem. In these cases, while it is relatively easy to align the teeth it may not be possible to produce ideal occlusal relationships (Fig. 11.4).

If the asymmetry is more marked and is of concern to the patient, surgery to reposition the maxilla/mandible is indicated which allows the orthodontist to produce the best possible occlusal relationships (Fig. 11.5).

SYNDROMIC CRANIOSYNOSTOSIS

The craniofacial morphology in the complex forms of craniosynostosis (mainly Apert and Crouzon syndromes) has been described by a number of authors, primarily using cephalometric analyses (Costaras-Volarich and Pruzansky 1984, Richtsmeier 1987, Kreiborg and Cohen 1992, Al-Qattan and Phillips 1996, Cohen and Kreiborg 1996, Kreiborg and Cohen 1998, Kreiborg et al 1999).

Cephalometric radiography is a standardised and reproducible form of skull radiography which is used extensively in orthodontics to characterise a patient's dental and skeletal relationships. Radiographs are acquired using specialised equipment, which includes a head positioning/stabilising device. There is a fixed distance between the X-ray source and the patient's mid-sagittal plane and also between the mid-sagittal plane and the X-ray film. This ensures standardisation and reproducibility of the resultant radiographs.

The maxilla, in all studies, has been shown to be hypoplastic in all three planes of space. Clinical experience shows that the degree of hypoplasia is very variable, i.e. from mild to

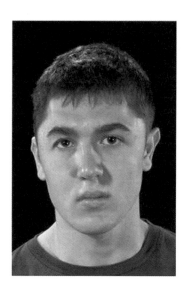
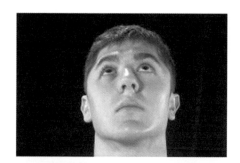
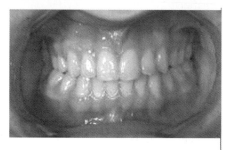

Fig. 11.4 Clinical photographs showing a patient with a mild facial asymmetry, which results from a right side coronal synostosis. The occlusion, which was asymmetric, has been corrected by orthodontic treatment.

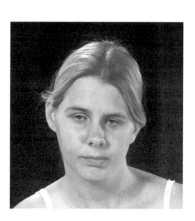
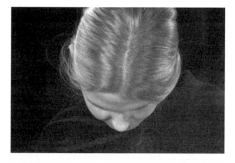
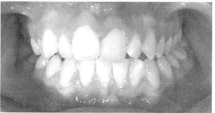

Fig. 11.5 Clinical photographs of a patient with a skull base asymmetry, which has resulted in a severe facial asymmetry. This type of facial asymmetry can occur following unicoronal synostosis. Orthognathic surgery is required to correct the underlying skeletal asymmetry to allow full correction of the occlusion.

severe, which in turn affects the relationship between the teeth in the antero-posterior, transverse and vertical planes. The mandible in Apert syndrome has been reported by Kreiborg et al (1999) as being of 'fairly normal size and shape but posteriorly inclined'. Costaras-Volarich and Pruzansky (1984) asked the question, 'Is the mandible intrinsically different in Apert and Crouzon syndromes?' Their findings agreed with those of Kreiborg et al (1999). In addition they suggested that there is a syndrome-specific mandibular malformation. We have undertaken a cephalometric analysis of the craniofacial morphology of patients with Crouzon syndrome and compared the data with age- and sex-matched controls. The mandible in Crouzon syndrome is not significantly different, in size, from that of unaffected individuals.

Richtsmeier and Lele (1990) used more complex methods to analyse craniofacial growth in Crouzon syndrome including finite element scaling, generalised procrustes and Euclidean distance matrix analyses. They showed, not surprisingly, general differences in the postnatal growth patterns between 'normal' children and children with Crouzon syndrome.

OCCLUSAL ABNORMALITIES

The relationship between the teeth (occlusion) is determined by a number of factors including the skeletal pattern (jaw size and position) and soft tissue influences. If the maxilla and mandible are of a correct size and normally positioned with reference to the cranial base and each other, the teeth will meet in class I or normal relationship.

In complex craniosynostosis the occlusal relationships most frequently seen include (Fig. 11.6):

- Class III incisor relationship, which is sometimes referred to as a mandibular overjet, i.e. the lower incisors are in front of the upper incisors in occlusion
- Class III molar relationship, which is sometimes referred to as a mesial molar relationship
- Anterior open bite
- Bilateral posterior crossbite

These features are primarily due to the deficient maxillary growth/development in all three planes of space and can vary in severity from mild to moderate to severe.

In the study carried out by Kreiborg and Cohen (1992) for Apert syndrome, mesial molar occlusion was observed in 68 per cent of the cases. In the general population the frequency of mesial molar occlusion is less than 5 per cent (Helm 1970). Distal molar occlusion was observed in 19 per cent of the cases and the remaining 13 per cent had a normal molar occlusion. Mandibular overjet was registered in 81 per cent of the patients – however, this trait is extremely rare in the general population, occurring in less than 1 per cent (Helm 1970). A deviation of the mandibular midline is commonly seen in patients with Apert syndrome; this may be related to the crowded incisor region and to the frequently observed asymmetry of the cranial base (Cohen and Kreiborg 1996).

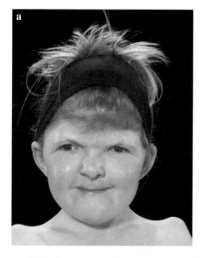

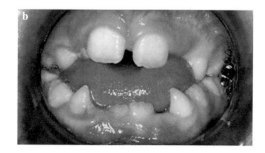

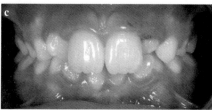

Fig. 11.6 (a) and (b) A 7-year-old girl with Apert syndrome. The occlusal features, i.e. class III incisor relationship, anterior open bite and posterior crossbite, are present. Compare with (c) which shows the occlusal relationships in an unaffected 7-year-old.

Orthodontic management for children with craniosynostosis.
How much can orthodontists achieve?

GENERAL CONSIDERATIONS

The extent, type and timing of orthodontic treatment will depend on the presenting malocclusion. For patients with the more complex forms of craniosynostosis the most important factor to consider is the interplay between orthodontic treatment and craniofacial and/or orthoganthic surgery which alters the position of the jaws. If the discrepancy between the maxilla and mandible, in all three planes of space, is within acceptable limits, orthodontic treatment in isolation is appropriate. However, if there is a significant 'skeletal' discrepancy, which necessitates surgery, orthodontic treatment is planned and executed to facilitate the surgery. This is an important distinction because the aims of orthodontic treatment when carried out in isolation, as opposed to as an adjunct to surgery, are completely different. Planning is carried out with the orthodontist and surgeon(s) working closely together with supporting records, i.e. dental study models, cephalometric analysis, stereolithographic model(s), extra- and intra-oral photographs and CT data. It is important to emphasise the multidisciplinary nature of the planning process to ensure agreement.

220

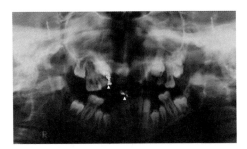

Fig. 11.7 A DPT radiograph of a patient with Apert syndrome showing bonded attachments and gold chains which are used to align impacted or displaced teeth.

SPECIFIC CONSIDERATIONS

To facilitate the eruption and alignment of teeth which are impacted or displaced, orthodontic treatment involving extractions and exposure of displaced teeth, for the attachment of bonded attachments (gold chains) which allow traction to be applied for alignment, may be necessary (Fig. 11.7). This can be considered as interceptive treatment, i.e. with specific, limited aims – not correcting all occlusal problems.

If the position of the maxilla and mandible is within normal limits and no surgery is planned to alter the jaw position, comprehensive orthodontic treatment can be carried out with the aim of correcting all aspects of the malocclusion and producing the best possible aesthetic and functional occlusion. This may be appropriate for the 'milder' or less affected forms of Saethre–Chotzen and Crouzon syndrome.

ORTHODONTIC PREPARATION FOR CRANIOFACIAL SURGERY

For most patients with complex (syndromic) craniosynostosis, surgery to reposition the jaws is required in order to produce a satisfactory dental occlusion, i.e. orthodontic treatment in isolation cannot correct all aspects of the malocclusion. Orthodontic treatment for this group of patients involves 'setting the teeth up for surgery' and follows three basic principles:

- Decompensation – correcting dento-alveolar compensation, i.e. if the maxilla is deficient in size and is posterior to the mandible, the upper incisors tend to become proclined ('lean forward') and the lower incisors retroclined ('lean back') in an attempt to produce occlusal contact (tooth–tooth contact).
- Dental alignment – if the dentition is crowded, teeth may need to be extracted to align (straighten) the teeth.
- Dental arch co-ordination – the transverse arch widths may need to be adjusted to produce the best possible occlusal interdigitation post-surgery. This involves transverse expansion of the maxillary dentition and possible transverse contraction of the mandibular dentition. Depending on the amount of transverse expansion of the maxillary dentition needed, surgery to widen the maxilla may be required.

All of the above means that comprehensive fixed appliance therapy is required using two-arch fixed appliances. The majority of the orthodontic preparation is completed before

221

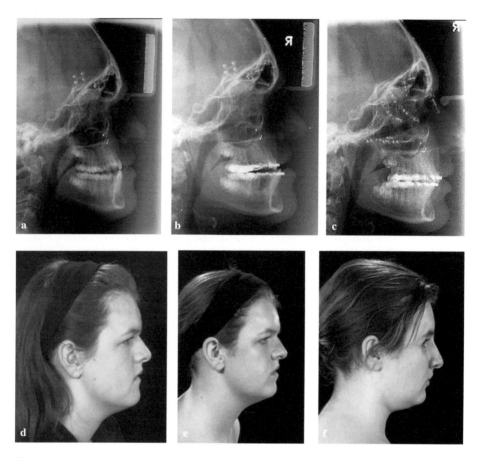

Fig. 11.8 Lateral cephalogram radiographs and right profile clinical photographs to illustrate the process of presurgical orthodontic preparation. The incisor relationship has 'worsened', i.e. made more class III and then corrected by the Le Fort III midface advance.

surgery (Fig. 11.8). The appliances are left on during surgery for the attachment of the intermaxillary wafer (a device used to locate the teeth/jaws) and are then used post-surgery to control the intermaxillary relationships and detail the occlusion.

FACIAL BIPARTITION
(For details of the surgery itself, see Chapter 19.)

Orthodontic preparation
Within the field of craniofacial surgery the facial bipartition requires special attention during presurgical orthodontic preparation. The surgical procedure has been described by Posnick (1996) and involves a midline maxillary osteotomy.

The orthodontic preparation prior to surgery includes the following:

- A space is created, whenever possible, between the maxillary central incisors and the roots are moved into a divergent position to allow the osteotomy to proceed without involving the teeth or the adjacent periodontal tissues (Fig. 11.9).
- The maxillary arch is expanded transversely during the bipartition. Contracting or narrowing the maxillary arch prior to surgery is helpful but will not always accommodate the surgical expansion.

Postoperative orthodontic treatment

Depending on the extent of the movement of the orbits, which may or may not be symmetrical, postoperative orthodontic treatment is needed to:

- Close the space created between the maxillary central incisors. It is not possible to start space closure immediately postoperatively. A period of time (approximately 3–6 months) is required to allow either an alveolar bone graft to consolidate or new bone to form if not grafted. A periodic radiographic review is needed to check on the amount and quality of bone before starting space closure.
- Produce an acceptable buccal segment occlusion or interdigitation using a series of intermaxillary elastics (Fig. 11.10).

Dental and orthodontic complications of craniofacial surgery

Major craniofacial surgery, e.g. monobloc, Le Fort III or facial bipartition, when carried out during the development/eruption of the dentition, may produce adverse effects which can broadly be divided into two groups. First, osteotomies which involve the tooth-bearing part of the maxilla, e.g. pterygomaxillary disjunction or maxillary midline 'split', may dislodge/displace developing teeth and cause problems such as loss of vitality, root resorption, ankylosis or the loss of attachment. In some cases the long-term prognosis of the teeth affected is compromised (Figs 11.11 and 11.12).

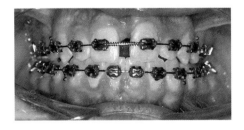

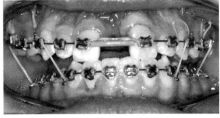

Fig. 11.9 Clinical photographs of a patient who is undergoing orthodontic treatment in preparation for a facial bipartition. A space has been created between the central incisors (and between their roots) to allow the midline osteotomy to be performed.

Fig. 11.10 Clinical photographs illustrating the use of intermaxillary elastics to control the occlusion post-facial bipartition.

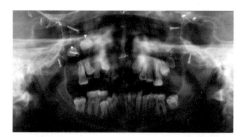

Fig. 11.11 DPT radiograph of a patient who has undergone a Le Fort III midface advance. The developing molars in the right posterior maxilla (arrowed) have become displaced to such an extent that they will not now erupt and may need to be removed at a later date.

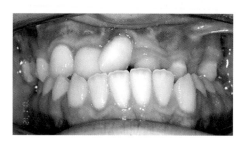 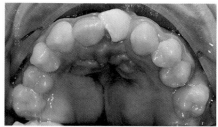

Fig. 11.12 The upper left central incisor has become ankylosed and cannot be moved, i.e. there is a fusion between the surface of the tooth root and surrounding bone. This tooth will have to be removed as part of the orthodontic treatment prior to further surgery and eventually replaced with either a fixed bridge or an implant-retained crown.

The second group of dental complications involves a more generalised disruption to the developing dentition. Although, fortunately, this type of problem occurs relatively infrequently, patients require an extensive dental reconstruction/rehabilitation which includes bone grafts, implants and fixed/removable dental prostheses (Fig. 11.13).

There is little data published regarding the incidence and types of dental complication following major craniofacial surgery. As part of a multidisciplinary outcomes analysis we have looked at the dental complications following facial bipartition. The data were

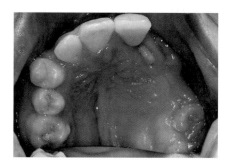 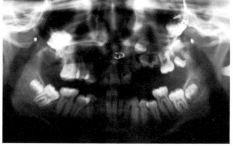

Fig. 11.13 The clinical photograph and DPT radiographs show that all the teeth in the upper left maxilla have been adversely affected, for reasons that are not clear, following a Le Fort III midface advance. None of the teeth can be 'saved' and an extensive reconstruction is planned.

collected in a retrospective case note/record audit including dental study models, intra-oral photographs and dental radiographs for a group of 25 patients. In 11 patients the following dental complications were found: ankylosis (3), root resorption (2), root canal sclerosis (2), loss of vitality (4), loss of periodontal support (4), disturbed/disrupted dental development (3). Our current practice is to create adequate space, orthodontically, to allow interdental (midline) osteotomies to be performed to reduce the risk to the teeth adjacent to the osteotomy.

Summary

- All possible steps should be taken to ensure that good general dental health is established and maintained.
- The development of the dentition/occlusion needs to be carefully monitored in conjunction with the growth of the craniofacial complex.
- Orthodontic treatment including extractions and fixed appliance therapy is invariably required to align the dentition.
- Orthodontic treatment is planned to support the 'surgical plan'.

REFERENCES

Al-Qattan MM, Phillips JH (1996) The cranial base angle and maxillary hypoplasia in unoperated Crouzon patients. *J Craniofac Surg* 7: 69–79.
Alvarez MP, Crespi PV, Shanske AL (1993) Natal molars in Pfeiffer syndrome type 3: a case report. *J Clin Paediatr Dent* 18: 21–24.
Cobourne M (1999) The genetic control of early osteogenesis. *J Orthod* 26: 21–28.
Cohen MM Jr, Kreiborg SA (1996) Clinical study of the craniofacial features in Apert syndrome. *Int J Oral Maxillofac Surg* 25: 45–53.
Costaras-Volarich M, Pruzansky S (1984) Is the mandible intrinsically different in Apert and Crouzon syndromes? *Am J Orthod* 85: 475–487.
Goho C (1998) Dental findings in Saethre–Chotzen syndrome (acrocephalosyndactyly type III): report of case. *ASDC J Dent Child* 65: 136–137.
Gorlin RJ, editor (1990) *Syndromes of the Head and Neck*, 3rd edn. Oxford: Oxford University Press.
Hagg U, Tarranger J (1986) Timing of tooth emergence. A prospective longitudinal study of Swedish urban children from birth to 18 years. *Swed Dent J* 10: 195–206.
Helm S (1970) Prevalence of malocclusion in relation to the development of the dentition. *Acta Odontol Scand* (suppl) 28: 58.
Kaloust S, Ishii K, Vargervik K (1997) Dental development in Apert syndrome. *Cleft Palate Craniofac J* 34: 117–121.
Kreiborg S, Cohen MM Jr (1992) The oral manifestations of Apert syndrome. *J Craniofac Genet Dev Biol* 12: 41–48.
Kreiborg S, Cohen MM Jr (1998) Is craniofacial morphology in Apert and Crouzon syndromes the same? *Acta Odontol Scand* 56: 339–341.
Kreiborg S, Pruzansky S (1981) Craniofacial growth in premature craniofacial synostosis. *Scand J Plast Reconstr Surg* 15: 171–186.
Kreiborg S, Aduss H, Cohen MM Jr (1999) Cephalometric study of the Apert syndrome in adolescence and adulthood. *J Craniofac Genet Dev Biol* 19: 1–11.
Mustafa D, Lucas VS, Junod P, Evans RD, Mason C, Roberts GJ (2001) The dental health and caries-related microflora in children with craniosynostosis. *Cleft Palate Craniofac J* 38: 629–635.
Posnick J (1996) Monobloc and facial bipartition osteotomies: a step by step description of the surgical technique. *J Craniofac Surg* 7: 229–250.

Proffit WR, editor (2000) *Contemporary Orthodontics*, 3rd edn. St Louis: Mosby.

Richtsmeier JT (1987) Comparative study of normal, Crouzon and Apert craniofacial morphology using finite element scaling analysis. *Am J Phys Anthropol* 74: 473–493.

Richtsmeier JT, Lele S (1990) Analysis of craniofacial growth in Crouzon syndrome using landmark data. *J Craniofac Genet Dev Biol* 10: 39–62.

Shaw WC, editor (1993) *Orthodontics and Occlusal Management*. London: Butterworth-Heinemann.

12

THE CHILD WITH CRANIOSYNOSTOSIS: PSYCHOLOGICAL ISSUES

Daniela Hearst

Introduction

'Don't go near Frog-eyes'
'Look at the Alien'
'Go away Fish Face'
'Why do you look like ET?'
'Here comes Runway Head'

Such are the remarks suffered all too often by the children seen in craniofacial clinics. We are left in no doubt of the enormous difficulties faced by many children with craniosynostosis and facial deformities.

This chapter describes the role of facial appearance in modern society, attitudes and behaviours towards the disfigured, and hence the psychological challenges for children and young people with craniofacial conditions and their families. These are outlined in a developmental framework together with the interventions the psychologist, as part of the craniofacial team, can offer, with illustrative case histories. The assessment and management of learning difficulties in craniosynostosis are then described. In conclusion, the role and contribution of the clinical psychologist to the craniofacial service are summarised with suggestions for future developments.

The psychosocial importance of facial appearance

> I am convinced that nothing has so marked an influence on the direction of a man's mind as his appearance and not his appearance in itself, so much as his conviction that it is attractive or unattractive.
>
> Tolstoy, *Childhood*, 1852

Facial appearance is fundamental to personal and social identity; it defines membership of the human species as well as the individual self and the presentation of that self to others. Facial appearance also acts as a powerful metaphor for social interactions. We speak of 'meeting face to face', 'showing one's face', 'facing up to problems' and 'falling flat on one's face'.

The importance of 'first appearances' may be just that; visual information is often the first available to the perceiver and remains continuously present throughout any social interaction (Kleck and Rubenstein 1975). Visual information processing by humans is not a neutral activity, but subject to processes of categorisation, attribution and judgemental inference by the perceiver – the basis of stereotyping (Miller 1982).

Research over the last 30 years has cited mounting evidence of the impact of an individual's facial appearance on social interaction and individual behaviour and, in particular, the benefits of possessing a face that is judged to be attractive (Bull and Rumsey 1988). While facial attractiveness is allusive to quantitative, 'objective' description, it would appear that the relative symmetry between facial components is particularly salient (Langlois 1995).

Attractive infants and young children may be judged more positively by their parents and caregivers in terms of likeability and adjustment, and elicit preferential treatment, including more nurturant behaviours and higher expectations of success (Dion 1972, 1974, Hildebrandt and Fitzgerald 1978, Field and Vega-Lahr 1984, Barden et al 1989, Barden 1990). Appearance can affect school performance (Clifford and Walster 1973, Richman 1978), legal proceedings (Sigall and Ostrove 1975), hiring and promotions (Landy and Sigall 1974, Dipboye et al 1975, Scheuerle et al 1982).

Facial appearance and expressions are crucial in the development of early relationships. Human infants appear to have a unique knowledge of and preference for faces and facial expressions (Bruce and Green 1990). Babies of 6 months can differentiate between attractive and unattractive faces and show significantly greater eye fixation to attractive faces (Langlois et al 1987, 1991). From as early as 3½ years and throughout childhood, children demonstrate a significant preference for attractive children as potential friends. Unattractive children may be judged by their peers as antisocial (Dion and Berscheid 1974). The face, over other body parts, holds primacy in conveying personality and communicating emotional and social messages, and is viewed as critically important in the development of social relationships and structures (Cole 1998). Facial appearance has all the more powerful an effect in a modern age in which we move, change job and are exposed to large numbers of unfamiliar people on a regular basis.

The development of self-concept and self-image is considered to be highly dependent on social interaction (Sommer 1969). The perceiver and the perceived are connected in a dynamic way (Gilligan 1989, Carey 1990, Lefebvre 1990). Self-concept may be constructed out of others' recognitions and judgements. Children learn what they live (Bennett and Stanton 1993). Equally, this feedback from social interactions may be interpreted on the basis of existing self-image (Kenny and De Paulo 1993). Whatever is cause or effect, as facial appearance has a strong effect on social interaction and self-concept, this will carry major implications for children who look facially different or disfigured.

There is a cross-culturally shared distress with facial difference, revealed throughout history, myth, legend and fiction (Shaw 1981). From Cicero to Walt Disney, deviant appearance has not escaped attribution and stereotyping. The very words 'abnormality', 'disfigurement', 'impairment', 'disability' and 'flaw' connote the negative attitudes attached to visible difference (MacGregor 1974). Facial difference continues to attract public curiosity and revulsion. (It was as late as 1974 that Chicago, among other American cities, repealed its Ugly Laws – part of the vagrancy legislation – which could impose fines on anyone appearing in public who was 'diseased, maimed, mutilated or in anyway deformed, so as not to be unsightly or disgusting objects' (Carey 1990).)

While for many children with simple craniosynostoses, surgical reconstruction will produce a more ordinary appearance, many children with syndromic craniosynostosis will be left with significant facial difference (Pertschuk 1990). The transformation is from the less to the more presentable (MacGregor 1990). Craniofacial disfigurement as the result of craniosynostosis may cause markedly disrupted head and facial symmetry as well as anomalies that may be stigmatising, i.e. affected children may not only be judged along an attractive–unattractive continuum but also along a normal–abnormal social dimension. Such stigmatisation may not confer automatic social rejection but ambivalence (Katz 1981). There are strong cultural traditions which dictate help and sympathy for the 'disabled', traditions that coexist with the social avoidance and discomfort also engendered by facial difference. The mixed messages conveyed by ambivalence in the observer – fear, hostility, rejection, competing with the desire to help, kindness and sympathy – may well threaten a disfigured child's self-esteem and self-protective mechanisms.

How does our society treat such children? The disfigured baby may be at increased risk of a disturbed attachment relationship with his/her primary caregivers: there is evidence of decreased parental responsiveness to and physical contact with a disfigured baby (Field 1995, Walters 1997). Disfigured children are subject to intrusive questioning, staring, teasing, harassment, hostility, ridicule and avoidance (Beuf 1990, Gerrard 1991, Bradbury 1996, Lansdown et al 1997). They are judged less popular, have fewer friends (Walters 1997, Broder et al 2001), tend to underachieve academically (Richman 1976, Broder et al 1998), and are subject to adverse differential treatment by teachers, who may underestimate their intelligence on the basis of their disfigured appearance (Richman 1978). Social interaction can be strained, at worst overtly hostile (MacGregor 1990). Facial disfigurement is consistently ranked among the least desirable of 'handicaps', by both children and adults (Hill-Beuf and Porter 1984, Sigelman et al 1986, Lansdown 1990, Harper 1995, Harper and Peterson 2001).

Facial difference cannot easily be hidden; the disfigured child with syndromic craniosynostosis does not usually blend into a crowd (Bull and Rumsey 1988, MacGregor 1990). The following extract from MacGregor (1990) is often quoted as it captures the essence of the experience of facial disfigurement:

> In their efforts to go about their daily affairs, they are subject to visual and verbal assault and a level of familiarity from strangers . . . including . . . naked stares, startled reaction, double takes, whispering, remarks, furtive looks, curiosity, personal questions, advice, manifestations of pity or aversion, laughter, ridicule or outright avoidance. Whatever form the behaviours may take, they generate feelings of shame, impotence, anger and humiliation in their victims.

In consequence, the disfigured child may be left with feelings of invaded privacy, powerlessness and loss of predictability over the outcome of social interactions, which in turn can lead to loneliness and despair (Bull and Rumsey 1988).

The potential for chronic psychological distress and disturbance would seem to be high. Children with syndromic craniosynostosis in particular, who may have additional sensory impairments, breathing and feeding difficulties and limb deformities, also have to cope with the extra stress of repeated medical investigations and interventions. Indeed what clearly arises from the research literature and clinical experience is that facially disfigured children are at greatly increased risk of social anxiety and behaviour problems (Pertschuk and Whitaker 1987, Pope and Ward 1997), dependence on significant adults, depression in adolescence (Pillemer and Cook 1989, Kapp-Simon et al 1992) and low self-esteem (Kapp 1979, Broder and Strauss 1989, Speltz et al 1993).

However, and it is a big 'however', risk and reality are not synonymous. Research has singularly failed to demonstrate consistent differences in overt psychopathology, social adjustment and self-esteem between groups of craniofacially disfigured and unaffected, 'normal' children and adolescents (MacGregor 1990, Speltz et al 1995, Speltz and Richman 1997). Facially disfigured children are remarkable for their lack of psychopathology. Adjustment is not equivalent to impairment.

Why is this? Several explanations have been proposed:

1   Facial disfigurement is not uniformly disturbing to society. Anomalies of the facial triangle (i.e. the area between the eyes, nose and mouth) provoke greater distress than less central features, e.g. jaw, ears.
2   'Objective' facial appearance is not a reliable predictor of subjective appraisal (Pruzinsky and Cash 1990). The extent and severity of facial disfigurement do *not* predict psychological adjustment (Heller et al 1985). Indeed, the evidence suggests that mild disfigurement can cause greater distress than more objectively severe disfigurement (Lansdown et al 1991, Robinson et al 1996).
3   Research findings have been based on small samples that are heterogeneous for type and severity of craniofacial disorders and the results are over-generalised (Cohen and MacLean 2000b). The specific contribution of associated problems including sensory impairment, feeding difficulties, etc. is frequently left unclear.
4   Measures of self-concept and self-esteem can be problematic, as hidden and unac-knowledged difficulties may be harder to tap. Studies reporting lower self-esteem in facially disfigured children, compared with unaffected peers (Lefebvre et al 1986, Pertschuk and Whitaker 1987, Broder and Strauss 1989, Pillemer and Cook 1989), are challenged by studies indicating equally high, if not higher, self-esteem in disfigured compared to non-disfigured peers (Leonard et al 1991, Kapp-Simon et al 1992). While it is important to emphasise that not all children are troubled by their facial disfigure-ment, failure to communicate and denial of distress may account for some children's reports of higher self-esteem compared to their unaffected peers (Lefebvre and Munro 1978). Additionally, the quality of children's social skills has a strong effect on the impact of disfigurement and the consequent social response (Kapp-Simon et al 1992).

Whatever the relative contribution of the above factors may be, the question Clifford posed in 1983, 'Why are they so normal?', has yet to receive a satisfactory answer. Until very recently, research has doggedly continued with its deficit-based model and focus on incidence of psychosocial disturbance. A frequently quoted figure for incidence of psychological difficulties with children with cleft lip and/or palate is around 30 per cent (Endriga and Kapp-Simon 1999). The figure for children with craniosynostosis, simple or syndromic, is harder to establish, owing to the much lower incidence in the general population, but clinical evidence would support a similar figure of around 30 per cent. As Eiserman (2001) remarks, there is a dearth of discussion on what researchers might learn of the special positive psychological characteristics of the 'normal' 70 per cent and the implications for helping the minority who have problems.

In the last two to three years, there has been an exciting sea-change in underlying assumptions and 'mantras' of health psychology research generally, and specifically in craniofacial issues. At last there is a move away from problem-focused outcome studies which highlight psychological dysfunction and disability, towards outcomes defined by a child and family's psychological strengths, resilience and coping strategies. Resilience is defined as successful adaptation to significant adversity (Beardslee et al 1998), using protective factors to respond to change. Resilience is not an innate, static personality trait but a dynamic state within and between individuals. Protective factors for individuals include high self-esteem, self-reliance, problem-solving skills, optimism, intelligence and sense of humour. Family protective factors include parental warmth, consistency and strong support for their children. Community protective factors include support from peers, teachers and other significant adults (Broder 2001, Place et al 2002). There is an increasing call for studies to explore psychological strengths and the unique contribution of facial difference to positive personal growth, health and success.

This has major implications for the delivery of psychosocial care to children with craniosynostosis and their families, offered by the clinical psychologist together with other craniofacial team members. The aim is to follow the child and family's developmental path, aware of the developmental 'tasks' at each stage, with particular attention to important transitions – starting and leaving school, starting work, ending treatment – as key challenges to psychological development. The focus is on promoting an individual child and family's strengths and coping styles as well as screening for potential vulnerabilities and difficulties as a result of craniosynostosis. Children and their families are part of wider social communities and networks and it is essential that the craniofacial team is sensitive to the different social, racial and cultural issues that families bring.

An important underlying ethical issue for psychological intervention is: who has the problem and therefore who needs treatment? Is it incumbent on the facially different or disfigured individual to seek to normalise their appearance to accede to society's demands for physical attractiveness (Strauss 2001)? Does offering treatment to improve the disfigured child's social skills place an extra and unjust burden on that child? It would seem more appropriate for the non-disfigured majority to change their attitudes and behaviours. However, as Clarke (1999) points out, it is professionally unethical to ignore a child and family's distress by not offering intervention. Rather than wait for society to change, one may be able to accelerate the pace of that change through enabling an individual child to be more socially successful and thereby acceptable.

In this context, the chapter now describes the psychosocial tasks at different developmental phases of development, the challenges imposed by craniosynostosis and the assessments and interventions designed to prevent or ameliorate psychological difficulties if they arise.

The early years: birth to 3 years

No baby is born into a psychological void; infancy can be a demanding time for any family, as it adjusts to the arrival of a new member. The developmental tasks at this stage include:

- establishing a secure attachment relationship
  Parents and their infants need to form their own unique and intimate transactional relationship, where a 'goodness of fit' between parent and infant characteristics can be established (Thomas and Chess 1980).
- promoting optimal emotional, behavioural and intellectual development
- growing infant individuation and communication

The impact of the birth of a baby with a craniofacial deformity may be profound, at least initially, confounding parents' expectations, hopes and fantasies of the 'perfect' child.

The psychological challenges include the following.

1 INITIAL REACTIONS AND EMOTIONAL RESPONSE

Feelings of anxiety, grief, confusion, depression, anger, rejection, hurt, inadequacy and stigmatisation have all been reported (Lansdown 1981, Bull and Rumsey 1988, Barden et al 1989, Pillemer and Cook 1989, Endriga and Kapp-Simon 1999). Parents are often shocked, even disgusted, by the appearance of their baby and there may be transitory rejection ('He looked like a monster. I could not bear to see him for several days' – report by a mother of a 6-month-old baby with Apert syndrome). The facial features associated with syndromes, such as Apert or Crouzon, may make it all the harder for parents to feel that their baby is truly theirs, as the baby may bear a greater resemblance to other children with Apert or Crouzon syndrome than to his/her parents and their families. Parents often report a preoccupation with how their child might have looked. While mourning the loss of 'what might have been' (Tomko 1983), parents may have to face their ambivalent feelings towards the 'imperfect' child they actually have (Fajardo 1987).

Facial disfigurement, particularly in complex syndromic conditions, cannot be hidden and may present a serious challenge to parental feelings of self-worth, competence and self-image, particularly if expectations of beauty are bound up in that self-image. There may be a sense of outrage – why me? – which can be difficult to share with close family members, let alone with a craniofacial team. As part of a society that strongly values beauty and perfection and that stigmatises disfigurement, parents may occupy an uneasy position in no man's land. They are the buffer between their disfigured child and the outside world, seeking to protect their child from potential rejection, while forced to confront their own reactions to disfigurement.

2 REACTIONS OF EXTERNAL FAMILY MEMBERS AND WIDER COMMUNITY

Grandparents and family friends are an important source of emotional and practical support to parents and siblings of a facially different child, which can facilitate parental feelings of social acceptance and adjustment (Bradbury and Hewison 1994). With non-judgemental acceptance, love and ability to contain their own anxieties and ambivalent feelings, the extended family can enhance the process of attachment between the new mother and baby (Fonagy et al 1991), providing a model for coping that promotes parental resilience.

Sometimes grandparents, extended family and friends have long-term adjustment difficulties themselves (they can feel stigmatisation by association), and the new parents then carry the extra burden of coping with their family's anxiety, sadness, shock, etc. as well as their own. As one grandmother of a 6-year-old with craniofrontonasal syndrome remarked, 'she is a funny little thing but I cannot come to terms with this. These things do not happen in our family.'

The challenge of public behaviour is in its unpredictability. While it may be an innate characteristic of humans to be highly alert to facial characteristics and instinctively drawn towards visible difference (Langlois 1995), the subsequent behaviour is a matter of voluntary choice. Looking may be automatic, staring is optional. There may be no ill intent – 'mere' curiosity, embarrassment or uncertainty as to how to act. Young children in particular are frequently only seeking information when they ask 'what's wrong with his face?' Particularly in the early days, parents can experience even a look or the most innocent question as a deeply intrusive and punishing experience. All too frequently, parents report highly distressing encounters with complete strangers or, worse, acquaintances. One mother of a toddler with Apert syndrome was approached in the street and told that she 'should get down on her knees and pray to God to forgive her her sins in producing such a child'. Another family with twin girls, one of whom has craniofrontonasal dysplasia, moved to a new estate; they immediately found themselves reported to the police and the NSPCC. A neighbour had seen the disfigured child and automatically assumed her father had assaulted her. A mother of twin boys, one of whom has severe Crouzon syndrome, was asked not to bring the affected twin along to a friend's birthday party, as he 'would spoil the photographs'. Parents are not necessarily being paranoid in their suspicion of a hostile world.

3 FAMILY INTERACTIONS

Attachment between parents and child

The development of an intimate and secure bond between parent and child is a prerequisite for future emotional health and successful social relationships (Bowlby 1969). This bond is built up from the mutual signalling and communication between parents and baby. Parents learn to 'read' and interpret their baby's facial and verbal messages – which cry means hunger, which cry means distress, fatigue, etc. – in order to identify and respond to those needs.

When craniofacial anomalies, particularly those of the eyes and mouth, affect a baby's expressiveness, it may be much harder for a baby to signal his/her needs and for parents to interpret those signals, more so when a parent has ambivalent feelings towards their child. There is, therefore, a potential risk, increased for children with craniosynostosis-related syndromes, that they receive less responsive and nurturant care (Barden et al 1989) and that attachment relationships are compromised (Field 1995, Walters 1997). Risk factors include maternal depression (Tronick and Field 1986, Oster and Rajvaidya 1996) and overprotective and intrusive parental anxiety (Speltz et al 1995).

Parental relationships
Parents adjust in different ways and at different rates. As many partnerships are strengthened by the birth of a disfigured baby as are put under severe stress. Difficulties may arise when parents feel guilty or blame the other, overtly or covertly, when they fail to acknowledge or understand each other's responses, or when a parent's attention is diverted away from his/her partner and given exclusively to the baby.

The developing child
During the first year of life, babies develop an awareness of physical self and separateness from others. By around 10 months of age, babies will recognise and smile at themselves in mirrors and, from about 1 year, start to notice changes to their own facial appearance. The age at which children become aware that they look different from others varies considerably; awareness and understanding of facial difference often precede ability to communicate these verbally. Children as young as 2 years have been observed to touch the different part of their face and then their mother's to signal acknowledgement of that difference. However, recognition of facial difference does *not* imply distress at that difference. Many young children only become aware that their face looks different from others' reactions.

Toddlerhood is a time for exploring independence and testing limits. Parents whose children have undergone early medical interventions, including craniofacial surgery, or who have experienced negative public reaction to their child, may be overprotective. In consequence, there is the potential for a child to be withdrawn, overdependent and clingy (Speltz et al 1995), particularly if there are accompanying sensory impairments.

Reactions of siblings
Like any new baby, the infant with a craniofacial problem can be the object of adoring sibling devotion as well as rivalrous jealousy. Parents often report that siblings quickly accept physical differences, appearing more concerned about the baby attending hospital. Siblings are a potential source of developmental stimulation and emotional support to a disfigured baby. However the disfigurement is also a potential risk factor for psychological problems, all the more so for being a visible, as opposed to a hidden, condition. Siblings may also suffer stigmatisation by association, at nursery and school (Lavigne and Ryan 1979). They may feel unable to express their jealousy and distress at the extra attention, indulgence and care the disfigured child appears to receive from their parents. Body image may be affected, particularly for unaffected twins of disfigured children (Walters 1997).

Siblings may also have to cope with disrupted care arrangements made necessary by frequent hospital attendance.

4 TREATMENT PLANS AND PREPARATION FOR SURGERY

The referral for the initial period of assessment, diagnosis and treatment planning at a specialist craniofacial centre can place high demands on a family, whether the referral occurs shortly after birth or several months later. Parents in the early phase of recovery after birth and adaptation to their new baby are required to meet a new set of professionals, absorb complex information, possibly adjust their perceptions and beliefs owing to prior inaccurate information, and participate in decision making with the team. It is unsurprising that, despite meticulous attention and care offered to new families, parents frequently report the early assessment phase as more stressful and anxiety-provoking than subsequent episodes of surgery.

The diagnosis itself can have great impact. In the case of complex craniosynostoses, the label 'syndrome' is not neutral, carrying an almost universal association with Down syndrome and an automatic assumption of concomitant global learning difficulties. Parents who are already anxious about their baby need reassurance that impaired cognitive functioning is not an automatic sequela of the craniosynostosis.

Conversely, a diagnosis may come as a relief. In the case of a 'simple' single suture craniosynostosis, parents may have suspected an abnormal head shape from birth but failed to convince their GP or health visitor of their concerns. Parents often report their frustration at being labelled 'over-anxious' or 'neurotic'.

In the absence of functional or sensory impairment, when the surgical reconstruction is 'elective', it can be hard for parents to take a decision on behalf of their child. On the one hand, they may perceive the head shape as acceptable and feel reluctant to allow their child to undergo a major procedure on cosmetic grounds 'only'. On the other hand, parents fear future teasing at school ('children are so cruel') and the consequences of not treating. In discussion with parents, it is striking how often the following remark is heard: 'I couldn't bear for him to turn round in years from now and ask why we did nothing when treatment was available.'

Other issues affecting decision making relate to the gender of the child – appearance still being considered as more important for girls – future marriageability, and need for secrecy from the wider family because of the family stigma of an 'imperfect' child, as well as fears associated with the surgery itself.

The timing of surgery can present a challenge: while many parents are shocked by the prospect of surgery in infancy, others who seek immediate intervention can find it very difficult when the recommendation is for surgery to be deferred.

Finally, surgical correction itself can be a challenge: parents need to adjust to their baby's altered appearance and reattune to their 'new' baby – not always a straightforward process.

5 Transition to Nursery

Starting nursery is an important developmental phase, marking separation from parents and growing individuation and independence, as well as entry to a wider social milieu. Parents who have acted as gatekeepers and buffers against a wider society have to prepare child and nursery for each other. Parents may not discuss facial difference with their child as a result of a conscious decision to reinforce normality and sameness. In turn, the child may not be aware of his/her facial difference. The family now faces a dilemma. What if anything should teachers and other children be told? And what should they, as parents, say to their own child? Do explanations and discussion of the anomalies merely emphasise the 'abnormalities' of the child and reinforce those differences parents seek to minimise?

Interventions

Interventions aim to promote positive family adjustment as the key to the development of resilience in the child, together with skills to manage anxiety and stress. A cognitive behavioural approach that emphasises the reciprocal relationship of individual thoughts, feelings and behaviours and social environment can be extremely effective in helping to develop and expand a strong repertoire of coping skills in the child and the family (Broder 2001).

It is important for the psychologist to routinely meet all new families soon after initial referral – not just those families presenting with difficulties – so that an early relationship can be established through which to identify and reinforce the family's strengths. A semi-structured interview is a useful and systematic means of noting the family's unique narrative and style, based on their account of events at the birth of their child, their subsequent actions, feelings, attitude and hopes for the future.

Subsequently, throughout the early years, interventions can be offered in the following areas.

Exploring the meaning and significance of disfigurement

Giving the opportunity to express anger, confusion, sadness, feelings of guilt, stigma and shame that can interfere with early attachment to the baby is important in order to normalise and legitimise such feelings before exploring effective strategies for change, which may differ for fathers and mothers.

Early indicators of difficulties can include a reluctance to take a baby out in public, prolonged distress, reluctance to take or show photos or videos of the child, and attitude to future children (Bradbury 1996). Initially, many parents say they could not tolerate the possibility of another similarly affected child, or conversely some parents want to have another child as soon as possible to prove their ability to have a 'normal' child ('I can't wait to have a proper baby', reported a mother of a child with Crouzon syndrome).

Regaining control

It is important that a craniofacial diagnosis does not define the child (e.g. a child with Apert syndrome rather than an Apert child). Regular developmental assessments can provide an effective way of highlighting a young child's developing skills, abilities and individual personality traits. Parents can easily feel distressed or deskilled when faced with unexpected, insensitive questioning in public. It can be useful to gently challenge or reinterpret 'faulty' parental beliefs (e.g. 'people blame me for my child's condition, my child will never be popular in school'), while helping parents develop personal 'scripts' of responses for use in various social situations, so that parents can feel assertive rather than aggressive in their responses.

A sense of control is heightened not just by the quality and the availability of social support but by the familiy's readiness to make use of such support (Crockenburg 1981). Arranging contact with craniofacial support groups or other organisations may be extremely helpful for some families.

Building self-esteem in parents and child

Good parental self-esteem is a necessary precursor for the development of confidence and strong self-worth in the child. Parents provide highly influential role models for their children: how a child copes with hospital visits or difficult social interactions is strongly influenced by parental example. In their response to others, parents implicitly convey their acceptance or otherwise of the disfigurement. A child's self-esteem is fostered through the parents establishing the craniofacial difference as one aspect, but not the defining aspect, of the child. Regularly showing the child the family photographs and baby pictures is one effective way of illustrating all the attributes that make up sameness and difference between family members.

Preparation for surgery and afterwards

The psychologist can facilitate the process of decision making, which can be very stressful for parents particularly if there is disagreement between partners. While awaiting surgery, the detailed information and preparation offered by other members of the craniofacial team can be supplemented with an exploration of parental hopes and expectations of their child's post-surgical appearance, to minimise possible disappointment and problems with adjustment. This is all the more important when the process of change is protracted (e.g. when a RED frame is used for midface distraction).

Preparation for nursery

Parents can be offered help with finding the most appropriate nursery placement for their child as well as help with preparing nursery staff and other families for the arrival of their child into the nursery. Members of the craniofacial team can also work directly with nursery staff to help educate them about craniofacial conditions and the impact on the young child.

TABLE 12.1
Summary: birth and early infancy

Issues	• mourning and acceptance
	• reactions of family and community
	• family reactions and interactions
	• reorganisation
	• treatment proposals
Interventions	• exploration of meaning and significance of diagnosis
	• regaining control
	• building parental and child self-esteem
	• coping strategies
	• preparation for surgery
	• adaptation to new appearance
	• preparation for nursery

Case study 1
L aged 4 years. Diagnosis: Pfeiffer syndrome

L, the second child of professional parents, was 2 weeks old when first admitted to the craniofacial unit. An older sibling was sent to relatives. The psychologist introduced herself and was told everything was fine; her visits were neither necessary nor welcome. L was a fretful, irritable baby who had sucking difficulties. Her mother was distraught at having to abandon breast-feeding. Even the bottle had to be replaced by a naso-gastric tube. The parents appeared shell-shocked: they asked questions but did not appear to hear the replies.

They sat for long hours looking at L, but rarely held her or talked to her. As the admission proceeded, L's mother became increasingly angry, complaining bitterly about the inefficiency and discomfort of hospital life. She felt she was in a goldfish bowl under permanent scrutiny. L's father appeared depressed and rarely spoke to staff. A crisis arose and L's mother threatened to make a formal complaint. The psychologist commiserated with her anger and commented how out of control everything might feel. In tears, the mother acknowledged what a shock L's arrival had been. The delivery had been prolonged and initially she thought L was dead. Someone mentioned 'syndrome' and she was convinced that implied Down syndrome. On first sight, she could not believe this was her child and refused to care for her for two days. In a second, unfamiliar hospital setting and guilty about not being with their other child, she was convinced that L would be intellectually retarded and rejected at school – 'who could ever want to play with her?' L's father said he could not overcome feelings of guilt although intellectually he knew no one was at fault.

L's mother began to confide her dread and guilt that she could never feel as close to L as she did to her first child. Both parents acknowledged how hard it was to feel so out of control. The ward staff negotiated a new care plan that afforded the parents the practical help they required to care for L while careful not to inadvertently undermine their confidence or feelings of competence. L's father became expert in all the practical aspects of L's care, including feeding her by naso-gastric tube. He chose not to discuss his feelings but gradually appeared less depressed. As L's mother began to cuddle and play with her baby, she began to comment on L's personality and behaviour, rather than focusing on her abnormalities. L first underwent surgery at 8 weeks; she remained frail and slow to thrive. She suffered ocular problems with proptosis and additionally required a nasal prong.

In her first two years L had eight hospital admissions with two further episodes of major craniofacial surgery. She was found to have moderate deafness in both ears. She had breathing difficulties with obstructive sleep apnoeas and repeated chest infections.

There were difficult medical decisions to be made. At this very early age, midfacial advancement was being recommended. Despite numerous consultations, the parents felt they did not have sufficient technical information to reach an informed decision and became very angry with the team. To the psychologist they described their mixed emotions: if L survived the operation, would she have later recall and suffer emotionally? How different would she look? L's parents had grown to love her and were frightened she would be unrecognisable, while feeling guilty that they also hoped that her facial appearance would be improved. For the first time L's mother revealed her distress and shame when taking L out in public. Her response to staring and questioning was helpless rage. She wondered how L would cope if she herself could not. She spoke about her older child who was showing some behavioural disturbance and admitted how important it was to have had a 'normal' child first, just to prove she could. The parents were to return to this theme many times. L was 2½ years old when she underwent major reconstructive surgery for the third time. There were postoperative complications but she survived and made a good recovery. After a short period of adjustment, the parents felt enormous relief and delight at L's new looks, especially when the nasal prong was removed. L began to thrive. Her parents could now envisage a future without constant hospital admission for their child and began to look at suitable local playgroups. L's mother consulted the psychologist on how to respond to public reactions and how to prepare teachers. This was the first of several sessions in which the mother reflected on the importance that physical attractiveness held for her and the stigma she felt because L looked so different from her. As her sense of shame diminished personally, she discussed various strategies to help herself and eventually to help L with intrusive comments or questions. She wanted to feel as competent as possible in order to set a good example for L. She practised relaxation techniques to use if she became uncomfortably anxious in public. She reported growing confidence and sense of control in public situations.

By the age of 4 years L was attending a local nursery school with additional help from a teacher for the deaf. A developmental assessment showed that L had normal intellectual ability with a slight delay in her language skills, attributed to her bilateral hearing loss. L was a lively and very sociable little girl. Her peers at nursery showed an initial reserve but that was quickly overcome with sensitive handling from the teacher. L's hearing aids tended to attract more attention than her different facial appearance.

More surgery awaited L but for now visits to the hospital were kept to a minimum. L herself had not yet commented on her appearance. Her older brother tended to be overprotective with L but was aggressive in school and tended to have outbursts of temper with his parents. He was seen with his parents by the psychologist to discuss his concerns and feelings, and this was followed by a referral for local psychological help. L's father had bouts of depression but was reluctant to seek help. L and her family continue to be offered regular follow-up.

Comment

This case illustrates the often long and complicated process of a family's psychological adaptation to the birth of a baby with syndromic craniosynostosis. Parents have to manage their own and their partner's emotions, including shock and grief, in the very public arena of a hospital ward, while simultaneously learning about their baby's condition and medical needs. Parental anger can all too easily become redirected towards the medical and ward staff and good liaison is essential so that parental expertise and autonomy are supported. Negative emotions including guilt, shame and stigma can persist over time and may only be acknowledged once a trusting relationship with the craniofacial team has been developed. It is, therefore, important for the psychologist to meet families early so that a relationship is established for any future intervention. Sibling reactions change over time and should be monitored.

Interventions included:

- exploration of parental reactions to diagnosis
- reduction of parental distress and anxiety
- coping strategies for public reactions
- assessment of developmental functioning and liaison with nursery regarding educational needs
- monitoring sibling adaptation
- facilitating communication between staff members and family to defuse conflict

Early childhood: 3 to 7 years

This is a time of increasing individuation, drive for autonomy and decreasing dependence on the immediate proximity of parents. These processes are mediated by the growing ability, with developing language skills, of the young child to understand their own and others' emotions – the basis of self-control.

Additional psychological challenges include the following:

1 SELF-IMAGE AND AWARENESS OF FACIAL DIFFERENCE

With developing concepts of self–other and growing awareness of themselves as social beings, young children with craniofacial difference are at heightened risk of excessive shyness and feeling self-conscious and conspicuous, particularly if sensitised by staring or parental distress in public. In contrast, some young children enter nursery completely unaware of their facial difference and entirely unprepared for other children's staring, comments and questions, which can come as a major shock, causing distress and negative self-image.

2 DEVELOPMENT OF PEER RELATIONSHIPS

It is not inevitable that problems will arise but making friends can certainly be more difficult. There is a heightened risk of early unpopularity, avoidance and rejection by peers, based on their judgements about physical appearance, which can cause anxiety, social inhibitions and withdrawal in the affected child.

If the child arrives at nursery already shy and withdrawn in anticipation of problems or rejection by peers (Richman and Elliason 1982), he/she may not initiate friendships or respond to peers' attempts to make friends. Parents can inadvertently contribute to this process: in their desire to minimise the opportunities for teasing, they may have limited the opportunities for their child to acquire and practise social skills. This then creates the potential for a vicious circle where a child, lacking age-appropriate skills, is perceived by peers as babyish and awkward and is consequently avoided.

3 DEVELOPING ACADEMIC COMPETENCE

Children with craniofacial anomalies may also be at a higher risk of learning difficulties (Broder et al 1998, Kapp-Simon 1998; see also later section), especially if compounded by sensory or functional impairment, e.g. ongoing hearing loss. Additionally, a child's social inhibitions can impact on academic achievement, reinforcing teachers' lowered expectations of academic performance (Richman 1978). Teachers may have their own distress or difficulty with disfigured appearance, which can negatively affect their relationship with the child and that child's consequent performance.

INTERVENTIONS

For parents

Parents can be offered ideas and support to help develop their child's strengths, abilities, self-esteem, confidence and social skills, as well as specific responses their child can give to direct questions or comments about appearance.

Parents frequently request advice on how best to enlist a school's help with prevention or control of teasing as well as how to support their child directly.

For the child

Direct work with a young child using age-appropriate play and materials, e.g. drawings, dolls and puppets, can foster self-confidence and help desensitise to aspects of appearance or altered functioning, e.g. poor speech, that may negatively impact upon social situations. Body image and fantasies about disfigurement can be explored and any misperceptions about causation corrected (e.g. 'This happened to me because I was bad'). The child can also be helped with how to answer questions on their appearance. Being ready with a 'script' of simple answers to questions increases control over potentially awkward situations, by removing the element of surprise, and facilitating responses. Early formal assessment of intellectual functioning can be vital to identify not only strengths in cognitive functioning but also any early deficits or delays so that educational intervention can be sought at the earliest opportunity.

For the family
Intervention can be offered to help promote continued family adjustment and cohesiveness, particularly where siblings are experiencing difficulties in relation to the disfigurement, either at home or at school.

For the school
The craniofacial team can perform a very useful external advocacy role, working directly with teachers and their classes to increase knowledge of and sensitivity to craniofacial conditions and their surgical treatment. Written information, care guidelines, and training have all been found to be helpful.

TABLE 12.2
Summary: early childhood

Issues	• awareness of facial difference
	• understanding treatment protocol
	• social behaviour
	• cognitive functioning
Interventions	• parental concerns
	• enhancing social skills and assertiveness
	• strategies for enhancing self-esteem
	• family adaptation, e.g. siblings
	• assessment of intellectual functioning

Middle childhood: 7 to 11 years
Developmental tasks at this stage include academic attainment at school and the development of effective and positive peer relationships and social behaviour. The main psychological challenges include the following.

1 INCREASING AWARENESS AND SELF-CRITICAL EVALUATION OF APPEARANCE
Distress with appearance is not directly related to the 'objective' severity or visibility of disfigurement. What medical professionals and the public regard as an insignificant problem can still cause the child major distress and desire for early treatment. A child with a craniofacially asymmetric appearance or abnormal head shape can often be more distressed than a child with a major craniofacial syndrome.

2 PEER RELATIONSHIPS

Most of the child's social life takes place at school. Belonging to and acceptance by the developing peer group is all-important at this time. The child with craniosynostosis needs, not just wants, to be just like the others. If a facial difference is accompanied by sensory or functional impairment, e.g. poor speech intelligibility, children are all the more at risk of psychological distress and problems. Children may be moving from the more protected environment of infant school to junior school where they are the youngest and physically smallest group and may face repeated questioning and name-calling.

Feelings of social isolation, compounded by repeated absences from school, can prevent the child from acquiring the social skills needed for the formation of satisfactory relationships in adult life, as well as impacting adversely on learning, particularly in a group. Teasing among all children reaches a peak at 7–8 years when the child is least able to manage it. The child may be reluctant to confide in his/her parents, wanting to protect and not upset them. Equally, they may be nervous about letting teachers know of their plight. Instead they show their distress in less adaptive ways, e.g. reluctance to go to school, physical symptoms or disruptive behaviour.

3 TRANSITION TO SECONDARY SCHOOL

Leaving the familiar primary school setting for a larger and unfamiliar secondary school community is daunting for most children. It is all the more anxiety-provoking for facially different children who face a reprise of the curiosity and questioning on a magnified and less controllable scale.

4 ACADEMIC PERFORMANCE

Some children with craniosynostosis are at heightened risk of having specific learning difficulties (see later section) that can impact on the acquisition of key academic skills, hindering progress but also self-confidence.

INTERVENTIONS

For the child

As the child matures, it becomes increasingly important to ascertain perceptions and feelings about diagnosis, proposed treatment, its timing, appearance and functioning, not only to promote adherence to treatment and participation in decision making, but also because the child's views may differ markedly from parental concerns, yet remain unexpressed. A child may be extremely distressed about his/her appearance and treatment may feel unbearably far off. Conversely, a child may be happy with his/her looks but accede to strong parental pressures for improvement. All children can be highly anxious about hospitalisation, invasive medical procedures and the outcome of surgery. All these concerns demand careful exploration using developmentally appropriate play materials, e.g. board games, drawing, stories, scrapbooks, etc.

A variety of problem-solving, cognitive-behavioural techniques can be offered to develop and expand the child's existing repertoire of coping strategies for questions, comments or teasing. Using modelling, rehearsal, goal setting and distraction, the child can be encouraged to build on his/her sense of humour, assertiveness and empathy to enhance confidence, self-esteem and interpersonal skills. Such intervention may be particularly useful at the two times of major transition, i.e. moving to primary and secondary schools.

For parents and siblings
Parents remain important role models for their children at this stage. The manner in which families discuss the child's increasingly complex and demanding questioning becomes a template for the child when on his/her own in school or out in the community. Parents can be helped to maintain open communication with their child, especially on treatment issues where there may be disagreement among family members. Parents can also be encouraged to actively foster their child's friendships, talents, enthusiasms and achievements.

The use of role-play in families to help a disfigured child develop and practise responses and coping strategies can be highly effective on many levels. By taking turns at playing tormentor and victim, the siblings, especially, can identify with problems and devise creative solutions for their brother or sister. Parents sometimes express their concern that role-playing difficult social situations may sensitise the disfigured child to future problems that may never arise. However, clinical experience indicates that this kind of 'safe', home-based preparation empowers the child and promotes self-confidence.

For the school
Teachers can be offered expert advice and consultation both for individual children with social or learning difficulties and for the school community as a whole: e.g. developing programmes and projects aimed at increasing knowledge and tolerance of facial difference and the integration of disfigured children.

TABLE 12.3
Summary: middle childhood

Issues	• appearance • peer relationships • academic attainments • educational transitions • treatment decisions
Interventions	• enhancing social skills • raising self-esteem • management of teasing • understanding treatment decisions • obtaining assent • preparation for surgery

Case study 2
B, aged 9 years. Diagnosis: sagittal craniosynostosis

Since her birth, B's parents had been concerned that her head shape was abnormal, but this was attributed to moulding, by their GP and health visitor. B's mother remembered being told not to be so 'over-anxious'. Still concerned nine months later, B's parents sought a private paediatric opinion. Radiological investigation confirmed a diagnosis of sagittal craniosynostosis. This was described as a purely cosmetic problem, with no functional consequences for intellectual development. Surgical reconstruction was not recommended, which greatly relieved the parents.

From the age of 6 years, B became increasingly aware of and preoccupied by her head shape. She complained to her parents that she was continually stared at and called 'egg head' or 'peanut head' by her peers. The school took her complaints seriously and carefully monitored the class. Her teachers felt that she was not being singled out and in fact often avoided the friendly overtures of other children. Over the next three years, B's complaints intensified: for every birthday and Christmas, she asked for her present to be 'big surgery'. B's schoolwork deteriorated; she began to sleep badly and frequently complained of headaches.

After repeated visits to the GP, a referral to the craniofacial centre resulted in an in-patient multidisciplinary assessment. B appeared delighted and relieved to be in hospital. She was eager to tell the psychologist just how much she hated her head shape, how she was teased at school and had no friends, and how she dreaded going to secondary school. B said the whole trouble was her mum who was too frightened to let her have surgery. She wished she could cast a spell to make her mother change her mind. A formal assessment of intellectual functioning showed B to be of well above average intelligence, but with specific cognitive deficits indicative of mild dyslexia. Interviewed on their own, B's parents recognised how desperately B hated her head shape. For their part, they were delighted with her appearance and terrified of the risks of elective surgery. They acknowledged how difficult it was becoming to ignore B's pleadings for treatment and just prayed that the surgeons would refuse to operate.

B underwent intracranial pressure monitoring. She had already observed another child undergoing the procedure; when she thought she was unobserved, she jumped up and down, in an attempt to increase the readings. She frequently asked, 'is it high enough for surgery?' All test results, including ICP, were normal. There were no neurosurgical indications for surgery.

B was present with her parents to discuss the results. The surgical procedure with its attendant potential risks was explained. B's understanding of this was checked. Again, she asked for surgery, a request supported by her parents, albeit reluctantly. The psychological findings were considered and surgery was agreed. B was elated.

Three months later, she was admitted for surgical reconstruction, after careful preparation by the psychologist and play specialist. Surgery proceeded uneventfully. On regaining consciousness, B demanded to know how she looked. She was carefully prepared for the changes to her appearance. Despite the bruising and swelling, she appeared delighted with the outcome. The nurses noted she made an exceptionally quick recovery. Liaison with the school resulted in the provision of extra help with literacy skills. Six months later, B's parents described her as a 'new child' in every sense. B was more settled and self-confident, her headaches had disappeared, she was catching up academically and able to maintain friendships.

Comment

Deformity, as well as beauty, is in the eye of the beholder; severity is as much a subjective experience as an objective measure. The cosmetic deformity produced by a simple craniosynostosis was of minor significance to the parents but caused major and chronic distress in the child. School contributed a helpful and not uncommon observation that the girl's inability to make friends was as much a product of her own awkward behaviour as of being teased. Her poor academic performance could have been attributed entirely to her emotional distress. However, it was important to investigate underlying learning difficulties as a correlate of the single suture craniosynostosis, and indeed psychometric assessment revealed specific cognitive deficits that required remedial educational help. The psychological assessment of the child's distress made an important contribution to the multidisciplinary assessment and treatment plan. The decision to proceed with surgical reconstruction, reluctantly reached by the parents, was of immense benefit to the subsequent emotional well-being of the child.

Psychological interventions included:

- exploration and clarification of the child's wishes and expectations of surgery
- family therapy to ameliorate distress
- liaison with the school to suggest interventions to control teasing
- psychometric assessment with recommendations for remedial help

Adolescence to early adulthood

The age boundaries of this stage are increasingly hard to peg, particularly in a western society, where improving nutrition and health have lowered the onset of puberty, while continuing education and longer economic dependence on parents have stretched the upper limit. Perhaps adolescence is a stage better described by its outcomes? Preparation for occupation, potential for economic independence, acquiring a social group, establishing sexual partnerships, and accepting responsibility for participation in society.

The developmental tasks facing all adolescents in a period dominated by self-doubt and insecurity include: acquiring a sense of individual identity to separate from the family (which includes an acceptance of physique and appearance), securing positive intimate peer relationships, achieving interdependence with family and acquiring a sense of autonomy, an individual value system and conscience (Bloom 1980).

Achieving these tasks can be even more of a challenge for an adolescent with a craniofacial difference, as follows:

1 FACIAL APPEARANCE AND IDENTITY

The process of rapid physical growth, with bodily and emotional changes, can produce feelings of insecurity, confusion, self-doubt and extreme self-consciousness. The peer group becomes the criterion against which to judge physical 'normality'. It is all the harder for a young person who looks different to integrate his/her appearance into an overall body image and identity, particularly if facial appearance is likely to change owing to imminent reconstructive surgery.

2 ACCEPTANCE BY PEERS

The peer group is all-important; social acceptance and acceptability are key to an individual's judgements of personal success or failure. Similarly the peer group provides the social context for the development of an individual's personal value system. A history of unsatisfactory peer relationships, with few friendships and experience of teasing, bullying or rejection, can make the adolescent feel socially isolated and highly vulnerable to anxiety, loneliness and inhibition, which may impact upon the later development of intimate and sexual relationships.

3 TREATMENT DECISIONS

The opinions, wishes and needs of the child, always important to decision making about surgery, now become paramount, as the adolescent and family approach the long-desired (and/or dreaded) craniofacial surgery that has awaited completion of facial bone growth. From the age of 16 it is the adolescent him/herself who will need to give informed consent. The adolescent will need to engage with the craniofacial team, to seek and process information that will guide decision making. There may be conflicting goals ('I want to look different but I am terrified of being unrecognisable'), as well as conflict between the adolescent and parents, in this time of challenge to parental authority. The craniofacial team members themselves may be perceived as authoritarian, parental figures, as well as authoritative professionals, against whom to rebel. Additionally, an outward show of defiant independence in the form of rejecting surgical recommendations can mask an adolescent's need to gain parental approval and acceptance.

INTERVENTIONS

Enhancing social skills and coping strategies

Many adolescents feel themselves to be passive victims of others' responses to them, but the behaviour of the disfigured adolescent him/herself is all-important. Studies suggest that social skills training can be effective in increasing self-awareness and empathy, which in turn has a positive impact on peer acceptance and popularity (Kapp-Simon and Simon 1991).

Interventions aimed at extending the repertoire of strategies are based on:

- creating a positive self-belief
- enhancing self-image
- improving sense of control in awkward situations
- enhancing perception of available social support
- increasing initiative taking in social situations

Such social skills training addresses problem solving, body language – particularly making eye contact – and conversational skills (Kapp-Simon and Simon 1995, Bradbury 1996, Kish and Lansdown 2000), and can be augmented by desensitisation to teasing (Gerrard 1991) based on cognitive-behavioural and social learning theory and techniques.

Research evidence on efficacy, both in the short and longer term, is as yet scant but clinical experience suggests encouraging outcomes.

Adolescents can be reluctant customers for help, and great flexibility and patience can be required. Some young people prefer to seek help outside the specialist centre and can be referred to local resources or specialist organisations (e.g. Changing Faces, a UK-based charity). Other adolescents prefer telephone contact alone or written information (Kish and Lansdown 2000). Small group sessions create the opportunity for young people to meet others facing similar challenges, as well as a place to practise newly acquired techniques for social interaction. However, many adolescents find the idea of groups threatening, and meeting others with similar diagnoses can reinforce their feelings of difference. A more indirect approach may be equally successful. A series of adventure weekend camps for young people with a craniofacial disorder, organised by ward staff at Great Ormond Street Hospital, offering supervised outdoor activities and sports, has been well received by participants, who reported increased feelings of confidence and self-efficacy following participation.

Treating anxiety and depression
Treatment in specialist craniofacial centres from birth creates the opportunity for the psychologist to get to know the child and family well and monitor any changes in emotional well-being. It is important to get as full a picture as possible of an individual's functioning within the family and at school, and to discuss interests, talents, hobbies and ambitions for the future.

Levels of distress, anxiety, self-esteem and depression in an individual should be carefully and regularly monitored, using interviews, clinical scales and questionnaires and, where possible, direct observation. The adolescent's views, concerns and feelings should be ascertained. Any indication of high distress, anxiety, depression or low esteem needs to be carefully monitored. If there is suspicion of increased risk of deliberate self-harm or suicide, the adolescent should be asked directly about this (Walters 1997). The difficulties should be acknowledged directly with the adolescent and appropriate psychological management instigated, including referral to other professionals or resources where appropriate.

School, college, work
Monitoring intellectual functioning and academic attainments to identify cognitive strengths and interests as well as weaknesses informs interventions that can be offered to augment educational or vocational help, in order to maximise the young person's chances of achieving their full potential at school, college or in the workplace. Liaison with community educational resources is essential.

Treatment decisions
Adolescents can find a face-to-face interview with the craniofacial team extremely daunting, embarrassing or generally difficult and may remain monosyllabic throughout the consultation, making it hard for team members to ascertain different family views and expectations of reconstructive surgery and/or further treatment.

It is very important that the adolescent should be offered consultation on his/her own to try to gain a clear understanding of how family decisions for or against surgery have been reached. Understanding individual family members' positions can then aid communications with parents, which is important when there is apparent conflict or disagreement. Adolescents can be helped to elucidate their expectations and fears of change (e.g. 'Will I be recognisable to myself and my friends, will I be a different person, how will I look, can't they love me as I am?'). Fears of surgery can also be addressed and anxiety management techniques offered, as appropriate, for procedural fears. Work with parents can focus on issues involving protectiveness, anxiety, desire to retain control over decision making, perceived fulfilment of obligations of treatment to their child. 'Shuttle diplomacy' between family members and the team can be helpful to clarify different viewpoints and empower individuals to say yes or no to surgery (Kapp-Simon and Simon 1995). It is important that the family should arrive at a treatment plan that is acceptable to all members, even if this runs counter to elective treatment possibilities.

Where surgery is sought and accepted, it is extremely important that both adolescents and their families have as realistic expectations as possible of what surgery can achieve. There is a near universal demand for pre- and post-surgical changes to be described or illustrated, and pre- and post-surgery photographs can be helpful in the absence of appropriate computer technology.

After surgery, there is a period of reorganisation and accommodation to the changes for both the adolescent and the family. The loss of the old person and the old face may have to be mourned; there may be some initial early disappointment and interventions need to be offered both to the adolescent and family members, as appropriate.

As part of the gradual preparation for ending of treatment and discharge from the craniofacial service, genetic counselling should be offered to adolescents routinely, although many may wish to defer this until some years later when they are nearer to having their own children.

TABLE 12.4
Summary: adolescence to early adulthood

Issues	
	• defining sense of identity
	• establishing positive peer relationships
	• establishing interdependence and autonomy
	• accepting appearance
	• decisions on further treatment
	• discharge from craniofacial service
Interventions	
	• enhancing social skills
	• coping strategies for public hostility
	• treating anxiety and depression
	• liaison with school, college, workplace
	• facilitating family's treatment decisions
	• preparation for surgery and aftermath

Case study 3
R, aged 17 years. Diagnosis: Crouzon syndrome

R had attended the craniofacial unit since his infancy, undergoing surgical recon-struction at 3 months and 12 years. Over the years, R's parents had repeatedly requested further surgery to improve his facial appearance but had been advised that a midface advancement should be postponed until facial growth was complete. Now aged 17, the craniofacial surgeons were recommending midface advancement to improve appearance and functioning. However, since the age of 13, R had vehemently refused to contemplate further surgery as he held terrible memories of the last hospital stay. He insisted he was happy as he was. His father was upset and angry with R for not listening to medical advice, well aware that he could not force his son to consent to surgery against his will. After several failed appointments, R attended a consul-tation with the team; he appeared highly embarrassed and distant, answering questions monosyllabically with his head averted. R agreed that his teeth were in poor condition and alignment, causing him chewing difficulties and adversely affecting speech intelligibility. Nevertheless he declined any offer of treatment. The psychologist suggested a separate meeting to explore his views. R was non-committal but turned up with his father at the agreed time. R's father stated how bitter he felt that 'nothing had been done'; he wished surgery had been possible when R was younger and his consent not needed. He thought R did not know what was in his own best interests and was being ungrateful. R smiled ruefully and shrugged. He said he appreciated his father wanting the best for him, but could not agree to surgery. In subsequent individual sessions with the psychologist, R described his traumatic memories of his previous surgical admission; he said it felt like extreme punishment.

R had questions about the proposed surgery; he knew he had been told everything in detail but could not remember anything said. He said that he hated thinking about anything to do with hospitals and indeed handled all potentially difficult situations,

250

e.g. exams, by avoiding thinking about them until forced to do so. R was offered techniques to help him control his anxiety so as to be able to think things over more effectively. R diffidently agreed. He was taught guided imagery and relaxation, which he appeared to enjoy and find useful. His questions regarding surgery received written answers, and after discussions with the specialist nurse he became able to retain information. It was put to R that perhaps further surgery was not the right course of action for him at this time – others, including his parents, might be mistaken.

R then began to question what difference surgery would make to his appearance and requested to see pre- and post-surgery photographs. Spontaneously, he began to talk about his life: how he had a group of close friends but no girlfriend, how he was enjoying college and his sporting activities. He had suffered teasing as a young boy but this had now stopped, although the public's staring upset him. He now began to contemplate the pros and cons of surgery. Pleasing his father and improving his looks were at the top of the 'in favour' list. 'Against' were his fear of hospitals and adverse reactions of his friends. Usually softly spoken, R became suddenly angry, asking, 'Why do I need to look better? Aren't I good enough for them? Can't they love me as I am?' He said he was obsessed with the idea that the surgery would involve 'breaking me down and taking my face apart'. Would he be recognisable to himself and others after surgery? Could he remain the same person? What would happen if he did not look better? R described his guilt that he could not bring himself to conform to his parents' wishes. Without prompting, R sought the opinions of individual friends whose views, though differing, he found reassuring and supportive. Without warning, R announced that he had decided to pursue the surgical option, although his doubts remained. Now that he had reached a decision, he was sticking to it. His parents were delighted. In fact, because R needed extensive orthodontic preparation, surgery had to be postponed for one year. R was relieved: 'It's a weight off my shoulders.' He regularly attended all his orthodontic appointments and coped well with a brief admission to hospital to remove some teeth, using the psychological techniques he had learned to master his anxiety. Subsequently, he underwent two reconstructive surgical procedures and declared himself pleased with the outcome and reassured that he had retained his identity.

Comment

In his opposition to parental wishes and surgical recommendations, R presented as an awkward customer. Midface surgical reconstruction in late teen-age had always been part of the long-term treatment plan and would bring aesthetic and functional improvements. Why should R refuse what 'objectively' was in his best interest? It was essential to create the opportunity for R to elaborate on his views and feelings, with no attempt made to persuade or influence him. In time, R revealed his painful struggles for identity, social acceptance and predictability over what change in facial appearance would mean for him.

In suggesting a 'no treatment' option, R was enabled to examine the alternatives. Fears about changing his appearance were separated from specific anxieties about hospitals and invasive or unpleasant procedures, for which he was offered coping strategies. His experience of previous surgery as traumatic and punishing was a salutary reminder that, despite the most careful preparation, some children are highly stressed by hospitalisation, though they may not show it at the time. Helping parents and adolescent to understand each other's position was a precursor to their finding a mutually satisfactory solution. In the end, R's need to please his parents may have been overriding. The extended presurgical orthodontic treatment was psychologically beneficial in allowing a gradual preparation for major change.

Psychological interventions included:

- enabling and empowering decision making without prejudice
- resolution of family differences
- reduction of procedural anxiety and desensitisation to aversive medical procedures
- exploration of expectations of surgery
- preparation for surgery and aftermath
- pre- and post-audit of satisfaction with appearance and quality of life

Cognitive development and learning difficulties in children with craniosynostosis

Clearly, functional outcome in terms of intellectual functioning is of prime importance; certainly for parents, a major fear is that craniosynostosis, whether simple or syndromic, will result in global learning disability.

Learning disability (formerly called mental retardation or mental deficiency) is a developmental disorder, characterised by significantly below average intelligence (social, practical and conceptual) and limitations in the adaptive skills demanded by society.

The criterion for a diagnosis of global learning disability has typically been set at a point two standard deviations below the mean on a standardised measure of intelligence. The prevalence of global learning disability in the general population is estimated at around 1.5 to 2 per cent (Reschly 1992).

Specific learning problems, in the absence of global learning disability, can also occur, caused by specific cognitive deficits, e.g. expressive and/or receptive language, memory (visual and/or verbal, short-term, long-term recall), conceptual reasoning, visuo-perceptual skills, non-verbal problem solving and motor co-ordination.

AETIOLOGY
For the craniosynostoses, potential causes of cognitive deficits leading to a global or specific learning disability include:

- direct effect of the genetic mutation underlying the craniosynostosis
- raised intracranial pressure
- primary brain malformations

- secondary brain malformations resulting from distorted brain growth in an abnormally shaped skull (Renier et al 1982, Camfield et al 2000)

Associated factors include:

- effects of associated sensory impairment, e.g. hearing loss, poor vision
- poor levels of stimulation related to attachment difficulties between parent and child and/or low levels of expectation
- reduced academic demands by teachers, based on low expectations of academic potential (Richman 1978)
- interrupted schooling owing to hospital visits, in-patient treatment

As surgical reconstruction alters the intracranial pressure and skull shape, the timing and effect of surgery on intellectual functioning are pertinent.
    Questions to be answered include:

- Is global intellectual functioning impaired in single suture craniosynostoses, e.g. metopic, sagittal, unicoronal?
- Is intellectual functioning impaired in syndromic conditions?
- Is impairment of intellectual functioning specific or global?
- Does surgical construction and its timing influence intellectual outcome?

Studies to date have many methodological limitations:

- differing definitions of learning disability
- differing or unspecified methods of testing intellectual functioning
- anecdotal reporting of outcome
- small sample size
- heterogeneous or biased sampling
- pooled pre- and post-surgery cases
- presence of additional complex medical problems, e.g. prematurity, primary brain malformation
- cross-sectional versus longitudinal data
- no reporting of data on contributory factors, e.g. hearing loss

This has resulted in a research literature that has provoked lively and contentious debate but no definitive answers (Kapp-Simon et al 1993, Kapp-Simon 1994, 1998).

SIMPLE, ISOLATED CRANIOSYNOSTOSES
In the absence of other congenital abnormalities, e.g. primary brain malformations, there is no conclusive evidence of global learning disability as a direct result of craniosynostosis (Camfield et al 2000). It is thought that the risk of global learning disability may increase when there is a synostosis of more than one suture (Chumas et al 1997).

However, there *is* increasing evidence of specific and often subtle cognitive impairments that:

- develop over time and may only become apparent with increasing age
- require careful, detailed, multidisciplinary differential evaluation and neuropsychological assessment (Sidoti et al 1996, Speltz et al 1997, Kapp-Simon 1998, Virtanen et al 1999)

For example, in a recent study at Great Ormond Street Hospital of 76 children with isolated sagittal synostosis, there was a high prevalence rate (37 per cent) of specific speech and/or language impairment – the expected rate in a normal population is 6 per cent (Law et al 1998) – in the absence of global learning disability and unaffected by surgical status (Shipster et al 2003).

SYNDROMIC SYNOSTOSES

For children with Crouzon, Pfeiffer 1 and Saethre–Chotzen syndromes, in the absence of other malformations, intelligence in usually normal (Cohen and MacLean 2000a), although cases of mild to moderate learning disability have also been reported (Bartsocas et al 1970).

In other syndromes with accompanying brain anomalies, e.g. Apert, Pfeiffer III, Carpenter and Antley–Bixler syndromes, the risks of learning disability may be increased (Cohen 2000, Shprintzen 2000). For example, global learning disability is commonly considered to be an integral feature of Apert syndrome (Cohen and Kreiborg 1990). Evidence is emerging to suggest a more complex picture of individual and specific learning problems. Again, in a recent study at Great Ormond Street Hospital of 10 children aged 4–6 years with Apert syndrome, all children for whom a non-verbal IQ was obtained had non-verbal abilities within the average range, with IQs considerably higher than those reported in previous studies. Eight out of 10 children had moderate to severe language problems, not associated with a global learning disability. All the children had ongoing hearing losses, and problems with attention, speech and oro-motor skills (Shipster et al 2002).

The same cohort of 10 children, now aged 8–9 years, was seen for assessment follow-up using an extensive battery of cognitive and speech and language tests to monitor developmental progress. Again, no evidence of global learning disability emerged but a complex pattern of individual learning strengths and difficulties was found, including attentional problems in group situations and poor use of pragmatic language in social situations (Shipster et al, in preparation).

ASSESSMENT

The aim of a neuropsychological assessment of a child with craniosynostosis is to obtain a detailed picture over time of the development of that child's cognitive functioning and attainments, (a) to determine the changing profile of intellectual strengths and weaknesses and (b) to recommend appropriate interventions and educational support in the community. This assessment should form part of a broad-base multidisciplinary assessment protocol by the craniofacial team: in particular it is essential that concurrent measures of audiological and visual status are available.

Neuropsychological evaluation should be performed by an experienced psychologist with appropriate expertise and should include assessment of specific cognitive processes as well as overall intellectual functioning, i.e.:

- memory – visual and auditory
- associative reasoning (verbal and non-verbal)
- visuo-spatial skills
- visuo-motor functioning
- academic attainments in literacy and numeracy
- attention control in individual and group settings

Tests should be selected to take account of any problems with fine motor skills (e.g. the use of certain timed tests for children with Apert syndrome may adversely affect their performance scores). Testing should be repeated to coincide with key stages in a child's development, e.g. before starting nursery and primary school, transition to secondary school, end of secondary education.

MANAGEMENT

The neuropsychological assessment, as part of a multidisciplinary protocol, forms the basis of subsequent interventions.

For parent and child

Providing a regular and detailed profile of current intellectual strengths and attainments helps to promote a positive and optimistic outlook to enhance family resilience and adaptation to the craniofacial condition. With syndromic conditions, particularly Apert syndrome, parents often report their delight at seeing developmental progress that has exceeded their expectations, based on early and pessimistic prognoses. Assessment allows the early identification of potential learning problems so that the appropriate interventions can be implemented.

Assessment reports from a specialist craniofacial centre strengthen parents' applications to educational authorities for statementing and remedial help.

For schools

Specialised assessment and recommendations can contribute to learning support programmes and teaching strategies for the child in school as well as help raise teachers' expectations of academic success.

For the craniofacial team

The inclusion of intellectual assessment in follow-up protocols can alert team members to any early problems in the context of other contributory factors. Longitudinal data on developmental outcome may generate new interventions, e.g. early intervention programmes for young children with Apert syndrome and their parents to enhance verbal and non-verbal social interaction skills. Finally, systematic collection of data can generate new care protocols and stimulate the craniofacial centre to engage in collaborative research to improve research design, and increase sample size – and hence the generalisability of results.

Conclusion

This chapter has aimed to highlight the particular psychological challenges of craniosynostosis in childhood, within a developmental, non-pathologising framework.

However excellent the technical quality of surgery and outcomes of medical treatment, ultimately outcome is defined in the long term by the individual's psychosocial well-being and quality of life. Craniofacial disfigurement is potentially an extremely socially stigmatising disability – 'the last bastion of discrimination' in this country (McGrowther 1997). Despite this, many children with craniosynostosis will follow an entirely normal developmental trajectory; other children will experience cognitive, emotional and behavioural difficulties, of a severity to cause distress and require intervention.

As a key member of the craniofacial team, the psychologist aims to offer a proactive, preventative and comprehensive service to the child and family, from birth to maturity, to:

- identify individual family strengths and competences and thereby promote optimal psychosocial adaptation, autonomy and control
- identify specific risk and protective factors throughout childhood and adolescence
- assess and treat specific problems associated with craniofacial difference, including bullying, teasing and social rejection, using cognitive-behavioural therapies and social skills training
- assess readiness for and expectations of surgical treatment
- assess psychosocial well-being, self-esteem and any behavioural and emotional difficulties
- monitor development, intellectual functioning and educational attainments
- provide consultation to the multidisciplinary craniofacial team in relation to psychological issues
- participate in audit and research within the team and across national and international craniofacial centres

The provision of a multidisciplinary craniofacial team approach has been identified as highly important to families as a means of communicating optimism and commitment (Chibbaro 1999, Kelton 2001). Using a theoretical model of normal developmental tasks and challenges and family strengths and vulnerabilities to underpin service delivery, the psychologist can influence the team's delivery of holistic child and family care – care that looks beyond symptoms and syndromes alone.

In the longer term, the psychologist can work with the team to provide long-term outcome studies and new models, interventions and protocols of care based on better understanding of resilience and adaptation. Contributing to service planning and training can influence professional and public awareness and help reduce prejudice and social stigmatisation. Ultimately, the goal is to produce a society where a 9-year-old child with craniofacial anomalies will not have to say, 'I don't want surgery for me. I like me. But I do want surgery so that other people will feel better about me and like me more.'

REFERENCES

Barden RC (1990) The effects of craniofacial deformity, chronic illness, and physical handicaps on patient and familial adjustment. In: Lahey B, Kazdin A, editors. *Advances in Clinical Psychology 13*. New York: Plenum Press, pp 343–375.

Barden R, Ford M, Jenson A, Rogers-Salyer M, Salyer K (1989) Effects of craniofacial deformity in infancy on the quality of mother–infant interactions. *Child Dev* 60: 819–824.

Bartsocas CS, Weber AL, Crawford OD (1970) Acrocephalosyndactyly type 111: Chotzen's syndrome. *J Pediatr* 77: 267–272.

Beardslee WR, Versage EM, Gladstone TRG (1998) Children of affectively ill parents: a review of the past 10 years. *J Am Acad Child Adolesc Psychiatry* 37: 1134–1141.

Bennett E, Stanton M (1993) Psychotherapy for persons with craniofacial deformities: can we treat without theory? *Cleft Palate Craniofac J* 30: 406–410.

Beuf A (1990) *Beauty is the Beast: Appearance Impaired Children in America*. Philadelphia: University of Pennsylvania Press.

Bloom MV (1980) *Adolescent Parental Separation*. New York: Gardner Press.

Bowlby J (1969/1982) *Attachment and Loss. Vol. 1 Attachment*. New York: Basic Books.

Bradbury ET (1996) *Counselling People with Disfigurement*. Leicester: British Psychological Society.

Bradbury ET, Hewison J (1994) Early parental adjustment to visible congenital disfigurement. *Child: Care Health Dev* 20: 251–266.

Broder HL (2001) Using psychological assessment and therapeutic strategies to enhance well-being. *Cleft Palate J* 38: 248–254.

Broder HL, Strauss RP (1989) Self-concept of early primary school age children with visible or invisible defects. *Cleft Palate J* 26: 114–117.

Broder HL, Richman LC, Matheson PB (1998) Learning disability, school achievement and grade retention among children with cleft: a two-center study. *Cleft Palate J* 35: 127–131.

Broder HL, Smith FB, Strauss RP (2001) Developing a behaviour rating scale for comparing teachers' ratings of children with and without craniofacial anomalies. *Cleft Palate J* 38: 560–565.

Bruce V, Green P (1990) *Visual Perception: Physiology, Psychology and Ecology*. 2nd edn. London: Erlbaum Associates.

Bull R, Rumsey N (1988) *The Social Psychology of Facial Appearance*. New York: Springer-Verlag.

Camfield PR, Camfield CC, Cohen MM (2000) Neurologic aspects of craniosynostosis. In: Cohen MC, MacLean RE, editors. *Craniosynostosis. Diagnosis, Evaluation and Management*. New York: Oxford University Press, pp 177–183.

Carey J (1990) The Quasimodo complex: deformity reconsidered. *J Clin Ethics* 1(3): 212–222.

Chibbaro PD (1999) Living with craniofacial microsomia: support for the patient and family. *Cleft Palate J* 36:40–42.

Chumas PD, Cinnall G, Arnaud E, Marchac D, Renier D (1997) Classification of previously unclassified cases of craniosynostosis. *J Neurosurg* 86:177–181.

Clarke A (1999) Psychological aspects of the facial disfigurement: problems, management and the role of a lay-led organisation. *Psychol Health Med* 4: 127–142.

Clifford E (1983) Why are they so normal? *Cleft Palate J* 20(1): 83–84.

Clifford M, Walster E (1973) Research note: The effect of physical attractiveness on teachers' expectations. *Soc Educ* 46: 248–258.

Cohen MM, Kreiborg S (1990) The central nervous system in the Apert syndrome. *Am J Med Genet* 35: 36–45.

Cohen MC, MacLean RE, editors (2000a) *Craniosynostosis. Diagnosis, Evaluation and Management*. New York: Oxford University Press.

Cohen MC, MacLean RE (2000b) Anatomic, genetic, nasologic, diagnostic, and psychological considerations. In: Cohen MC, MacLean RE, editors. *Craniosynostosis. Diagnosis, Evaluation, and Management*. New York: Oxford University Press, pp 119–143.

Cole J (1998) *About Face*. Cambridge, MA: MIT Press.

Crockenburg S (1981) Infant irritability, mother responsiveness, and social influences on the security of the infant–mother attachment. *Child Dev* 52: 857–865.

Dion KK (1972) Physical attractiveness and evaluation of children's transgressions. *J Pers Soc Psychol* 24: 207–213.

Dion KK (1974) Children's physical attractiveness and sex as determinants of adult punitiveness. *Dev Psychol* 10: 772–778.

Dion K, Berscheid E (1974) Physical attractiveness and peer perception among children. *Sociometry* 37: 1–12.

Dipboye RL, Franklin HL, Wiback K (1975) Relative importance of applicant sex, attractiveness and scholastic standing in evaluation of job application résumés. *J Appl Psychol* 60: 39–43.

Eiserman W (2001) Unique outcomes and passive contributions associated with facial difference: expanding research and practice. *Cleft Palate J* 38: 236–244.

Endriga MC, Kapp-Simon KA (1999) Psychological issues in craniofacial care: state of the art. *Cleft Palate J* 36: 3–11.

Fajardo B (1987) Parenting a damaged child: mourning, regression and disappointment. *Psychoanal Rev* 74(1): 19–43.

Field T (1995) Early interaction of infants with craniofacial anomalies. In: Eder RA, editor. *Craniofacial Anomalies. Psychological Perspectives.* New York: Springer-Verlag, pp 99–110.

Field T, Vega-Lahr N (1984) Early interactions between infants with craniofacial anomalies and their mothers. *Infant Behav Dev* 7: 527–530.

Fonagy P, Steele H, Steele M (1991) Intergenerational patterns of attachment: maternal representations of attachment during pregnancy and subsequent infant–mother attachment. *Child Dev* 62: 891–905.

Gerrard J (1991) Beating the teasing syndrome. In: Caronni EP, editor. *Craniofacial Surgery. Proceedings of the Second International Conference of the International Society of Cranio-Maxillo-Facial Surgery.* Bologna: Mondozzi Editore, pp 429–432.

Gilligan C (1989) Mapping the moral domain: new images of self in relationship. *Cross Currents* 39.

Harper DC (1995) Children's attitudes to physical differences among youth from western and non western cultures. *Cleft Palate J* 32: 114–119.

Harper DC, Peterson DB (2001) Children of the Philippines: attitudes toward visible physical impairment. *Cleft Palate J* 38: 566–575.

Heller A, Rafman S, Zvagulis I, Pless IB (1985) Birth defects and psychological adjustment. *Am J Dis Child* 139: 257–263.

Hildebrandt KA, Fitzgerald HE (1978) Adults' responses to infants varying in perceived cuteness. *Behav Processes* 3: 159–172.

Hill-Beuf A, Porter JD (1984) Children coping with impaired appearance: social and psychologic influences. *Gen Hosp Psychiatry* 6: 294–301.

Kapp K (1979) Self-concept of the child with cleft lip and/or palate. *Cleft Palate J* 16: 171–176.

Kapp-Simon KA (1994) Mental development in infants with nonsyndromic craniosynostosis with and without cranial release and reconstruction. *Plast Reconstr Surg* 94: 408–410.

Kapp-Simon KA (1995) Psychological interventions for the adolescent with cleft lip and palate. *Cleft Palate J* 32(2): 104–108.

Kapp-Simon KA (1998) Mental development and learning disorders in children with single suture craniosyn-ostosis. *Cleft Palate J* 35: 197–203.

Kapp-Simon KA, Simon D (1991) *Meeting the Challenges: A Social Skills Training Program for Adolescents with Special Needs.* Chicago: University of Illinois.

Kapp-Simon KA, Simon D (1995) Psychological interventions for the adolescent with cleft lip and palate. *Cleft Palate J* 32: 104–108.

Kapp-Simon KA, Simon PJ, Kristovich S (1992) Self-perception, social skills, adjustment, and inhibition in young adolescents with craniofacial anomalies. *Cleft Palate J* 29: 352–356.

Kapp-Simon KA, Figuera A, Jocher CA, Schafer M (1993) Longitudinal assessment of mental development in infants with nonsyndromic craniosynostosis with and without cranial release and reconstruction. *Plast Reconstr Surg* 92: 831–839.

Katz I (1981) *Stigma: A Social Psychological Analysis.* Hillsdale, NJ: Erlbaum.

Kelton RW (2001) Facing up to stigma: workplace and personal strategies. *Cleft Palate J* 38: 245–247.

Kenny DA, De Paulo BM (1993) Do people know how others view them? An empirical and theoretical account. *Psychol Bull* 114: 145–161.

Kish V, Lansdown R (2000) Meeting the psychological impact of facial disfigurement: developing a clinical service for children and families. *Clin Child Psychol Psychiatry* 5: 497–512.

Kleck R, Rubenstein C (1975) Physical attractiveness, perceived attitude similarity, and interpersonal attraction in an opposite-sex encounter. *J Pers Soc Psychol* 31: 107–114.

Landy D, Sigall H (1974) Beauty is talent: task evaluation as a function of the performer's physical attractiveness. *J Pers Soc Psychol* 29: 299–304.

Langlois JH (1995) The origins and functions of appearance-based stereotypes: theoretical and applied implications. In: Eder R, editor. *Craniofacial Anomalies, Psychological Perspectives*. New York: Springer-Verlag, pp 22–47.

Langlois JH, Roggman LR (1990) Attractive faces are only average. *Psychol Sci* 1: 115–121.

Langlois JH, Roggman LA, Casey RJ, Ritter JM, Rieser-Danner LA, Jenkins VY (1987) Infant preferences for attractive faces: rudiments of a stereotype? *Dev Psychol* 23: 363–369.

Langlois JH, Ritter JM, Roggman LA, Vaughn LS (1991) Facial diversity and infant preferences for attractive faces. *Dev Psychol* 27: 79–84.

Lansdown R (1981) Cleft lip and palate: a prediction of psychological disfigurement. *Br J Orthod* 8: 83–88.

Lansdown R (1990) Psychological problems of patients with cleft lip and palate: discussion paper. *J R Soc Med* 83: 448–450.

Lansdown R, Lloyd J, Hunter J (1991) Facial deformity in childhood: severity and psychological adjustment. *Child: Care Health Dev* 17: 165–171.

Lansdown R, Rumsey N, Bradbury E, Carr T, Partridge J, editors (1997) *Visibly Different: Coping with Disfigurement*. Oxford: Butterworth-Heinemann.

Lavigne JV, Ryan M (1979) Psychological adjustment of children with chronic illness. *Paediatrics* 63: 616–626.

Law J, Boyle J, Harris F, Harkness A, Nye C (1998) Screening for speech and language delay: a systematic review of the literature. *Health Technol Assess* 2: 11–15.

Lefebvre A (1990) Commentary on Carey, J. (1990) The Quasimodo complex: deformity reinforced. *J Clin Ethics* 1(3): 226–227.

Lefebvre A, Munro I (1978) The role of psychiatry in a craniofacial team. *Plast Reconstr Surg* 61: 564–569.

Lefebvre A, Travis F, Arndt E, Munro I (1986) A psychiatric profile before and after reconstructive surgery in children with Apert's syndrome. *Br J Plast Surg* 39: 510–513.

Leonard BJ, Brust JD, Abrahams G, Sielaff B (1991) Selfconcept of children and adolescents with cleft lip and/or palate. *Cleft Palate J* 28(4): 347–353.

MacGregor F (1974) *Transformation and Identity: The Face and Plastic Surgery*. New York: Quadrangle/New York Times Books.

MacGregor FC (1979) *After Plastic Surgery: Adaptation and Adjustment*. New York: Praeger.

MacGregor F (1990) Facial disfigurement: problems and management of social interaction and implications for mental health. *Aesthetic Plast Surg* 14: 249–257.

McGrowther DA (1997) Facial disfigurement: the last bastion of discrimination. *BMJ* 314: 991.

Miller A (1982) *In the Eye of the Beholder: Contemporary Issues in Stereotyping*. New York: Praeger.

Oster H, Rajvaidya S (1996) The signal value of positive and negative facial expressions in infants with craniofacial anomalies. Presented at the Annual Meeting of the American Cleft Palate Association. San Diego, CA.

Pertschuk M (1990) Reconstructive surgery: objective change of objective deformity. In: Cash TF, Pruzinsky T, editors. *Body Images: Development, Deviance and Change*. New York: Guilford Press, pp 237–252.

Pertschuk MJ, Whitaker LA (1987) Psychosocial considerations in craniofacial deformity. *Clin Plast Surg* 14(1): 163–168.

Pillemer FG, Cook KV (1989) The psychosocial adjustment of paediatric craniofacial patients after surgery. *Cleft Palate J* 26(3): 201–208.

Place M, Reynolds J, Cousins A, O'Neill S (2002) Developing a resilience package for vulnerable children. *Child Adolesc Ment Health* 7: 162–167.

Pope AW, Ward J (1997) Factors associated with peer social competence in preadolescents with craniofacial anomalies. *J Pediatr* 22: 455–469.

Pruzinsky T, Cash TF (1990) Integrative theses in body image developments, deviance and change. In: Cash TF, Pruzinsky T, editors. *Body Images: Development, Deviance and Change*. New York: Guilford Press, pp 337–349.

Renier D, Sainte Rose C, Marchac D (1982) Intracranial pressure in craniosynstosis. *J Neurosurg* 57: 370–377.

259

Reschly DJ (1992) Mental retardation: conceptual foundations, definitional criteria, and diagnostic operations. In: Hooper SR, Hynd GW, Mattison RE, editors. *Developmental Disorders: Diagnostic Criteria and Clinical Assessment*. Hillsdale, NJ: Erlbaum.

Richman L (1976) Behaviour and achievement of the cleft palate child. *Cleft Palate J* 13: 4-10.

Richman LC (1978) The effects of facial disfigurement on teachers' perceptions of ability in cleft palate children. *Cleft Palate J* 15: 155–160.

Richman L, Eliason M (1982) Psychological characteristics of children with cleft lip/palate: intellectual achievement, behavioural and personality variables. *Cleft Palate J* 19: 249–257.

Robinson E, Clarke A, Cooper C (1996) *The Psychology of Facial Disfigurement: A Guide for Health Professionals*. London: Changing Faces.

Scheuerle J, Guilford AM, Garcia S (1982) Employee bias associated with cleft lip/palate. *J Appl Rehabil Couns* 13: 6–8.

Shaw KC (1981) Folklore surrounding facial deformity and the origins of facial prejudice. *Br J Plast Surg* 34: 237–246.

Shipster C, Hearst D, Dockrell JE, Kilby E, Hayward R (2002) Speech and language skills and cognitive functioning in children with Apert syndrome: a pilot study. *Int J Lang Commun Disord* 37: 325–343.

Shipster C, Hearst D, Somerville A, Stackhouse J, Hayward R, Wade A (2003) Speech, language and cognitive development in children with isolated sagittal synostosis. *Dev Med Child Neurol* 45: 34–43.

Shprintzen RJ (2000) Speech and language disorders in syndromes of craniosynostosis. In: Cohen MM, MacLean R, editors. *Craniosynostosis. Diagnosis, Evaluation and Management*. New York: Oxford University Press, pp 197–203.

Sidoti EJ Jr, Marsh JL, Marty-Grames L, Nuetzel MJ (1996) Long-term studies of metopic synostosis: frequency of cognitive impairment and behavioural disturbances. *Plast Reconstr Surg* 97: 276–281.

Sigall H, Ostrove N (1975) Beautiful but dangerous: effects of offender attractiveness and nature of the crime on juridic judgement. *J Pers Soc Psychol* 31: 410–414.

Sigelman CK, Miller TE, Whitworth LA (1986) The early development of stigmatizing reactions to physical differences. *J Appl Dev Psychol* 7: 17–32.

Sommer R (1969) *Personal Space: The Behavioural Basis of Design*. Englewood Cliffs, NJ: Prentice Hall.

Speltz ML, Richman L (1997) Progress and limitations in the psychological study of craniofacial anomalies. *J Pediatr Psychol* 22: 433–438.

Speltz ML, Morton K, Goodell EW, Clarren SK (1993) Psychological functioning of children with craniofacial anomalies and their mothers: follow-up from late infancy to school entry. *Cleft Palate J* 30(5): 482–489.

Speltz ML, Galbreath H, Greenberg MT (1995) A developmental framework for psychosocial research on young children with craniofacial anomalies. In: Eder R, editor. *Craniofacial Anomalies. Psychological Perspectives*. New York: Springer-Verlag, pp 258–286.

Speltz ML, Endriga MC, Mouradian WE (1997) Presurgical and postsurgical mental and psychomotor development of infants with saggital synostosis. *Cleft Palate J* 34: 374–379.

Strauss RP (2001) 'Only skin deep': health, resilience, and craniofacial care. *Cleft Palate J* 38: 226–230.

Thomas A, Chess S (1980) *Dynamics of Psychological Development*. New York: Brunner-Mazel.

Tomko B (1983) Mourning the dissolution of the dream. *Soc Work* 28: 391–393.

Tronick EZ, Field T, editors (1986) *Maternal Depression and Infant Disturbance*. New Directions for Child Development, no. 34. San Francisco: Jossey-Bass.

Virtanen R, Korhonen T, Fagerholm J, Viljanto J (1999) Neurocognitive sequelae of scaphocephaly. *Pediatrics* 103: 791–795.

Walters E (1997) Problems faced by children and families living with visible differences. In: Lansdown R, Rumsey N, Bradbury E, Carr T, Partridge J, editors. *Visibly Different: Coping with Disfigurement*. Oxford: Butterworth-Heinemann, pp 112–120.

13
NEUROLOGICAL PROBLEMS IN THE CHILD WITH CRANIOSYNOSTOSIS AND THE ROLE OF THE PAEDIATRICIAN IN OVERALL MANAGEMENT

Lucinda J. Carr

Introduction

In the preceding chapters many of the medical and psychological aspects of the craniosyn-ostoses have been discussed. It is clear that the child with craniosynostosis may present with a multitude of symptoms and signs, particularly those with the complex and syndromic forms, where there is early fusion of multiple cranial sutures. In addition these complex forms are often accompanied by other extracranial manifestations, most often in the hands and feet. However, even the child with fusion of a single suture (simple craniosynostosis) is at risk of medical and developmental difficulty. This chapter will discuss some of the specific neurological problems reported in these groups of children.

The chapter will also discuss the important role of the paediatrician in the overall management of the child with craniosynostosis. While the specialist craniofacial clinic aims to maintain a holistic perspective of the child with craniosynostosis, there is a risk that in focusing on the individual medical problems the comprehensive overview is compromised. The child's local paediatrician, with the support of the specialist nurse for the craniofacial clinic, is ideally placed to overcome this, recognising and responding to the individual and specific needs of each child and their family in their own environment. A key worker may be invaluable in such cases.

Neurological problems in craniosynostosis

The published literature contains few references to the neurological outcome in children and young adults with craniosynostosis, the greatest emphasis being on the emerging genetics of the condition, descriptions of the diverse phenotypes and discussion of the many issues related to surgical management. Classical neurological symptoms and signs may however be a manifestation of a number of the well-recognised physical features and will be discussed below. Furthermore a number of anecdotal but consistent neurological and developmental concerns are raised by parents and confirmed on observation in the clinic. Table 13.1 summarises the recognised neurological problems in this group of children.

TABLE 13.1
Neurological features of the craniosynostoses

	Symptom/sign	Patient subgroup most at risk	Diagnosis and management
Intracranial hypertension	Often asymptomatic. Early morning headache, drowsiness, vomiting. Papilloedema and optic atrophy.	All groups, particularly the complex craniosynostoses, Crouzon syndrome and cloverleaf skull.	Neuroimaging. Direct measurement of intracranial pressure. May require vault expansion or ventricular shunt. Ongoing monitoring, especially vision, indicated.
Chronic cerebellar tonsillar herniation	Often asymptomatic. Symptoms/signs of intracranial hypertension and/or syringomyelia: parasthesiae particularly in upper limbs, early loss of deep tendon reflexes, occasional bulbar and long tract signs.	All the complex craniosynostoses, particularly Crouzon syndrome and cloverleaf skull.	Monitor/treat intracranial hypertension. Symptoms of herniation and syringomyelia often resolve spontaneously. Ongoing monitoring indicated.
Learning disability	Delayed acquisition of developmental, particularly cognitive, milestones.	All the complex craniosynostoses, particularly Apert syndrome.	Define difficulties with standardised assessments. Institute appropriate multidisciplinary therapy.
Specific learning difficulties	Difficulties in circumscribed areas such as reading, spelling. School failure.	Simple craniosynostoses, particularly metopic and sagittal synostosis.	Define difficulties with standardised assessments. Liaise with education. Institute appropriate support.

As with other systems, it is helpful to divide the synostoses into the simple (non-syndromic) and complex (syndromic) forms. The experience of specialist craniofacial clinics would concur that the simple craniosynostoses comprise around 85 per cent of the children referred, the commonest being premature fusion of the sagittal suture (see Renier et al 2000, Hayward, personal communication).

SIMPLE CRANIOSYNOSTOSIS
Fusion of a single suture usually presents with cosmetic concerns and this is the most common reason for surgical intervention. The described skull shapes include scaphocephaly (secondary to sagittal synostosis), plagiocephaly (secondary to fusion of a single coronal suture) and trigonocephaly (secondary to metopic synostosis). Raised intracranial pressure is well recognised in this group of children, reported in around 15 per cent of patients formally monitored (Thompson et al 1995, Renier et al 2000). However, its clinical significance is uncertain since the connection with visual problems is less secure than in children with syndromic forms of craniosynostosis (see 'Crouzon syndrome' below and

also Chapter 8). Hydrocephalus is rare – seen in only 0.3 per cent of 1447 patients in a retrospective study by Cinalli et al (1998). Cerebellar tonsillar herniation has not been reported in this group.

The majority of studies indicate that developmental delay and particularly specific learning difficulties are more common in this group of children when compared with their unaffected peers (Arnaud et al 1995, Sidoti et al 1996, Speltz et al 1997, Bottero et al 1998, Kapp-Simon 1998, Renier et al 2000, Panchal et al 2001, Magge et al 2002). This appears to be independent of increased intracranial pressure. The developmental benefits of early surgery remain contentious. Some authors suggest that early surgery may improve developmental outcome (Speltz et al 1997, Bottero et al 1998, Renier et al 2000) but this observation has not been supported by the majority of other studies (see also Chapter 7).

Mild to moderate learning disability appears to be more common in children with metopic synostosis, particularly if this is associated with other extracranial abnormalities (Sidoti et al 1996, Bottero et al 1998). Sidoti's study suggested that of 32 children, 4 had significant learning difficulties and a further 8 had mild to moderate cognitive or behavioural problems (Sidoti et al 1996). Sagittal and coronal synostosis are generally perceived as more benign; however a recent study from Yale found that, despite normal intelligence, 8/16 children with sagittal synostosis had specific difficulties with reading and/or spelling (Magge et al 2002). Torticollis may be a particular feature of plagiocephaly (Raco et al 1999) – particularly those forms labelled as 'positional' in origin (where it may also have a causative role). Careful longitudinal follow-up is therefore indicated in all these children, actively looking for evidence of raised intracranial pressure and developmental problems.

COMPLEX/SYNDROMIC CRANIOSYNOSTOSIS
Premature fusion of cranial sutures is a recognised feature of over 100 described syndromes (see Chapter 2). All are rare; however the four most common (Apert, Crouzon, Pfeiffer and Saethre–Chotzen) comprise over two-thirds of the cases of syndrome-associated synostoses and are individually discussed below. In all of the complex craniosynostoses there are greater risks of developmental problems and intracranial hypertension. The incidence varies according to the specific syndrome.

Apert syndrome
Characteristic features include irregular craniosynostosis with particular involvement of the coronal sutures and skull base. Fusion of cervical vertebrae primarily at C5–C6 is seen in around two-thirds of patients. Midfacial hypoplasia is characteristic as is extensive symmetrical syndactyly of the hands and feet. Cases are usually sporadic although autosomal dominant inheritance is also seen. An incidence between 1 in 42,000 and 1 in 160,000 live births is quoted (Blank 1960, Renier et al 1996).

Developmental problems are particularly common in Apert syndrome. Studies consistently show that a significant number of these children will have moderate learning disability, with an IQ between 50 and 70. Special educational needs may be compounded by associated hearing and visual problems. Of the three definitive studies, Lefebvre et al (1986) found a mean IQ of 73 in 20 children under 15 years of age. Patton et al (1988) found that of 29 affected children and young adults, 15 had an IQ <70. Renier et al (1996) studied 60 patients and estimated that 68 per cent had an IQ <70. Only a minority showed severe learning disability (IQ <50). All studies considered the role of early surgery, and Renier (1996) combined his study with magnetic resonance imaging (MRI). Only 16 (28 per cent) children had normal neuroimaging; the remainder showed one or more abnormalities; in particular abnormalities of the corpus callosum in 30 per cent (generally hypoplasia), ventriculomegaly in 43 per cent, and anomalies of the septum pellucidum in 55 per cent. The septum pellucidum was absent in just over half of these children; the remainder showed a cavum septum pellucidum. No gyral or white matter abnormalities were seen. Logistic regression analysis suggested that poor developmental outcome was significantly associated with septal anomalies and late cranial surgery (after 1 year of age). At least 90 per cent of children will indeed require cranial surgery, often in more than one stage. However other studies have not demonstrated that early surgery improves cognitive outcome.

A more recent study of 41 children by Sarimski (1998) found that, despite the intensive medical intervention and the recognised cognitive difficulties, children with Apert syndrome were generally socially well adjusted. No behavioural phenotype specific to Apert syndrome was identified although around 20 per cent of nursery and school-aged children showed emotional lability, hyperactivity and poor attention. Parents attending the specialist craniofacial clinic at Great Ormond Street Hospital, also report a lack of empathy in their children. These behavioural traits, along with the facial disfigurement, were identified as a significant source of stress for parents, for whom support and counselling were recommended.

The complications of hydrocephalus and chronic cerebellar tonsillar herniation are particularly seen in Crouzon syndrome and are discussed below. Renier's study of 60 children with Apert syndrome (1996) reported hydrocephalus in 8.3 per cent and tonsillar herniation in one case only.

Crouzon syndrome
This contrasts with Apert syndrome in that it involves only the face and skull; there are no major abnormalities of the hands and feet. The facial features are characteristic; when compared with Apert syndrome the ocular proptosis and maxillary hypoplasia are more severe. The synostosis is often progressive, appearing at around 12 months. The basal and coronal sutures are most commonly affected and this leads to the characteristic brachy-cephalic skull shape. Around 25–50 per cent of cases are sporadic, the rest being dominantly inherited, to give an incidence of around 1 in 25,000 live births.

Of greatest neurological significance is the well-recognised association with hydro-cephalus and chronic cerebellar tonsillar herniation. The diagnosis and management of increased intracranial pressure are discussed in detail in Chapter 8. In the syndromic craniosynostoses the overall incidence of hydrocephalus is around 12 per cent but is as high as 60 per cent in Crouzon syndrome (Cinalli et al 1998). Papilloedema is reported in around one-third of these children, with resulting optic atrophy in 10 per cent. Cinalli et al (1998) found that all children with Crouzon syndrome and progressive hydrocephalus also showed chronic tonsillar herniation.

Chronic cerebellar tonsillar herniation constitutes a Chiari 1 malformation where the lower cerebellum, particularly the tonsils, shows downward displacement with elongation of the fourth ventricle and lower brainstem. It is rarely symptomatic in childhood, although it is known to be associated with hydrocephalus and syringomyelia. Fig. 8.4 (see page 145) shows the MR image of a child with Pfeiffer syndrome associated with hydrocephalus and a Chiari 1 malformation.

Cinalli et al (1995) evaluated the incidence of chronic cerebellar tonsillar herniation in Crouzon and Apert syndromes by performing MRI on 44 and 51 patients respectively. The mean age was 42 months (3 months to 30 years). Cinalli found chronic tonsillar herniation in 72.7 per cent of children with Crouzon syndrome and 1.9 per cent of children with Apert syndrome. Six of the 32 affected children were symptomatic; in four cases this was related to an associated syringomyelia, with the characteristic complaints of sensory disturbances of the upper limbs. Two subjects presented with painful torticollis. One presented with cranial nerve signs and one with respiratory symptoms. Three children subsequently underwent posterior fossa decompression. Cinalli postulates that the early fusion of the sagittal and lambdoid sutures (seen in Crouzon but rarely in Apert syndrome) results in a small posterior fossa, predisposing to cerebellar displacement. Thompson et al (1997) studied 27 cases of complex craniosynostosis and confirmed that both small posterior fossa size and raised intracranial pressure were significantly correlated with the extent of hindbrain herniation.

Pfeiffer syndrome

This is closely related to Apert syndrome, but its effects are more variable. Cases follow an autosomal dominant pattern of inheritance. There are three types, type 1 being the most common. This is characterised by bicoronal synostosis, middle ear abnormalities, broad thumbs and great toes, and partial syndactyly of the hands and feet. In type 2 the skull takes on a characteristic cloverleaf shape (see Fig. 2.12, p. 38); and type 3 is also a severe form but without the cloverleaf shape. A recent study suggests that most type 2 patients die shortly after birth (Plomb et al 1998), but this has not been our experience, although our knowledge is of course confined to those children who have survived long enough to be referred to our unit.

Saethre–Chotzen syndrome

Presentation is very variable even within affected families and as a result is probably underdiagnosed (Dollfus et al 2002). The most consistent features comprise coronal synostosis, hypertelorism, ptosis, nasal septal deviation and mild syndactyly of the hands and feet. Cervical fusion is often seen at the C2–C3 vertebral level. Both TWIST and FGFR mutations have been reported in this group. These mutations are also found in both Pfeiffer and Crouzon syndromes (Paznekas et al 1998).

MISCELLANEOUS NEUROLOGICAL PROBLEMS

The well-recognised problems of learning disability, intracranial hypertension and chronic tonsillar herniation have been discussed above. A number of other neurological problems have been reported, although they are less well documented.

Epilepsy has a higher incidence in this group of patients (Elia et al 1996), although the seizures are usually easy to control.

A significant number of children attending the specialist craniofacial clinic at Great Ormond Street Hospital complain of intractable headaches which affect their daily lives. The headaches are not consistently related to intracranial hypertension or previous shunt surgery. It is obviously important to exclude any provoking factors, in particular raised intracranial pressure or hypercarbia secondary to chronic respiratory problems. In practice many children respond to standard proprietary treatment.

Many parents attending the specialist craniofacial clinic at Great Ormond Street Hospital comment on their child's poor co-ordination and clumsiness. This may be related to the abnormalities (often subtle) seen in the hands and feet in children with complex craniosynostosis (Anderson et al 1997a, 1997b). Shipster et al (2002) found poor oro-motor skills and difficulties in expressive language in a subgroup of children with Apert syndrome attending the clinic. We suspect that many children with complex craniosynostosis have a more general problem with developmental dyspraxia. The occupational therapist is valuable in assessment and treatment and can provide useful advice to the child's school.

Finally, respiratory, ophthalmological and ENT complications may on occasion present to a neurologist. For example, chronic airway obstruction may lead to poor quality sleep and carbon dioxide retention. This may result in headaches and drowsiness and inattention in the daytime. Deafness may also present with inattention and distractibility. Failing vision secondary to optic atrophy may be mistaken for clumsiness in the young child.

The role of the paediatrician

The second section of this chapter discusses the role of the paediatrician in the management of the child with craniosynostosis. The local team is often the first point of contact before and during the process of diagnosis and can provide a key co-ordinating role for the package of management and support thereafter.

The specialist multidisciplinary clinic is likely to play a pivotal role in the management of a child with a rare multisystem disorder such as a complex craniosynostosis. Management advice and direct intervention are provided. While the collective expertise of the team generally provides an important source of information and support to families, occasionally the nature of the clinic can prove intimidating to the child and their family. The team is sensitive to this and at all times aims to maintain an holistic view of each individual child and their family, aware that issues may arise in any area of health, education and social well-being. These may or may not be directly related to the child's medical diagnosis. The local paediatrician can offer an additional point of contact for the child and family and is generally ideally placed to address many of the important issues that cannot be fully covered in the specialist clinic. Not only can the paediatrician offer rapid and flexible medical care but in addition they will have close working links with local education, social and voluntary services. Table 13.2 summarises some of the issues that may arise.

In order for the local team to be effective it is vital that the specialist clinic provides consistent and clear communication in terms of written clinic reports. This may be reinforced by direct liaison with the clinical nurse specialist (see Chapter 17).

TABLE 13.2
The role of the local paediatrician and child development team

Medical	Co-ordinate local services, both acute and community, and ensure effective communication within the team and with specialist centre.
	Provide rapid assessment and management of medical emergencies such as intercurrent infections, tracheostomy problems, etc. Liaison with specialist centre as required.
	Assessment and treatment of general medical problems such as atopy, constipation, etc.
	Advice in general paediatric management.
	Assessment and advice regarding developmental progress. Institute appropriate therapeutic input and support.
	Implement the advice from the specialist centre, such as initiating nasogastric feeding, etc.
	Co-ordinating recommended investigations and arranging these locally where appropriate to minimise travel to referral centre, e.g. videofluoroscopy, sleep studies, etc.
Educational	Liaison with local school.
	Provide Statement of Special Educational Needs if required and ensure that needs are being met.
	Involvement of specialist peripatetic teachers (vision and hearing) if required.
Social	Support and information for child and family and advice to respective agencies regarding the medical diagnosis.
	Practical support with day-to-day issues such as arranging travel, respite care, provision of specialist equipment (feeds and feeding pumps, etc.).
	Ensuring benefit entitlements are offered.

The extent of local and specialist paediatric involvement will be largely dictated by the medical needs of the child. The ability of local resources to provide for the medical needs of the child will vary from area to area. The distance and ease of travel will also influence the degree of involvement with the local and specialist teams. The child is generally seen regularly in local clinics where problems can be identified and prioritised. Investigations and interventions can be discussed and co-ordinated and future plans clarified.

Often a multitude of professionals from different agencies will become involved in the child's care. This can easily result in conflicting advice and confusion, with the family overwhelmed with appointments. A key worker (such as a clinical nurse specialist – see Chapter 17) may play an important role in co-ordinating and rationalising the respective inputs and ensuring effective communication between all those involved. Regular multidisciplinary team meetings that include the family can also help to prioritise any interventions to allow a needs-led approach. This results in more effective management that is responsive to the individual family's needs and wishes.

The key to effective management is good communication between all involved in the child's care, including the family themselves. The common aim is that there is a seamless package of care appropriate for each individual child.

To optimise the outcome and fulfil the potential of children with craniosynostosis, the full spectrum of their difficulties needs to be recognised, and appropriate, timely intervention instituted. As with all rare conditions, large-scale studies are hard to conduct and evaluating 'best management' can be difficult. However, modern genetic techniques continue to unravel the underlying mutations associated with the craniosynostoses. The diversity of the resulting phenotypes is increasingly recognised. The establishment of specialist craniofacial clinics further enhances expertise among professionals, allowing dissemination of knowledge and improving the comprehensive management of children with craniosynostosis.

REFERENCES

Anderson PJ, Hall CM, Evans RD, Jones BM, Hayward RD (1997a) Hand anomalies in Crouzon syndrome. *Skeletal Radiol* 26: 113–115.

Anderson PJ, Hall CM, Evans RD, Jones BM, Hayward RD (1997b) The feet in Crouzon syndrome. *J Craniofac Genet Dev Biol* 17: 43–47.

Arnaud E, Renier D, Marchac D (1995) Prognosis for mental function in scaphocephaly. *J Neurosurg* 83: 476–479.

Blank CE (1960) Apert's syndrome (a type of acrocephalosyndactyly): observations on a British series of 39 cases. *Ann Hum Genet* 24: 151–164.

Bottero L, Lajeunie E, Arnaud E, Renier D, Marchac D (1998) Functional outcome after surgery for trigonocephaly. *Plast Reconstr Surg* 102: 952–958.

Cinalli G, Renier D, Sebag G, Sainte-Rose C, Arnaud E, Pierre-Kahn A (1995) Chronic cerebellar tonsillar herniation in Crouzon's and Apert's syndromes: the role of premature synostosis of the lambdoid suture. *J Neurosurg* 83: 575–582.

Cinalli G, Sainte-Rose C, Kollar EM, Zerah M, Brunelle F, Chumas P, Arnaud E, Marchac D, Pierre-Kahn A, Renier D (1998) Hydrocephalus and craniosynostosis. *J Neurosurg* 88: 209–214.

Dollfus H, Biswas P, Kumaramanickavel G, Stoetzel C, Quillet R, Biswas J, Lajeunie E, Renier D, Perrin-Schmitt F (2002) Saethre–Chotzen syndrome: notable intrafamilial phenotypic variability in a large family with Q28X TWIST mutation. *Am J Med Genet* 109: 218–225.

Elia M, Musueci SA, Ferri R, Greco D, Romano C, Del Gracco S, Stefanini MC (1996) Saethre–Chotzen syndrome: a clinical, EEG and neuroradiological study. *Childs Nerv Syst* 12: 699–704.

Kapp-Simon KA (1998) Mental development and learning disorders in children with single suture craniosynostosis. *Cleft Palate Craniofac J* 35: 197–203.

Lefebvre A, Travis F, Arndt EM, Munro IR (1986) A psychiatric profile before and after reconstructive surgery in children with Apert's syndrome. *Br J Plast Surg* 39: 510–513.

Magge SN, Westerveld M, Pruzinsky T, Persing JA (2002) Long-term neuro-psychological effects of sagittal craniosynostosis on child development. *J Craniofac Surg* 13: 99–104.

Panchal J, Amirsheybani H, Gurwitch R, Cook V, Francel P, Neas B, Levine N (2001) Neurodevelopment in children with single-suture craniosynostosis and plagiocephaly without synostosis. *Plast Reconstr Surg* 108: 1492–1498.

Patton MA, Goodship J, Hayward R, Lansdown R (1988) Intellectual development in Apert's syndrome: a long term follow up of 29 patients. *J Med Genet* 25: 164–167.

Paznekas WA, Cunningham ML, Howard TD, Korf BR, Lipson MH, Grix AW, Feingold M, Goldberg R, Borochowitz Z, Aleck K, Mulliken J, Yin M, Jabs EW (1998) Genetic heterogeneity of Saethre–Chotzen syndrome, due to TWIST and FGFR mutations. *Am J Hum Genet* 62: 1370–1380.

Plomb AS, Hamel BC, Cobben JM, Verloes A, Offermans JP, Lajeunie E, Fryns JP, de Die-Smulders CE (1998) Pfeiffer syndrome type 2: further delineation and review of literature. *Am J Med Genet* 23: 245–251.

Raco A, Raimond AJ, De-Ponte FS, Brunelli A, Bristot R, Bottoni DJ, Ianetti G (1999) Congenital torticollis in association with craniosynostosis. *Childs Nerv Syst* 15: 163–168.

Renier D, Arnaud E, Cinalli G, Sebac G, Zerah M, Marchac D (1996) Prognosis for mental function in Apert's syndrome. *J Neurosurg* 85: 66–72.

Renier D, Lajeunie E, Arnaud E, Marchac D (2000) Management of craniosynostoses. *Childs Nerv Syst* 16: 645–658.

Sarimski K (1998) Children with Apert's syndrome: behavioural problems and family stress. *Dev Med Child Neurol* 40: 44–49.

Shipster C, Hearst D, Dockrell JE, Kilby E, Hayward R (2002) Speech and language skills and cognitive functioning in children with Apert syndrome: a pilot study. *Int J Lang Commun Disord* 37: 325–343.

Sidoti EJ Jr, Marsh JL, Marty-Grames L, Noetzel MJ (1996) Longterm studies of metopic synostosis: frequency of cognitive impairment and behavioural disturbances. *Plast Reconstr Surg* 97: 276–281.

Speltz ML, Endriga MC, Mouradian WE (1997) Presurgical and postsurgical mental development of infants with sagittal synostosis. *Cleft Palate Craniofac J* 34: 374–379.

Thompson DN, Malcom GP, Jones BM, Harkness WJ, Hayward RD (1995) Intracranial pressure in single-suture craniosynostosis. *Paediatr Neurosurg* 22: 235–240.

Thompson DN, Harkness W, Jones BM, Hayward RD (1997) Aetiology of herniation of the hindbrain in craniosynostosis. An investigation incorporating intracranial pressure monitoring and magnetic resonance imaging. *Paediatr Neurosurg* 26: 288–295.

14
SPEECH AND LANGUAGE CHARACTERISTICS OF CHILDREN WITH CRANIOSYNOSTOSIS

Caroleen Shipster

Introduction

There are few reports in the literature on the speech and language characteristics of children with syndromic craniosynostosis. Existing literature focuses primarily on the articulation and resonance characteristics related to the structural abnormalities found in syndromic craniosynostosis (Peterson and Pruzansky 1974, Elfenbein et al 1981, Peterson-Falzone and Vallino 1993, Shprintzen 2000). There is a real paucity of studies on language development, with only two studies identified (Elfenbein et al 1981, Shipster et al 2002).

One of a child's most remarkable developmental achievements is the acquisition of speech and language skills. These skills emerge in a predictable sequence which starts at birth and develops most rapidly in the first five years of life. Speech and language involve a great deal more than just the ability to make sounds and understand and produce spoken language. They are also our primary means of communication, socialisation and the cornerstone of academic achievement. Any disruption to the developmental process of speech and language skills will have far-reaching consequences socially, emotionally and academically. Research has shown that failure to develop adequate language levels in the preschool years is a risk factor for later language difficulties (Whitehurst and Fischel 1994), literacy impairment (Snowling and Stackhouse 1983, Stark et al 1984, Stackhouse and Wells 1997, Tallal et al 1997, Snowling et al 2000), numeracy impairment (Fazio 1994, Grauberg 1998) and socio-behavioural aspects of development (Benaisch et al 1993, Botting and Conti-Ramsden 2000, Lindsay and Dockrell 2000).

Within the craniofacial unit at Great Ormond Street Hospital (GOSH) in London, the speech and language skills of all children with syndromic craniosynostosis are routinely assessed at regular intervals from infancy to maturity as part of the multidisciplinary follow-up protocol. This has provided an opportunity to follow their speech and language development longitudinally and to consider the broad array of factors that impact on this developmental process. There are currently 194 children being followed. This routine documentation has revealed a high prevalence of speech and language impairments in this cohort of children. This is not surprising as many factors specific to syndromic craniosynostosis (oral structural anomalies, hearing loss, visual impairment, cognitive difficulties and psychosocial factors) predispose this population to speech and language impairments.

The four most commonly occurring syndromes with craniosynostosis are Apert syndrome, Crouzon syndrome, Pfeiffer syndrome, and Saethre–Chotzen syndrome (see Chapter 2), and these constitute the main focus of this chapter. However, as other more rare syndromes with craniosynostosis have craniofacial features and functional problems similar to those in these four syndromes, they also have similar patterns of speech and language impairment. Therefore the assessment and management of these syndromes can be approached using a similar paradigm.

This chapter discusses the predisposing risk factors for speech and language impairment in syndromic craniosynostosis and describes the speech and language characteristics of this population as reviewed from the literature and local evidence. Children with single suture craniosynostosis are not vulnerable to the same predisposing risk factors for speech and language impairment, but, interestingly, some of our research has shown that there is a high prevalence rate of speech and language impairment in isolated sagittal synostosis, and this is discussed. The prevalence of speech and language impairment in other isolated single suture conditions has not been investigated. Lastly, general assessment and management principles of speech and language impairment for children with craniosynostosis are described.

Factors influencing the development of speech and language skills in children with syndromic craniosynostosis

This section discusses the predisposing interrelated risk factors for speech and language impairment in children with syndromic craniosynostosis, which are diagrammatically represented in Fig. 14.1.

ABNORMAL ORO-FACIAL STRUCTURES

The altered oro-facial structures which can affect dentition, occlusion, the configuration of palate, and the patency and dimensions of the oronasopharynx in syndromic craniosynos-

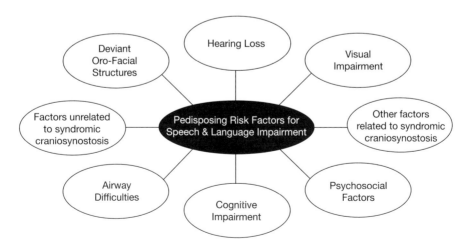

Fig. 14.1 Predisposing risk factors for speech and language impairment.

TABLE 14.1

Oro-facial characteristics of Apert, Crouzon, Pfeiffer and Saethre–Chotzen syndromes

Syndrome	Occlusion	Dentition	Palatal	Pharyngeal	Other
Apert	Class III malocclusion secondary to midface hypoplasia causing a relative mandibular prognathism Anterior open bite (73%) Mandibular overjet (81%) Bilateral posterior crossbite (63%) Unilateral posterior crossbite (22%) Midline deviation (57%)	V-shaped dental arch. Delayed dentition is common (68%) Ectopic eruption (50%) Shovel-shaped incisors (30%) Crowding of teeth, more severely in the maxilla (96%) than in the mandible (87%) Mesial molar occlusion (68%)	Hard palate is highly arched, constricted and usually has a median furrow which has the appearance of a pseudocleft (94%) Bulging alveolar ridges Lateral palatal swellings which can increase with age Short hard palate Long thick soft palate Cleft palate/bifid uvular occurs in 75% and is more common in Ser252Trp mutation	Nasopharynx and oropharynx are reduced in height width and depth	Lips often assume a trapezoidal configuration in a relaxed state particularly during infancy because the upper lip is lifted in the midline secondary to extreme reduction in upper facial height Decreased patency or stenosid of the posterior nasal choanae
Crouzon	Class III malocclusion secondary to midface hypoplasia causing a relative mandibular prognathism Anterior open bite Mandibular overjet Unilateral or bilateral posterior crossbite in two-thirds	Crowding of maxillary teeth common Crowding of mandibular anterior teeth common Ectopic eruption of maxillary first molars in 47%	Cleft palate (3%) Bifid uvular (9%) Lateral palatal swellings (50%) but only in a few are they large enough to produce a median pseudocleft	Nasopharynx and oropharynx are reduced in height, width and depth	Cleft lip (2%) Occasional choanal stenosis or atresia Deviation of the nasal septum in 33%
Pfeiffer	Class III malocclusion secondary to midface hypoplasia causing a relative mandibular prognathism	* (see below)	* (see below)	Nasopharynx and oropharynx are reduced in height width and depth	* (see below) Occasional choanal stenosis or atresia
Saethre–Chotzen	Class III malocclusion secondary to midface hypoplasia causing a relative mandibular prognathism	Supernumerary teeth Enamel hypoplasia and other dental defects	Narrow or highly arched palate Cleft palate on occasion	* (see below)	Deviation of the nasal septum

Source: Summarised from Cohen and Maclean (2000).

* Abnormalities were not reported. Variable abnormalities noted within our population at GOSH.

tosis create the most obvious hazard to speech production and resonance (see Chapters 9 and 11). Table 14.1 provides a summary of the reported findings of abnormal oro-facial characteristics in each syndrome (Cohen and MacLean 2000). How the deviant anatomy impacts on resonance and speech production in syndromic craniosynostosis is described in the sections on 'Resonance' and 'Speech impairment' in the next part of this chapter.

RESPIRATORY DIFFICULTIES

Upper airway obstruction is a common feature of children with syndromic craniosynostosis secondary to the abnormal oro-facial structures. These effectively reduce the volume of the nasal cavity, the oropharynx and the nasopharynx. The upper airway may be compromised further by choanal stenosis or atresia, the long thick soft palate found in Apert syndrome (see Table 14.1), and the presence of tonsils and adenoids even when these are of a normal size. The upper airway obstruction may present differing degrees of severity, from nasal obstruction to obstructive sleep apnoea to severe respiratory distress, which can be fatal. Lower respiratory airway difficulties related to tracheal abnormalities have also been reported in both Crouzon and Apert syndromes (Cohen and MacLean 2000).

When respiratory difficulties are severe they can result in extreme daytime fatigue and impact cognitive functioning (Stradling 1982). In the developing child, airway obstruction can cause developmental delay, suboptimal neurological development and failure to thrive (Sculerati et al 1998), any or all of which may affect speech and language acquisition. A commonly observed finding is that children with respiratory difficulties often make dramatic general developmental progress, including progress in language development, when respiratory difficulties have been dealt with effectively. For a detailed discussion of airway obstruction, its sequelae and the management of respiratory difficulties see Chapter 9.

HEARING LOSS

Numerous studies indicate that hearing loss is frequently associated with syndromic craniosynostosis (Table 14.2). The most common finding is conductive hearing loss. Sensorineural hearing loss is infrequent but occurs with an increased prevalence rate compared with the normal population. The conductive hearing loss may be acquired as a result of otitis media with effusion (OME), which is the most common otological manifestation in craniosynostosis, or congenital as a result of structural abnormalities of the outer and/or middle ear, or the two types of conductive loss can co-occur. Conductive hearing loss can cause a mild to moderate hearing loss.

Effect of hearing loss on speech and language development

It is well recognised within the literature that untreated permanent hearing loss can have a significant impact on the development of speech and language (Bamford et al 1985, Northern and Downs 2002). Northern and Downs (2002) describe the effects of the different degrees of hearing loss on speech and language development (Table 14.3). The effects of hearing loss will depend on the configuration of the loss, the degree of loss, and the age of onset. Age at onset is an especially important factor in speech and language development. A loss

TABLE 14.2
Studies reporting hearing loss in syndromic craniosynostosis

Syndrome	Acquired conductive hearing loss	Congenital conductive hearing loss	Sensorineural hearing loss
Apert	OME and its sequelae is an almost universal finding. Can be unrelenting and persist into adulthood (Gould and Calderelli 1982, McGill 1991). It may be related to the high frequency of cleft palate in Apert syndrome (Selder 1973, Crysdale 1981, Gould and Calderelli 1982, Philips and Miyamoto 1986).	Due to ossicular anomalies such as stapes fixation (Bergstrom et al 1972, Lindsay et al 1975, Gould and Calderelli 1982, Philips and Miyamoto 1986).	Sensorineural hearing loss is rare (McGill 1991).
Crouzon	OME and its sequelae is common. Kreiborg (1981) reported its presence in 55%. Prevalence may increase with age (Corey et al 1987).	Atresia of the external auditory canals in 13% (Kreiborg 1981). Fixation of middle ear ossicles (Cremers 1981).	May be a significant sensorineural component (Orvidas et al 1999).
Pfeiffer	OME (Vallino-Napoli 1996).	Meatal atresia and ossicular fixation (Cremers 1981, Vallino-Napoli 1996).	
Saethre–Chotzen	Most common type of loss reported (Pantke et al 1975, Konigsmark and Gorlin 1976, Ensink et al 1996).		May have a sensorineural component (Pantke et al 1975, Konigsmark and Gorlin 1976, Ensink et al 1996).

which is present at birth or within the first few months of life will have a much greater effect than a loss after language has been acquired.

There is also a growing consensus that fluctuating mild to moderate losses as a result of OME also affect speech and language skills. Haggard et al (1993) undertook a literature review on the impact of recurrent otitis media on speech and language development. Nine out of 13 studies reviewed reported detrimental effects on both receptive and expressive language. Those that had also collected data on speech reported that this was adversely affected too. Overall, early age of onset, long duration and recurrent episodes made speech and language difficulties more likely. This evidence suggests that OME in syndromic craniosynostosis is also likely to be a significant contributory factor to speech and language impairment.

All degrees of hearing loss and fluctuating hearing loss can affect the development of attention, which is the ability to focus on and remain focused on salient features of a situation (Northern and Downs 2002). Lewis (1976) suggests that inefficient listening strategies, developed during periods of conductive loss, persist well beyond the episodes of active middle ear disease and affect levels of attention. The development of attention is an essential prerequisite to all types of learning, particularly the acquisition of speech and language skills. The ability to attend is present from birth and progresses through clearly defined developmental stages to about 6 years of age, when children develop 'two-channelled' attention control, which means they can easily assimilate new directions while carrying out

TABLE 14.3
Effects of hearing loss on speech and language development

Type of loss and possible condition	Effect on speech and language if not treated in the preschool years
15–25 dB (slight loss) Conductive hearing losses, some sensorineural hearing losses	Mild auditory dysfunction in language learning. Inattention
25–30 dB (mild loss) Conductive or sensorineural hearing loss	Auditory learning dysfunction. Mild speech and language impairment. The short unstressed words and less intense speech sounds (such as voiceless stops and fricatives) are inaudible. Inattention
30–50 dB (moderate loss) Conductive hearing loss from chronic middle ear disorders; sensorineural hearing losses	Speech and language impairment. Will have difficulty perceiving short unstressed words and morphological word endings. This reduction in information can lead to limited vocabulary and confusion of grammatical rules, omission of articles, conjunctions and prepositions. Speech production includes omitted and distorted consonants. Learning dysfunction. Inattention
50–70 dB (severe loss) Sensorineural or mixed losses due to a combination of middle ear disease and sensorineural involvement	Severe speech and language impairment. Learning dysfunction. Inattention
70+ dB (profound loss) Sensorineural or mixed losses due to a combination of middle ear disease and sensorineural involvement	Severe speech and language impairment. Learning dysfunction. Inattention

Source: Modified from Northern and Downs (2002).

another task and sustain attention without being distracted (Cooper et al 1978). Attainment of this level of selective attention control is essential for language learning in older children, particularly in classroom situations.

Local evidence has shown that poor development of auditory attention skills is a common feature in syndromic craniosynostosis and is most prevalent in Apert syndrome. In a recent study of children with Apert syndrome, Shipster et al (2002) reported that all the children had difficulties with attention control and/or concentration span and parents and teachers commented that these were aspects of the children's development that they were particularly concerned about. Sarimski (1998) in his study of 41 preschool- and school-age children with Apert syndrome reported that 20 per cent of the children had poor attention.

Crysdale (1978) and McGill (1991) both report that fluctuating or permanent hearing loss in children with craniofacial conditions is often not diagnosed and dealt with effectively in the preschool years because of the presence of more severe craniofacial and neurosurgical considerations, or the attributing of poor performance to learning difficulties. Unfortunately, local evidence suggests that this is often the case for some children with syndromic craniosynostosis.

275

VISUAL IMPAIRMENT

Visual problems in relation to speech and language development in this population are often overlooked. Visual impairment is usually caused by raised intracranial pressure causing pressure on the visual pathway, and if left untreated can lead to permanent damage to the vision. In rare cases proptosis may also contribute to visual loss if corneal ulceration occurs. Less overt causes are refractive errors, and more common causes are astigmatism with hypermetropia (longsightedness) or myopia (shortsightedness). A higher percentage of children with craniosynostosis have astigmatism when compared to children in the normal population. Uncorrected astigmatism causes blurring of vision and inability to focus fully.

In the young child visual impairment leads to difficulties perceiving and focusing on the human face, objects and pictures. A great deal of language learning takes place through vision. For example, children learn vocabulary by following a caregiver's eye gaze, or finger-point, to the pictures/objects it relates to. Thus, visual impairment can reduce language learning opportunities in the young child. In the older child it affects the acquisition of literacy and other aspects of academic work, unless the difficulties are recognised and addressed.

Also common in children with craniosynostosis are abnormal eye movements caused by missing eye muscles or malpositioning of the muscles on the globe of the eye and orbital excyclorotation. These difficulties prevent the child from using both eyes simultaneously (binocular single vision). This can result in abnormal head position such as turning the head sideways in order to use the preferred eye. During social exchanges, this can be interpreted as 'rudeness', inability to make good eye contact or gaze avoidance. Indeed, there have been suggestions of some children having pragmatic language disorders or autistic spectrum disorder as a result of these undiagnosed visual difficulties. Poor eye contact as a result of visual impairment has also been interpreted as poor attention within the classroom.

COGNITIVE IMPAIRMENT

Cognitive impairment has been found in varying degrees of frequency and severity in Apert, Crouzon, Pfeiffer and Saethre–Chotzen syndromes. This is often reported to be secondary to CNS abnormalities and damage, raised intracranial pressure and hydrocephalus. It is most consistently associated with Apert syndrome. Language impairment is a predictable consequence secondary to cognitive impairment.

However, as relatively few studies of intellectual functioning have been carried out (see Chapter 13) the prevalence rate of cognitive impairment in syndromic craniosynostosis is not known. There are also some limitations with existing studies, which may make their results questionable. These include not stating how subjects were selected, and the study samples may therefore be a biased selection; in some studies informal assessments have been used and, in several studies, assessment measures are not reported which makes interpretation of the results difficult.

Most assessments of cognition comprise three scales from which an intelligence quotian (IQ) can be derived. These are a Non-Verbal or Performance Scale, a Verbal Scale and a Full Scale, the latter being a combination of the scores from the Performance and Verbal

Scales. A further flaw of some studies in the literature is the tendency to only report the Full Scale IQ scores, and thus the overall IQ may be unduly lowered if language impairment is present. Shipster et al (2002), in a study of the language and cognitive skills of children with Apert syndrome, discussed these issues. Eight children in this study were assessed using IQ tests which clearly differentiated Performance IQ from Verbal IQ and did not penalise them for fine motor deficits secondary to hand deformities. A Performance IQ standard score within the average range was obtained for all the children (range of scores: 88–107; mean score: 96). These IQ scores were substantially higher than the ranges and mean IQ scores quoted in the three largest studies of cognitive impairment in Apert syndrome (Lefebvre et al 1986, Patton et al 1988, Renier et al 1996). These results highlight the importance of appropriate test selection and differentiating between performance and verbal IQ scales.

PSYCHOSOCIAL FACTORS

Local evidence suggests that a variety of negative psychosocial factors can restrict many speech and language learning opportunities for children with syndromic craniosynostosis, and this is substantiated by reports in the literature. Infancy can be a particularly stressful period for parents. They have to come to terms with having a child with special needs and are often 'grieving' for the loss of a normal child. Additionally, they may be coping with feeding difficulties, sleeping disturbances, which are more prevalent than in the normal infant, and frequent hospital admissions and appointments. Consequently, focusing on early communication skills in children with syndromic craniosynostosis may be difficult. Field (1995) reports that there is a tendency for young facially disfigured children to receive less physical contact and less expressive interaction. As early speech and language milestones are often very delayed, it is often falsely assumed that they will have great difficulty learning to talk or be unable to speak, and less demand is placed on them to produce speech and language. Children who are developing speech and language need responsive and available communication partners to help reinforce their attempts to communicate and to provide appropriate levels of language input. These partners may not be available for the reasons described above.

As the children develop, the opportunity to use language in social situations is often adversely affected. Adults and siblings may speak for the children to spare them the discomfort of negative reactions from listeners, particularly when these are strangers. Other children may avoid interacting with them and children with hand and limb abnormalities find it difficult to fully partake in peer group activities such as sport. The children themselves may avoid social interactions owing to awareness of their differences from other children or because of teasing and bullying. Because of these restricted opportunities for social interaction many children with syndromic craniosynostosis do not learn at a young age how to engage in social situations, taking this learned pattern of behaviour with them to new social situations, and this compounds the problem. Kapp-Simon and McGuire (1997) reported that children with facial disfigurement initiated and received fewer social approaches than those without facial differences and their strategies for engaging with peers were less effective and more tentative than those of the comparison group. Rumsey and Bull

277

(1986) reported that individuals with facial differences received negative reactions from others in social situations and this may adversely affect social interaction.

It is often assumed that a child who has an abnormal facial appearance (particularly when this is associated with a syndrome) has a cognitive impairment. The communication demands placed on them may be fewer than the normal peer group as a result of low expectations. Owing to the relative rarity of the conditions and the paucity of information on the development of children with syndromic craniosynostosis, parents/carers and professionals have few resources on which to base their expectations for the children in their care.

OTHER PREDISPOSING RISK FACTORS

Frequent hospitalisations, clinic and hospital appointments, recovery periods after surgery, particularly in the preschool years, can disrupt emotional stability, normal routines and opportunities to socialise (such as home routines; play opportunities; interaction with family members and peers; and regular attendance at nursery) which are essential to provide speech and language learning opportunities and the opportunity to develop communication skills.

Additionally, a few children fail to thrive as a consequence of severe feeding difficulties (see Chapter 16). Children with syndromic craniosynostosis often take longer to recover from upper respiratory tract infections when these occur. These factors will affect general well-being and may also slow overall development including speech and language development.

FACTORS UNRELATED TO SYNDROMIC CRANIOSYNOSTOSIS

Children with syndromic craniosynostosis are at risk for speech and language impairment for the same reasons that may occur in any child and these may coexist with other predisposing risk factors specific to syndromic craniosynostosis. Law et al (1998) conducted a systematic review of prevalence studies of speech and language development. They concluded that 6 per cent of children have speech and language impairments in the general population. These impairments can occur for a variety of reasons. A few examples are: the presence of perinatal risk factors such as prematurity; a positive familial history of speech and language impairment; external factors such as low socioeconomic status and the quality of the linguistic input children are exposed to (Bishop and Butterworth 1980, Bishop and Edmundson 1986, Saigal et al 1991, Walker et al 1994, Bishop et al 1995, Spitz et al 1997, Cherkes-Julkowski 1998, Luoma et al 1998, Resnick et al 1998, Tomblin and Buckwater 1998, Weindrich et al 1998, Gopnik 1999, Wolke and Meyer 1999, Locke et al 2002). Clinicians need to be aware that communication impairments may result from other factors unrelated to syndromic craniosynostosis and take these into account when diagnosing and managing speech and language impairments.

In summary, all the predisposing factors described can influence the development of communication in children with syndromic craniosynostosis and will have most impact in the preschool years when a child's speech and language skills are emerging. Coexistence of predisposing factors also makes children more vulnerable to speech and language impairments. For example, a hearing loss will have far less impact on the development of speech and language in a child of normal cognitive ability than in a child with cognitive impairment. Peterson-Falzone et al (2001) make two important points, which are very relevant when considering the aetiology of speech and language impairments of children with syndromic craniosynostosis. First, there is often a poor correlation between the severity of expression of the physical manifestations of a condition and various aspects of developmental, cognitive, communicative and psychosocial function. Children who have mild craniofacial abnormalities may have severe functional difficulties and, conversely, some children with relatively severe physical findings exhibit cognitive, social and communicative skills within normal limits. Second, there may be a tendency to focus on the visible problems and not give enough consideration to less obvious factors such as hearing loss and psychosocial adjustment.

Speech and language impairment in syndromic craniosynostosis
This section discusses the aspects of speech and language development that are most vulnerable to impairment: resonance, speech, language and voice. Specific management considerations related to each of these areas are also discussed.

RESONANCE
In speech production, resonance refers to the supraglottic modulation of the noise produced by the vocal cords in the hypopharynx, oropharynx, nasopharynx, oral cavity and nasal cavity, by changing the height and width of the pharynx and opening and closing a series of valves above the vocal cords (Shprintzen 2000). The most common resonance characteristic associated with syndromic craniosynostosis is hyponasality, which is caused by lack of nasal resonance for the three nasal consonants /m,n,ng/ resulting from a partial or complete obstruction in the nasal tract. The abnormal structural features in syndromic craniosynostosis which can combine to cause hyponasality have been described by Shprintzen (2000) and are summarised below:

- The height, width and depth of the oropharynx and nasopharynx are reduced. Access to the nasal cavity is often compromised by the small nasopharynx. There is therefore less airflow through the pharynx, which reduces nasal resonance.
- The nasopharynx may be further reduced in volume by even a normal amount of adenoidal tissue.
- The soft palate often sits in close approximation to the adenoids even in its rest position; thus hyponasalitiy is unavoidable.
- Tonsils may obstruct the oropharynx even when they are of normal size because of the abnormal configuration of the pharynx.
- Choanal stenosis or atresia where present also contribute to hyponasality.
- Children with Apert syndrome usually have a long, thick soft palate, which crowds the nasopharynx, and this tends to become more severe with age (Peterson and Pruzansky 1974, Peterson-Falzone et al 1981, 2001).

Local evidence suggests that, prior to midface advancement, hyponasality of varying degrees of severity is consistently present in all children with Apert syndrome, Pfeiffer syndrome types 2 and 3, and in cases of Crouzon syndrome with severe midface hypoplasia, and is invariably present in Saethre–Chotzen syndrome and in milder cases of Crouzon syndrome even when the tonsils and adenoids have been removed. Upper respiratory tract infections also contribute to the hyponasality.

Other abnormalities of resonance may also occur. Resonance is frequently more muffled in quality than in normal individuals because of the altered oral structure, which dampens sound. Shprintzen (2000) attributes this to a possible combination of a smaller oral cavity, a soft palate which tends to hang straight down into the pharynx instead of gently curving, and soft tissue hypertrophy of the lateral palatal shelves, found in Apert syndrome and some cases of Crouzon syndrome.

Clefts of the soft palate, submucous cleft or bifid uvula have been reported in 75 per cent of children with Apert syndrome (Kreiborg and Cohen 1992). However, even when cleft palate is unrepaired (often to help maintain the airway), resonance is usually still hyponasal rather than hypernasal (an excessively undesirable amount of perceived nasal cavity resonance during phonation) which is the resonance characteristic commonly associated with cleft palate.

When glasses are worn to correct some visual impairments, it can be difficult to keep them in place owing to facial deformities such as a depressed nasal bridge. A common finding is that they slip down and occlude the nostrils to a degree that contributes to hyponasality.

Management considerations
Muffled resonance is often an irreversible feature in syndromic craniosynostosis when present. Removal of tonsils and adenoids may improve hyponasality to a degree but usually it is a consistent feature in many cases of syndromic craniosynostosis until midface advancement surgery occurs.

Midfacial advancements are undertaken to 'normalise' the appearance of the facial complex and for functional reasons such as improving the airway and vision (see Chapter 19). These procedures are usually at a Le Fort III level and move the midface forward, and are accompanied by a differential downward displacement of the palate in relation to the posterior pharyngeal wall. Additionally, the complex three-dimensional skeletal movements in facial bipartition modify the properties of the palate and nasal airways with combinations of advancement, differential vertical movements and alterations in width. The degree to which the midface can be brought forward in a Le Fort III procedure is illustrated in Chapter 19 (page 389).

There has only been one paper (Cedars et al 1999) that has looked at the impact of Le Fort III level procedures on nasality and velopharyngeal function in syndromic craniosyn-ostosis. The authors reported a decrease in hyponasality and a transient velopharyngeal insufficiency in 5 out of 10 cases. Other studies which have looked at the effects of midface advancement on resonance are at a Le Fort I level in children with cleft palate. (See Sell 2001 for a review of the studies looking at the effects of this procedure on resonance.)

Pereira et al (2002) report on one boy with Crouzon syndrome, who developed significant hypernasality or velopharyngeal insufficiency immediately following distraction at a Le Fort III level. The acquired velopharyngeal insufficiency was permanent even 12 months postoperatively.

SPEECH IMPAIRMENT

Speech may be disrupted for a variety of reasons and the three types of speech impairment commonly associated with syndromic craniosynostosis are discussed in this section. These are articulatory, phonological and neurological impairments, all of which may co-occur.

Structural articulation impairment

These are speech impairments that occur as a result of structural malformations in the physical structures involved in speech production (Grundy 2001). In syndromic craniosynostosis, articulation impairment occurs as an obligatory feature secondary to the presence of some of the oral malformations described in Table 14.1. These structural malformations are most frequently found in Apert syndrome, severe Crouzon syndrome and Pfeiffer syndrome types 2 and 3, and are variably found in mild Crouzon syndrome and Saethre–Chotzen syndrome and Pfeiffer syndrome type 1.

The articulatory impairments associated with the occlusal and dental malformations are summarised below.

Class III malocclusion and anterior open bite. In normal occlusion the tongue rests within the oral cavity against the maxillary alveolus and palate. In class III malocclusion the tongue rests in the floor of the mouth past the maxillary incisors. Approximating the tongue tip anterior to the retruded maxillary alveolus is not possible, particularly when the maxillary arch is often constricted. Additionally, retraction of the tongue into the oral pharynx may inhibit the airway. The severity of the class III malocclusion can vary greatly (see Figs 14.2 and 14.3). Articulatory patterns associated with class III malocclusion are as follows:

- It usually causes blade production of tongue tip consonants /t,d,n,l,s,z,sh, ch as in *chair* and ge as in *jam*/ (the body of the tongue articulates against the top teeth instead of the tongue tip behind the top teeth).
- Mild cases of class III malocclusion will only lead to dental production of tongue tip sounds (the tip of the tongue against the teeth instead of behind the teeth).
- It can lead to lingualabial production of the bilabial consonants /p,b,m/ (the tongue against the top lip instead of the lower and upper lip together).
- It usually causes reverse production of labiodental consonants /f,v/ (the mandibular incisors against the top lip instead of the maxillary incisors against the lower lip).

Posterior crossbite. This can cause lateralisation of sibilants and affricates, giving sounds such as s, z, sh and ch a 'slushy' quality.

Dental anomalies. Rotated anterior teeth and ectopic teeth may also contribute to oral distortion of tongue tip sounds, particularly s, z, sh and ch.

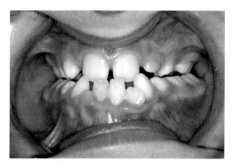 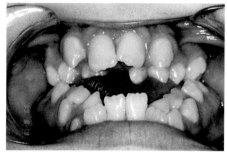

Fig. 14.2 Mild class III malocclusion and bilateral posterior crossbite.

Fig. 14.3 Severe class III malocclusion. Anterior open bite and bilateral posterior crossbite. Malaligned and ectopic teeth.

In syndromic craniosynostosis, when a cleft palate is left unrepaired it may have no adverse effect on speech production and the characteristic structural articulatory impairments associated with unrepaired cleft palate are not evident.

Phonological impairment
Phonology refers to the ability to use speech sounds and sound combinations to signal meaningful contrasts between words. Phonological impairment occurs when there is a reduction in the child's ability to signal differences in meaning. In the normal child, speech sounds within a language emerge in a predictable developmental sequence through progressive stages from about 9 months to about 4 years 6 months, when most of the speech sounds in a child's language have been acquired. This developmental progression in speech enables the child to signal increasing differences in meaning in a language. For example, many 2-year-olds may produce the words 'zoo, shoe, do and two' all as 'do', but at the age of 3 years they will be able to make the distinction in meaning when saying these words.

A common finding is that children under the age of 2 years with syndromic craniosynostosis have a more reduced range of consonants in their babble and early word attempts when compared to the normal child. Within our population of children with syndromic craniosynostosis there is an extremely high prevalence of phonological impairment due to a delay in the development of phonological skills. In a recent audit of the phonological skills of 6-year-olds with syndromic craniosynostosis 55/55 children with Apert syndrome, 25/30 with Crouzon syndrome, 12/18 with Pfeiffer syndrome and 12/20 children with Saethre–Chotzen syndrome all had varying degrees of phonological delay. Some commonly observed patterns in the children were as follows:

- Stopping of fricatives and affricates, for example, /s/ or /sh/ may be realised as /t/.
- Word final consonant deletion.
- Voicing of voiceless consonants, for example, /t/ may be realised as /d/.
- Fronting of velars and palatoalveolar sounds, for example, /k/ or /ch/ may be realised as /t/.

Additionally, local evidence suggests that phonological impairment is characteristic of a high proportion of school-age children with syndromic craniosynostosis.

The high prevalence of phonological impairments and in particular phonological delay in children with syndromic craniosynostosis has not previously been reported in the literature. Phonological impairment can have a greater impact on the intelligibility of speech than the articulatory errors related to structural impairments. This is because the majority of articulatory errors related to structure primarily 'visually' distort rather than 'acoustically' alter speech production. In other words, they do not have a particularly negative effect on intelligibility as they do not alter the acoustic qualities of speech sounds, but they do have a negative impact on the visual perception of speech as the children look 'different' when they speak. In contrast, phonological errors have a far greater effect on the acoustic perception of speech, making it more difficult to understand.

Neurological impairment

Neurological impairment is caused by damage to the central nervous system. Shprintzen (2000) reports that both dysarthria (impairment of movement and co-ordination of the muscles required for speech, due to abnormal muscle tone (Grundy 2001)) and dyspraxia (a disorder of the performance of an action (Ozanne 1995)) are found in Apert syndrome and Pfeiffer syndrome.

Local evidence suggests that mild dysarthria is observed in some children with Apert syndrome. The most commonly observed symptoms of dysarthria include mild hypotonia and decrease in sensation in the oro-facial musculature which affects the production of bilabial sounds /p,b,m/ and the consonants /w/ and /sh/ which require lip rounding. Children with Apert syndrome also drool more severely than other children with similar class III malocclusions and respiratory difficulties. Shipster et al (2002) in a study of ten children with Apert syndrome reported continued drooling in eight of the children well into childhood. Drooling is a normal phenomenon of infancy that subsides in early childhood, usually by 15–18 months of age (Blasco 1996).

Overall speech intelligibility

As well as articulation, phonological and neurological impairment, intelligibility of speech may also be affected by the additional presence of several other factors. These may include elision and omission of consonants and weak syllable deletion in connected speech (these patterns are usually related to hearing loss), hyponasality, abnormal voice quality and reduced voice volume where present.

Management considerations

Articulation errors related to abnormal structure will not improve spontaneously or respond to speech therapy until midface advancement surgery and corrective orthodontic treatment have been carried out to improve the relationship between the mandible and the maxilla (Bloomer 1971, Witzel et al 1980, Vallino 1990). However, correct production of bilabial consonants /p,b,m/ is a realistic therapeutic goal, prior to midface surgery, even in cases of severe class III malocclusion and respiratory difficulties. Improved production of these bilabial consonants will improve the 'visual' appearance of speech and may help the child socially.

Preliminary results from an ongoing research study (Pereira et al 2002) examining the effects of midfacial advancement on speech, nasality and velopharyngeal function in syndromic craniosynostosis suggest improved articulation for sounds that involve dental-occlusal relationships and improved nasal resonance. Articulation therapy may also be indicated after midface surgery in order to maximise the benefits of the altered oral structure.

Unlike structural articulation impairment, phonological impairment can be addressed in the preschool and primary school years (if hearing loss is managed effectively) prior to surgery and orthodontic treatment. Children with syndromic craniosynostosis benefit from therapy being initiated at an early age, aimed at developing their phonological skills and direct speech work to increase the range of speech sounds they are using. When dyspraxia/dysarthria are also present, then therapy to improve articulation and oro-motor skills will also be beneficial.

LANGUAGE IMPAIRMENT

In this section receptive language (comprehension of spoken language), expressive language (spoken language) and pragmatic language (social use of language) are discussed.

Receptive and expressive language impairment

Local evidence and a study by Shipster et al (2002) conducted on children with Apert syndrome suggest that the following patterns of language development are common in children with syndromic craniosynostosis:

- Both receptive and expressive language skills are frequently delayed, particularly in the preschool years. This delay can affect the understanding and production of grammatical structures (morphology and syntax) and/or vocabulary.
- Expressive language skills are usually significantly more impaired than receptive language skills.
- Language impairment is more common in Apert syndrome, Pfeiffer syndrome types 2 and 3, and severe Crouzon syndrome than in mild Crouzon syndrome, Saethre–Chotzen syndrome and Pfeiffer syndrome type 1.
- There is often a significant discrepancy between the child's levels of language functioning and the child's non-verbal cognitive levels, indicating specific difficulty with the attainment of language skills rather than global cognitive impairment.
- The quantity of verbal output may be significantly reduced in situations outside the home.

In a recent audit at GOSH of 150 children with syndromic craniosynostosis aged between 4 and 18 years, 148 had developed spoken language as their primary means of communication. The remaining two children, who both had Apert syndrome, were reliant on basic signing. They both had severe cognitive impairment and moderate to severe hearing losses that had not been aided until after the age of 3 years. Peterson-Falzone et al (2001) report that children with type 2 or 3 Pfeiffer syndrome do not develop adequate means of expressive language and often require alternative means of communication such as basic sign language and communication boards. In contrast, the GOSH audit has shown that all 12 of the children with type 2 or 3 Pfeiffer syndrome have spoken language and are not reliant on signing. However, they often have severe expressive language impairment.

Pragmatic language impairment
This refers to difficulties in using language to interact socially with others. There is a non-verbal and a verbal component to effective use of social language. Bray et al (1999: 46) describe these two components as follows: non-verbal pragmatic language skills refer to 'norms' of communication such as turn taking, eye contact, use of gesture, facial expression, and use of spatial and postural adjustments for different contexts. Verbal pragmatic skills refer to the ability to converse by making statements, asking questions, making requests, responding appropriately, knowing what kind of information is required and how much information to give. Both of these aspects may be disrupted in children with syndromic craniosynostosis, particularly verbal pragmatic skills secondary to the psychosocial factors previously described, which restrict opportunities for social interaction and the development of social use of language.

Eye contact may also be poor, secondary to visual impairment. Use of facial expression is limited in some children with Apert syndrome who have facial weakness.

Tracheostomy
When a tracheostomy is required as a management option for respiratory difficulties, this has an appreciable impact on the development of language. Tracheostomy placement disrupts the normal expiratory airflow with air passing out of the tracheostomy tube instead of passing up through the larynx and out of the mouth/nose. The child may be unable to achieve voice, or, when present, it may be of variable quality and efficiency, which can affect speech intelligibility.

Research has shown that children with tracheostomies are most at risk for speech and language impairment when they have a tracheostomy *in situ* during the linguistic stage of development (Simon et al 1983, Locke and Pearson 1990). Reported difficulties are mild receptive language delay with more marked expressive language delay, phonological impairment, and there is often a paucity of oro-motor skills. Figs 14.4 and 14.5 illustrate the redirection of airflow when a tracheostomy is in place.

Management considerations
The general assessment and management strategies discussed in the 'Principles of assessment and management' section of this chapter are all of fundamental importance when managing children who have language impairment or who are at risk for language impairment. Additionally, in young children, encouraging symbolic and social play will facilitate language development. Social integration from a young age to encourage social use of language in a variety of contexts and to build self-confidence is of paramount

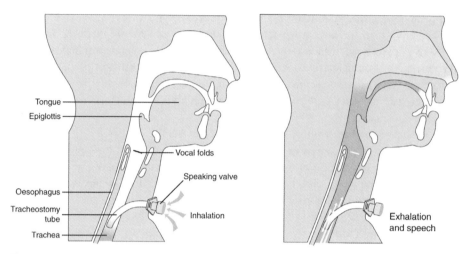

Fig. 14.4 Inhalation through the speaking valve and tracheostomy.

Fig 14.5 Exhalation with restored expiratory airflow.

importance. A detailed profile of the child's language skills across a range of functions is necessary to plan specific targets for remediation.

In children with tracheostomies, early intervention is essential in order to maximise communication development. The optimum method of management is a speaking valve. However a speaking valve is only a management option if there is an air leak around the valve and some children may not have a trachea of sufficient size for this to occur. A speaking valve may also not be viable (i.e. some children may not be able to cope with it). In these cases, the children will need to be assessed for suitability for alternative and augmentative communication systems.

VOICE IMPAIRMENT

This refers to any deviation in pitch, intensity, quality or other basic vocal attribute which consistently interferes with communication, draws unfavourable attention, adversely affects the speaker or listener, or is inappropriate to the age, sex, or perhaps the culture or class of the individual. The impairment may be the result of structural anomalies and/or behavioural problems.

Local evidence suggests that children with Apert syndrome frequently present with a variety of abnormal voice features. In a recent study perceptually analysing the voice quality of nine children with Apert syndrome, all had abnormal voice quality (Shipster et al 2002). Abnormal features included breathy voice quality, reduced vocal loudness and inappropriate habitual pitch. Also, abnormal features of 'wet' voice (the voice quality associated with laryngeal penetration in dysphagia) were identified in four of the children, and diplophonia (when two distinct pitches are perceived simultaneously during phonation) in two of the children.

Questions were raised during the perceptual analysis as to whether there was an organic aetiology contributing to the perceptual voice disorder for some of the subjects rated. None of the children in the study had undergone an ENT laryngeal examination, so it was not known whether there was an organic aetiology contributing to the perceptual voice disorder. However, Cohen and Kreiborg (1996) report the presence of abnormal calcification of the subglottic airway and larynx in Apert syndrome, which may well affect voice quality. Investigating laryngeal structure in conjunction with perceptual analysis would be an interesting area of study in the future. There are no other reports of abnormal laryngeal structure in the literature.

Clinically, a raised prevalence of voice disorders in the other craniosynostosis syndromes, apart from lowered voice volume, is not evident. Shprintzen (2000) reports that reduced voice volume is a common finding in syndromes of craniosynostosis which he attributes to conductive hearing loss. Local evidence also suggests that low voice volume can occur as a result of lack of confidence in speaking situations.

Management considerations
If low voice volume is related to hearing loss, this will usually be resolved when the hearing loss is effectively managed. If an organic cause of a voice impairment is suspected, then a child should be referred for an ENT examination of the larynx.

Speech and language impairment in children with sagittal synostosis
A study was undertaken recently at Great Ormond Street Hospital to investigate the occurrence, nature and severity of speech, language and literacy impairments in a consecutive series of 76 children (61 males and 15 females) with radiographically confirmed non-syndromic isolated sagittal synostosis (ISS) aged 9 months to 15 years 7 months (Shipster et al 2003). Additional aims of this study were:

- To establish the prevalence rate of cognitive impairment within the group.
- To ascertain if the speech and language impairments where present were related to global cognitive impairment or specific in nature.
- To establish if there was an association between surgery, age at surgery and raised intracranial pressure (ICP), and speech/language, and/or cognitive performance. (There has been considerable debate within the literature regarding the influence of surgery to release the suture, the age when the surgery is performed and the presence of ICP.)
- To establish if there were other factors present (unrelated to ISS) which could contribute to cognitive and/or speech and language impairments within the sample. The factors examined included perinatal risk factors, low socioeconomic status, a history of otitis media and a positive history of speech and language impairment.

A high prevalence rate of speech and/or language impairment, with 28 of the children (37 per cent) displaying impairment, was identified. This is significantly higher than the 6 per cent of children considered to have speech and language impairment in the normal population (Law et al 1998). Twenty of the 28 children with speech and language impairment (71 per cent) had moderate or severe impairments that fulfilled the criteria for specific disorders (that is a speech and/or language standard score that is below 85 and at least 20 standard score points (moderate impairment) or 30 standard score points (severe impairment) below the performance IQ. The speech, receptive and expressive impairments occurred in combinations, with expressive language impairments occurring most frequently. Thirteen children over the age of 7 years had their literacy skills (spelling, single word reading, and reading comprehension) assessed. Six of these children had literacy impairment and, of these, four also had specific speech and/or language impairment.

These speech and language impairments could not be accounted for by global cognitive impairment as there was no increased prevalence of global cognitive impairment (a Full Scale IQ score below 70) within the group. An interesting finding was that there was an increase of high average, high, and exceptionally high Full Scale IQ scores for children aged between 3 years 6 months and 15 years 7 months tested with the WPPSI and WISC when compared to the expected distribution of Full Scale IQ scores in the normal population. These findings are in contrast to findings in other studies (Noetzel et al 1985, Virtanen et al 1999) where the Full Scale IQ scores fell only in the average or low average range.

Low socioeconomic status could not account for the high prevalence of speech and/or language impairment as the study group had a social class mix that was similar to the UK population. Raised intracranial pressure, peri-neonatal risk factors, otitis media or having undergone surgery were not associated with impairment. Surgery at a later age and a family history of speech and language impairment were both associated with impairments but numbers were small. The findings suggest that children with ISS are at an increased risk of developing speech and language impairment. It is recommended that parents and professionals involved in the care of children with ISS are informed of this increased risk. Speech and language skills in children with ISS should be monitored throughout the preschool- and school-age years and also screened for literacy competence at regular intervals.

Principles of assessment and management
This section discusses the key principles of assessment and management of speech and language impairments in children with syndromic and non-syndromic craniosynostosis. Case history examples are given to illustrate these principles.

Assessment
The aim of assessment is to achieve the following goals:

- To establish which areas of communication (speech, resonance, voice, attention, receptive and expressive language, and pragmatic language skills) are impaired.
- To ascertain the extent and severity of the impairments.
- To compare the severity of the impairments across different areas of communication and to obtain a profile of the child's strengths and weaknesses.
- To provide a baseline assessment against which future progress can be measured.
- To identify those factors that may be contributing to the impairments so that these can be addressed.

- To identify any discrepancies between speech and language skills and other areas of development (i.e. are language skills significantly weaker than performance IQ and therefore indicative of a specific language impairment, or is the child globally delayed?)
- To enable planning and prioritisation of speech and language therapy goals.
- To inform the multidisciplinary team, other professionals involved in the child's care and the parents of the findings of the assessment and therapy goals.

At the initial assessment information is gathered from a variety of sources. These include: the initial referral letter; the medical records; assessment results from other members of the multidisciplinary team; reports from other medical and educational professionals who have seen the child; and the case history information. The case history provides vital information such as the parents'/caregivers' description of: the child's speech and language skills; the rate of speech and language acquisition; how the child communicates in a variety of settings; how the child compensates for any difficulties they have; the child's ability to attend to tasks; their perceptions of the child's overall developmental level; and the current concerns for the child.

This information, in conjunction with observation of the child's communication skills (attention control, listening ability, resonance and voice quality, social interaction skills, speech, expressive language and comprehension), guides the clinician as to which areas of speech and language need to be assessed in more detail. Observations can also be made of the child's functioning in other areas of development such as hearing, vision, fine and gross motor skills, and cognitive functioning. Klee et al (1998) report that parent/teacher questionnaires are an accurate and useful adjunct to provide additional detail about the child's speech and language skills in a variety of contexts. Once areas of suspected speech and language difficulty are identified, these are assessed using a combination of formal and informal assessment techniques (Lees and Urwin 1997, Kersner and Wright 2001). A selection of commonly used assessment procedures to assess speech and language skills is given in Table 14.4. Assessment procedures selected will depend on the age of the child, the child's developmental level and the presenting problem. Appropriate modifications will need to be made during assessment if the child has a visual or hearing impairment.

General Management Principles

The overall goal of management is to obtain the child's optimal level of speech and language functioning. The following management strategies will facilitate this goal.

Preventative work

Parents/caregivers of all children with syndromic craniosynostosis should be encouraged to focus on early communication and prelinguistic skills during infancy. These skills include behaviours such as vocalising, babbling, use of gestures, facial expressions, listening, turn taking and situational understanding. This focus may prevent some speech and language impairments from occurring; prevent existing problems from becoming exacerbated; and also heighten parents'/caregivers' awareness of when early speech and language skills are not emerging normally.

TABLE 14.4
Speech and language assessments

Speech/articulation vs phonology	South Tyneside Assessment of Phonology (Armstrong and Ainley 1988) PACSTOYS (Grunwell and Harding 1995) GOSPASS (Sell et al 1999)
Language (receptive/expressive)	Bzoch-League Receptive and Expressive Emergent Language Test-2 (REEL-2) (Bzoch and League 1991) 0–3 years questionnaire MacArthur Communicative Development Inventory (MacArthur and MacArthur 1993) Clinical Evaluation of Language Fundamentals – Pre-school UK Pre-school Language Scale-3 (PLS-3) 0–6 years Clinical Evaluation of Language Fundamentals – school-age British Picture Vocabulary Scale (BPVS) 2.6–18years Renfrew Action Picture Test (RAPT) 1988 Reynell Zinkin visual impairment
Voice	Vocal Profile Analysis (Laver et al 1981) Buffalo Profile III
Resonance	GOSPASS (perceptual) Naseometry Nasendoscopy Lateral view X-ray
Oro-motor skills	POSP Nuffield oro-motor assessment Brodsky Drooling Scale
Pragmatic skills	Pragmatic Profile Pre-school & School Age (Dewart and Summers 1995) – 9 months to 10 years (questionnaire)
Attention	Attention Scale (Cooper et al 1978)
Literacy	Phonological Assessment Battery (PhaB) (Frederickson et al 1997) – 6.14.11 Phonological Abilities Test (PAT) (Muter et al 1997)
Symbolic play	Symbolic Play Test (Lowe and Costello 1976)

Early intervention
When difficulties with speech and language are identified, intervention should take place as early as possible.

Working with parents and other professionals
Parents should always be active partners with therapists in any speech and language intervention. When this collaboration takes place the parents' insights and experiences of the child are combined with the therapist's knowledge of language acquisition and observations about the child, enabling strategies to be developed that will increase the rate of language development (Cummins and Hulme 2001). Therapists and parents should work closely with other professionals (i.e. teachers, specialist teachers, classroom assistants and other therapists) who are able to facilitate the development of the child's communication skills, to set speech and language targets and reinforce therapy goals.

It is also important that parents and professionals have accurate information about the child's craniofacial condition and what the implications of this are for all areas of development. Expectations for the child's functioning should also be based on accurate assessment across a broad range of functions.

Multidisciplinary team collaboration
Children with suspected difficulty in other areas of functioning should be referred for further investigations. Regular audiological, ophthalmic and orthoptic examinations are essential to detect hearing and visual impairments so that these can be treated appropriately. Where difficulties exist, input from specialist teachers for hearing-impaired children or visually impaired children may be necessary. Regular developmental and cognitive assessments are also essential, to compare speech and language functioning to other areas of development, and for educational planning. Children with fine and gross motor problems may need a neurological evaluation and input from occupational therapists and physiotherapists. For those children with hand and limb abnormalities, occupational therapists will also advise on suitable play materials and adaptations to allow the children to integrate as fully as possible in everyday living and peer group activities.

Developing listening and attention skills
Improving these skills and concentration are usually essential prerequisites for developing speech and language skills in children of all ages. Modifications may have to be made to the environment to aid development of these skills – such as reducing background noise.

Regular monitoring of speech and language skills
Children's speech and language skills change as they develop and therefore their needs will change over time. Additionally some children who are not identified at young ages may manifest problems at later ages (Silva et al 1987).

The following case histories illustrate some of the assessment and management principles and procedures discussed above.

Case study 1

Robert, who has Crouzon syndrome, was seen for routine speech and language assessment aged 6 years. At his 18-month, three-year and four-year assessments both his receptive and expressive language scores had been well above average. However, at school he was reportedly considered immature, to have poor listening skills, and to be in the lowest group academically within his class, but was not receiving any additional learning support. He reportedly had particular difficulty with numeracy and literacy, particularly recognition of numbers and letters. Observation and informal assessment revealed no difficulties with voice, resonance or speech. Receptive and expressive language skills were assessed using a battery of tests. His receptive language standard score was 90 and, while this was well within the normal range (standard scores between 85 and 115 represent the normal range of ability), it had dropped by 29 standard score points since his last assessment. His expressive language scores were also in the normal range but had dropped significantly. It was noted during the assessment that he had difficulty identifying details in the pictures he was presented with.

He was referred for audiological and visual assessment. He was found to have bilateral mild conductive hearing loss and was given grommets. Visual assessment revealed severe hypermetropia which makes small near objects (i.e. letters, numbers and small pictures) blurred. He was prescribed glasses, which corrected the problem. His school was contacted and was surprised to learn that his language skills were within the average range as they had felt that he was an immature child with low average abilities which accounted for his current poor academic performance. They were even more surprised to learn that at previous assessments his language skills were well above average. Strategies were discussed with the teacher to facilitate listening, increase understanding of language and participate verbally in school activities. Robert's mother met regularly with the teacher so that she could reinforce learning targets at home. At Robert's seven-year review, his language skills were once again well above average. He no longer had problems with literacy and numeracy. He was in the top group academically in the class and was reported to be a happier and more confident child.

Comment

This case illustrates how changes in performance can sometimes be indicative of other problems, and it highlights the value of monitoring a child's performance at regular intervals. Once the teacher was aware that Robert had average abilities and potential for improved performance it increased her expectations of him. When a child has normal speech and language development, and this is reported, it can be extremely helpful to give this to teachers to raise expectations about the child's abilities.

It also highlights the importance of detailed visual testing. Hypermetropia is unusual and would not have been identified in routine distance testing assessments. This child also had OME, which was not apparent until he was placed in the large noisy classroom where he had trouble listening. Parental and teacher co-operation is also an important factor in developing language skills and literacy.

<h1 style="text-align:center">Case study 2</h1>

Rachel, who has Pfeiffer syndrome with a cloverleaf skull (Pfeiffer syndrome type 2), was seen for speech and language assessment aged 4 years. She attended a mainstream school and had support from a classroom assistant for half of the week. Assessment showed that her speech and language skills were all at a 2-year level and her receptive and expressive language standard scores were both 50. She also had severe phonological speech impairment. During this hospital admission, a bilateral congenital moderate conductive hearing loss was diagnosed. She was given bone-anchored hearing aids and this was followed by monthly input in school from a teacher for the hearing impaired. Unfortunately, no speech and language therapy service was available locally. Therapy targets for speech, language and auditory skills were agreed between the hospital therapist, classroom teacher and assistant, teacher for hearing-impaired children, and parents. At 5 years of age, her local education authority recommended that she should attend a school for children with moderate learning disabilities, as this was the only school within her county that was suitable for her level of functioning. Reassessment at GOSH showed that although Rachel's auditory skills were noticeably improved, her speech and language skills were still severely delayed and only at a 2.6-year level. Her receptive and expressive language standard scores were both <50. At this point she was also seen for cognitive assessment in the hospital and she obtained a performance IQ of 105. This indicated that Rachel had normal non-verbal cognitive skills but severe specific difficulty with speech and receptive and expressive language development. On the basis of this assessment, it was argued that she should attend a Language Unit where she would be able to receive intensive daily speech and language therapy with specific language targets integrated into other aspects of the curriculum. Her local health authority subsequently funded her attendance at a Language Unit in an adjacent county. She made rapid and substantial progress in her speech and language skills in this placement, and at 11 years of age she was reintegrated back into mainstream school.

Comment
The late diagnosis of the congenital moderate conductive hearing loss is likely to have had a major impact on the development of Rachel's speech and language skills. An indirect therapy approach (unlike case study 1) was inadequate to address this child's needs and she required direct therapy on an intensive basis. The importance of differential cognitive assessment is highlighted. In this case, the child had normal non-verbal IQ and severe specific language impairment. Her needs would not have been met in a school for children with moderate learning difficulties, particularly as speech and language provision within this school was poor. Intensive daily speech and language therapy was required.

Case study 3

Billy, who has Apert syndrome, was seen at 6 months of age for initial multi-disciplinary team evaluation. Assessment revealed delayed pre-linguistic receptive and expressive skills with poor auditory and visual attention. He made very little sound and was an extremely undemanding, 'good' baby. Overall development was also delayed and was at a 2- to 3-month level. Billy's mother expressed her distress and grief at having a disabled child. Billy had three older siblings all under the age of 6 years. His mother stated how, prior to his birth, she felt she already had a 'perfect and complete' family. His birth had been unplanned and had caused a great strain within the family. The father was often away from the home. She expressed her desire for the child not to survive.

She also had the mistaken idea that all children with Apert syndrome have severe learning difficulties, and she felt that there was 'little point' stimulating him as he would be so disabled anyway. It also transpired that the mother gave Billy very little attention because of the demands of the other three siblings and also because Billy demanded so little attention. The team psychologist provided ongoing counselling support for the mother.

Billy's mother was also surprised to hear that many children with Apert syndrome make good developmental progress, despite often overall slow development in infancy, and usually attend normal school. She expressed a wish to meet other children with Apert syndrome and was put in contact with two local families with children with Apert syndrome. Social services were able to provide a disability allowance, which enabled the mother to purchase some weekly domestic help and childcare support.

After multidisciplinary assessment, the child's respiratory and feeding difficulties were addressed, and considerable improvement was achieved in both areas. The child had a bilateral moderate hearing loss and was prescribed hearing aids and was referred to a local teacher for hearing-impaired children, who subsequently visited the child on a monthly basis. Referral was made to the local SLT who saw the child once a month for therapy to facilitate both improved feeding patterns and early communication skills. The mother was also referred to Portage, a play scheme which provides ongoing weekly therapy aimed at facilitating all areas of development. Therapy goals were co-ordinated between the mother, the hospital speech and language therapist, the local therapist, the teacher for hearing-impaired children and the Portage worker.

At 18 months of age the child had made significant developmental strides. Speech and language skills were at a 14-month level, and the child was communicating verbally and highly interactive. The mother had also come to terms with the child's condition and was taking great pride and interest in the child's developmental progress.

Comment

This case illustrates the importance of multidisciplinary team working and liaison with local services to ensure that all the child's needs are met in order to obtain the best outcome developmentally for the child. In this case achieving this goal was also dependent on providing emotional and domestic support for the mother. Other parents and parent support groups can also be a valuable source of support. This case also highlights the importance and effectiveness of early and co-ordinated intervention.

Conclusion

When cognitive skills are normal and hearing losses where present are managed effectively, normal speech and language skills can be a realistic goal for children with craniosynostosis. Furthermore, good linguistic ability and social use of language are vital to help individuals cope with facial disfigurement (Rumsey et al 1986, Robinson et al 1996). Ongoing large-scale longitudinal multidisciplinary research is required to increase our knowledge of speech and language development in children with craniosynostosis.

REFERENCES

Armstrong S, Ainley M (1988) *South Tyneside Assessment of Phonolology (STAP)*. Bicester: Winslow Press.
Bamford J, Saunders E, Crystal D, Cooper J, editors (1985) *Hearing Impairment, Auditory Perception and Language Disability*. London: Edward Arnold.
Benaisch AA, Curtiss S, Tallal P (1993) Language, learning, and behavioural disturbances in childhood: a longitudinal perspective. *J Am Acad Child Adolesc Psychiatry* 32: 585–594.
Bergstrom L, Neblett LM, Hemenway WG (1972) Otologic manifestations of acrocephalosyndactyly. *Arch Otolaryngol* 96: 117–123.
Bishop DVM, Butterworth GE (1980) Verbal–performance discrepancies: relationship to birth risk and specific reading retardation. *Cortex* 16: 375–390.
Bishop DVM, Edmundson A (1986) Is otitis media a major cause of specific developmental language disorder? *Br J Dis Comm* 21: 321–338.
Bishop DVM, North T, Donlan C (1995) Genetic basis of specific language impairment: evidence from a twin study. *Dev Med Child Neurol* 37: 56–71.
Blasco P (1996) Drooling. In: Sullivan P, Rosenbloom L, editors. *Feeding the Disabled Child*. London: Mac Keith Press, pp 92–105.
Bloomer H (1971) Speech defects associated with dental malocclusions and related abnormalities. In: Travis L, editor. *Handbook of Speech Pathology and Audiology*. New York: Appleton-Century-Crofts.
Botting N, Conti-Ramsden G (2000) Social and behavioural difficulties in children with language impairment. *Child Lang Teach Ther* 16: 105–120.
Bray M, Ross A, Todd C (1999) *Speech and Language Clinical Process and Practice*. London: Whurr.
Bzoch K, League R (1991) *The Bzoch-League Receptive and Expressive Emergent Language Test – Second Edition (REEL-2)*. Austin, TX: Pro-Ed.
Cedars MG, Linck DL 2nd, Chin M, Toth BA (1999) Advancement of the midface using distraction techniques. *Plast Reconstr Surg* 103(2): 429–441.
Cherkes-Julkowski M (1998) Learning disability, attention-deficit disorder, and language impairment as outcomes of prematurity: a longitudinal descriptive study. *J Learn Disabil* 31: 294–306.
Cohen MM Jr, Kreiborg S (1996) A clinical study of the craniofacial features in Apert syndrome. *Int J Oral Maxillofac Surg* 25: 45–53.
Cohen MM Jr, MacLean RE (2000) *Craniosynostosis Diagnosis, Evaluation, and Management*, 2nd edn. New York and Oxford: Oxford University Press.
Cooper J, Moodley M, Reynell J (1978) *Helping Language Development: A Developmental Programme for Children with Early Language Handicaps*. London: Edward Arnold.

Corey JP, Caldarelli MD, Gould HJ (1987) Otopathology in cranial facial dysostosis. *Am J Otol* 8(1).

Cremers CW (1981) Hearing loss in Pfeiffers's syndrome. *Int J Paediatr Otolaryngol* 3(4): 343–353.

Crysdale WS (1978) Abnormal facial appearance and delayed diagnosis of congenital hearing loss. *J Otolaryngol* 7: 349–352.

Crysdale WS (1981) Otorhinolaryngologic problems in patients with craniofacial anomalies. *Otolaryngol Clin North Am* 14: 145–155.

Cummins K, Hulme S (2001) Managing pre-school children in community clinics. In: Kersner M, Wright JA, editors. *Speech and Language Therapy*. London: David Fulton, pp 53–62.

Dewart H, Summers S (1995) *The Pragmatics Profile of Everyday Communication Skills in Children*. Windsor: NFER-Nelson.

Dunn LM, Dunn LM, Whetton C, Pintilie D (1982) *British Picture Vocabulary Scale*. Windsor: NFER-Nelson.

Dunn LM, Wetton C, Burley J (1997) *British Picture Vocabulary Scale II*. Windsor: NFER-Nelson.

Edwards S, Fletcher P, Garman M, Hughes A, Letts C, Sinka I (1997) *Record Booklet Comprehension and Expressive Scales: The Reynell Developmental Language Scales III (RDLS)*. Windsor: NFER-Nelson.

Elfenbein JL, Waziri M, Morris HL (1981) Verbal communication skills of children with craniofacial anomalies. *Cleft Palate J* 18(1): 59–64.

Ensink RJH, Marres HAM, Brunner HG, Cremers CRWJ (1996) Hearing loss in the Saethre–Chotzen syndrome. *J Laryngol Otol* 110: 952–957.

Fazio B (1994) The counting abilities of children with specific language impairment: a comparison of oral and gestural tasks. *J Speech Hear Res* 37: 358–368.

Fenson L, Dale PS, Reznick JS, Thal D, Bates E, Hartung JP, Pethick S, Reilly JS (1993) *MacArthur Communicative Development Inventories*. California: Singular Publishing Ltd.

Field T (1995) Early interactions of infants with craniofacial anomalies. In: Eder RA, editor. *Craniofacial Anomalies. Psychological Perspectives*. New York: Springer-Verlag, pp 99–110.

Fredrickson N, Frith U, Reason R (1997) *The Phonological Assessment Battery*. Windsor: NFER Nelson.

Gopnik M (1999) Familial language impairment: more English evidence. *Folia Phoniatr Logop* 51(1–2): 5–19.

Gould HJ, Caldarelli DD (1982) Hearing and otopathology in Apert syndrome. *Arch Otolaryngol* 108: 347–349.

Grauberg E (1998) *Elementary Mathematics and Language Difficulties*. London: Whurr.

Grundy K (2001) Working with children with unclear speech: differentiating sub-groups of intelligibility impairment. In: Kersner M, Wright JA, editors. *Speech and Language Therapy*. London: David Fulton, pp 130–139.

Grunwell P (1995) *PACS*. Windsor: NFER-Nelson.

Grunwell P, Harding A (1995) *PACSTOYS*. London: NFER-Nelson.

Haggard M, Birkin J, Pringle D (1993) Consequences of otitis media for speech and language. In: McCormick B, editor. *Practical Aspects of Audiology*. London: Whurr, pp 79–101.

Kapp-Simon KA, McGuire DE (1997) Observed social interaction patterns in adolescents with and without craniofacial anomalies. *Cleft Palate Craniofac J* 34: 380–384.

Kersner M, Wright JA, editors (2001) *Speech and Language Therapy*. London: David Fulton.

Klee T, Carson DK, Gavin WJ, Hall L, Kent A, Reece S (1998) Concurrent and predictive validity of an early language screening program. *J Speech Lang Hear Res* 41(3): 627–641.

Konigsmark BW, Gorlin RJ (1976) *Genetic and Metabolic Deafness*. Philadelphia: W.B. Saunders.

Kreiborg S (1981) Crouzon syndrome. A clinical and roentgencephalometric study. *Scand J Plast Reconstr Surg Suppl* 18: 1–198.

Kreiborg S, Cohen MM Jr (1992) The oral manifestations of Apert syndrome. *J Craniofac Genet Dev Biol* 12: 41–48.

Laver J, Wirz S, Mackenzie J, Miller S (1981) A perceptual protocol for the analysis of vocal profiles. *Work Prog Univ Edinburgh* 14: 139–155.

Law J, Boyle J, Harris F, Harkness A, Nye C (1998) Screening for speech and language delay: a systematic review of the literature. *Health Technol Assess* 2(9): 11–15.

Lees J, Urwin S (1997) *Children with Language Disorders*, 2nd edn. London: Whurr.

Lefebvre A, Travis F, Arndt EM, Munro IR (1986) A psychiatric profile before and after reconstructive surgery in children with Apert syndrome. *Br J Plast Surg* 39: 510–513.

Lewis N (1976) Otitis media and linguistic incompetence. *Ann Otol* 102: 387–390.

Lindsay G, Dockrell JE (2000) The behaviour and self-esteem of children with specific speech and language difficulties. *Br J Educ Psychol* 70: 583–601.

296

Lindsay J, Black F, Donnelly W (1975) Acrocephalosyndactyly (Apert syndrome): temporal bone findings. *Ann Otol Rhinol Laryngol* 84: 174–178.

Locke J, Pearson D (1990) Linguistic significance of babbling. *J Child Lang* 17: 1–16.

Locke A, Ginsborg J, Peers I (2002) Development and disadvantage: implications for the early years and beyond. *Int J Lang Commun Disord* 37(1): 3–17.

Lowe M, Costello JA (1976) *Symbolic Play Test*, 2nd edn. Windsor: NFER-Nelson.

Luoma L, Herrgard E, Martikainen A, Ahonen T (1998) Speech and language development of children born at ≤ 32 weeks' gestation: a 5-year prospective follow-up study. *Dev Med Child Neurol* 40: 380–387.

MacArthur JD, MacArthur CT (1993) *The MacArthur Communicative Development Inventory*. San Diego, CA: Singular Publishing Group Inc.

McGill T (1991) Otolaryngological aspects of Apert ayndrome. *Clin Plast Surg* 18: 309–313.

Muter V, Hulme C, Snowling M (1997) *Phonological Abilities Test (PAT)*. London: The Psychological Corporation.

Noetzel MJ, Marsh JL, Palkes H, Gado M (1985) Hydrocephalus and mental retardation in craniosynostosis. *J Pediatr* 107: 885.

Northern JL, Downs MP (2002) *Hearing in Children*, 5th edn. Baltimore, MD: Lippincott Williams and Wilkins.

Orvidas LJ, Lee B, Fabry LB, Diacova S, Thomas J, McDonald TJ (1999) Hearing and otopathology in Crouzon syndrome. *Laryngoscope* 109(9): 1372–1375.

Ozanne, A (1995) The search for developmental verbal dyspraxia. In: Dodd B, editor. *Differential Diagnosis and Treatment of Children with Speech Disorder*. London: Whurr.

Pantke OA, Cohen MM Jr, Witkop CJ, Feingold M, Schaumann B, Pantke HC, Gorlin RJ (1975) The Saethre-Chotzen syndrome. *Birth Defects* 11(2): 190–225.

Patton MA, Goodship J, Hayward R, Landsdown R (1988) Intellectual development in Apert syndrome: a long term follow up of 29 patients. *J Med Genet* 25: 164–167.

Pereira V, Sell D, Dunaway D (2002) 'Seeing red'. Presented at 4th Asian Pacific Craniofacial Conference, Tokyo, 21–23 October.

Peterson SJ (1973) Speech pathology in craniofacial malformations other than cleft lip and palate. In: Wertz RT, editor. *Orofacial Anomalies: Clinical and Research Implications*. ASHA Reports no. 111.

Peterson S, Pruzansky S (1974) Palatal anomalies in the syndromes of Apert and Crouzon. *Cleft Palate J* 11: 394–402.

Peterson-Falzone SJ, Vallino LD (1993) A longitudinal perspective on communication development in 113 patients with 4 syndromes of craniofacial synostosis. Presented at 7th International Congress on Cleft Palate and Related Craniofacial Anomalies, Queensland.

Peterson-Falzone SJ, Pruzansky S, Parris PJ, Laffer JL (1981) Nasopharyngeal dysmorphology in the syndromes of Apert and Crouzon. *Cleft Palate J* 18: 237–250.

Peterson-Falzone SJ, Hardin-Jones MA, Karnell MP (2001) *Cleft Palate Speech*, 3rd edn. St Louis: Mosby.

Philips SG, Miyamoto RT (1986) Congenital conductive hearing loss in Apert syndrome. *Otolaryngol Head Neck Surg* 95: 429–433.

Renier D, Arnaud E, Cinally G, Sebag G, Kerah M, Marchac D (1996) Prognosis for mental functioning in Apert syndrome. *J Neurosurg* 85: 66–72.

Resnick MB, Shanti V, Gomatam SV, Carter RL, Ariet M, Roth J, Kilgore KL, Bucciarelli RL, Mahan CS, Curran JS, Eitzman DV (1998) Educational disabilities of neonatal intensive care graduates. *Pediatrics* 102(2): 308–314.

Robinson E, Rumsey N, Patridge J (1996) An evaluation of the impact of social interaction skills training for facially disfigured people. *Br J Plast Surg* 49: 281–289.

Rumsey N, Bull R (1986) The effects of facial disfigurement on social interaction. *Hum Learning* 5: 203–208.

Saigal S, Szatmari P, Rosenbaum P, Campbell D, King S (1991) Cognitive abilities and school performance of extremely low birth weight children and matched term control children at age 8 years: a regional study. *J Pediatr* 118(5): 751–780.

Sarimski K (1998) Children with Apert syndrome: behavioural problems and family stress. *Dev Med Child Neurol* 40: 44–49.

Sculerati N, Gottlieb MD, Zimbler MS, Chibbaro PD, McCarthy JG (1998) Airway management in children with major craniofacial anomalies. *Laryngoscope* 108(12): 1806–1812.

Selder A (1973) Hearing disorders in children with otocraniofacial syndromes. In: ASHA Report 8: *Orofacial Anomalies: Clinical and Research Implications*. American Speech and Hearing Association.

297

Sell D, Grunwell P (2001) Speech assessment and therapy. In: Watson ACH, Sell DA, Grunwell P. *Management of Cleft Lip and Palate*. London and Philadelphia: Whurr, pp 227–257.

Sell D, Harding A, Grunwell P (1999) GOS.SP.ASS.'98: an assessment for speech disorders associated with cleft palate and/or velopharyngeal dysfunction (revised). *Int J Lang Commun Disord* 34(1): 17–33.

Semel E, Wiig EG, Secord W (1987) *Clinical Evaluation of Language Fundamentals Revised (CELF-R)*. San Antonio, TX: The Psychological Corporation.

Shipster C, Hearst D, Dockrell JE, Kilby E, Hayward R (2002) Speech and language skills and cognitive functioning in children with Apert syndrome: a pilot study. *Int J Lang Commun Disord* 37(3): 325–343.

Shipster C, Hearst D, Somerville A, Stackhouse J, Hayward R, Wade A (2003) Speech, language, and cognitive development in children with isolated sagittal synostosis. *Dev Med Child Neurol* 45: 34–43.

Shprintzen RJ (2000) Speech and language disorders in syndromes of craniosynostosis. In: Cohen MM Jr, MacLean RE, editors. *Craniosynostosis Diagnosis, Evaluation, and Management*, 2nd edn. New York and Oxford: Oxford University Press, pp 197–203.

Silva PA, Williams SM, McGee R (1987) A longitudinal study of children with developmental language delay at age three: later intelligence, reading and behaviour problems. *Dev Med Child Neurol* 29: 630–640.

Simon B, Fowler M, Handler S (1983) Communication development in young children with long-term tracheostomy. *Int J Paediatr Otorhinolaryngol* 6: 37–50.

Snowling M, Stackhouse J (1983) Spelling performance of children with developmental verbal dyspraxia. *Dev Med Child Neurol* 25: 430–437.

Snowling M, Bishop DVM, Stothard SE (2000) Is preschool language impairment a risk factor for dyslexia in adolescence? *J Child Psychol Psychiatry* 41(5): 587–600.

Spitz RV, Tallal P, Flax J, Benasich AA (1997) Look who's talking: a prospective study of familial transmission of language impairments. *J Speech Lang Hear Res* 40(5): 990–1001.

Stackhouse J, Wells B (1997) How do speech and language problems affect literacy development? In: Hulme C, Snowling M, editors. *Dyslexia: Biology, Cognition and Intervention*. London: Whurr, pp 182–211.

Stark RE, Bernstein LE, Condino R, Bender M, Tallal P, Catts H (1984) Four-year follow-up study of language impaired children. *Ann Dyslexia* 34: 49–68.

Stradling J (1982) Obstructive sleep apnoea syndrome. *BMJ* 285: 528–529.

Tallal P, Allard L, Miller S, Curtiss S (1997) Academic outcomes of language impaired children. In: Hulme C, Snowling M, editors. *Dyslexia: Biology, Cognition and Intervention*. London: Whurr, pp 167–181.

Tomblin JB, Buckwater PR (1998) Heritability of poor language achievement among twins. *J Speech Lang Hear Res* 41(1): 188–199.

Vallino LD (1990) Speech, velopharyngeal function, and hearing before and after orthognathic surgery. *J Maxillofac Surg* 48: 1274–1281.

Vallino-Napoli LD (1996) Audiologic and otologic characteristics of Pfeiffer syndrome. *Cleft Palate Craniofac J* 33: 524–529.

Virtanen R, Korhonen T, Fagerholm J, Viljanto J (1999) Neurocognitive sequelae of scaphocephaly. *Pediatrics* 103(4): 791–795.

Walker D, Greenwood C, Hart B, Carta J (1994) Prediction of school outcomes based on early language production and socioeconomic factors. *Child Dev* 6: 606–621.

Weindrich D, Jennen-Steinmetz CH, Laucht M, Esser G, Schmidt MH (1998) At risk for language disorders? Correlates and course of language disorders in preschool children born at risk. *Acta Paediatr* 87: 1288–1298.

Whitehurst G, Fischel J (1994) Practitioner review: early developmental language delay: what, if anything, should the clinician do about it? *J Child Psychol Psychiatry* 35: 613–648.

Wiig EH, Secord W, Semel E (2000) *CELF-Preschool^{UK}*. London: The Psychological Corporation.

Witzel MA, Ross B, Munro IR (1980) Articulation before and after facial osteotomy. *J Maxillofac Surg* 83: 161–256.

Wolke D, Meyer R (1999) Cognitive status, language attainment, and pre-reading skills of 6-year-old very pre-term children and their peers: the Bavarian longitudinal study. *Dev Med Child Neurol* 41: 94–109.

Zimmerman IL, Steiner VG, Pond RE (1991) *Pre-school Language Scale – 3*. London: The Psychological Corporation; Harcourt Brace Jovanovich.

15
HEARING PROBLEMS IN CHILDREN WITH CRANIOSYNOSTOSIS

Tony Sirimanna

Audiological assessment and management of any hearing problems is an important part of the management of children with craniofacial disorders. The audiology department at Great Ormond Street Hospital has close links with the craniofacial unit, and an audiological assessment, and subsequent follow-up as necessary, forms an integral part of the initial assessment of all children presenting with complex (syndromic) forms of craniosynostosis, and also of children with non-syndromic forms when there are concerns about their hearing and educational progress.

Introduction

A patent external auditory canal, intact eardrum and fully developed middle ear structures are vital if day-to-day sounds are to be conducted to the inner ear. For normal hearing the inner ear must also be intact along with its central connections. Normal functioning of the middle ear cleft is dependent on an intact Eustachian tube function, which is responsible for maintaining the pressure within the middle ear cleft at normal atmospheric pressure. Any condition that affects the development of the head and neck may involve the external, middle and inner ear structures and their function, thus causing a hearing loss.

Development of the otic structures commences around the 23rd embryonic day and by the 12th week almost all the important components are in place. By the 8th month the inner ear is fully formed and is essentially similar to that seen in the adult. The first and the second pharyngeal arches contribute to the ossicles within the middle ear, which are vital for transmission of sound from the eardrum to the inner ear. The tissues between the first and the second arch develop into the eardrum while the tissues around the margins of the first groove develop into the external ear. This complexity of the development of the ear makes it vulnerable to many developmental abnormalities of the head and neck (Sulik and Cotanche 1995).

Otological manifestations

The commonest otological manifestation in craniosynostosis is otitis media with effusion (OME) (synonyms: middle ear effusions, 'glue ear'). Most of the other otological problems relate to complications of OME. Thus in some cases chronic middle ear disease such as chronic suppurative otitis media, tympanic membrane perforations, adhesive otitis media and, rarely, cholesteatoma can be found. In addition, congenital ossicular fixation with or without external auditory meatal atresia and abnormalities of the pinna can be seen in some patients. Sensorineural hearing loss is not a common finding but can be seen on occasions, with a prevalence greater than in the general population.

APERT SYNDROME

Low-set ears are commonly seen with pre-auricular tags on occasions (Cohen and Gorlin 1995). Hearing loss is normally mild to moderate and conductive, found in almost all children and usually due to OME (Gould and Calderelli 1982) and therefore fluctuating, although permanent conductive hearing loss due to fixation or hypomobility of the middle ear ossicles (usually the stapes) is not an uncommon feature in Apert syndrome (Lindsay et al 1975). An occasional sensorineural component of the hearing loss has also been noticed. As a significant proportion of these children have learning difficulties (Renier et al 2000) their hearing loss may go unnoticed for some time, partly due to difficulties in audiologically testing them as well as late presentation to audiology departments.

CROUZON SYNDROME

Congenital meatal atresia is a common feature seen in about 13 per cent, with conductive hearing loss reported in over half of the cases (Kreiborg 1981). There is also some outward rotation of petrous pyramids from cranial base dysplasia and also varying degree of fixation of middle ear ossicles in addition to meatal atresia or narrowing (Cremers 1981). Ossicular fixation in Crouzon syndrome includes fixation of incudo-malleal joint, ankylosis of malleus into the outer wall of the epitympanum and underdevelopment of the first arch components of the ossicular chain. These result in a conductive hearing loss of mild to moderate degree that can be fluctuating on occasions due to superadded OME (Corey et al 1987). Sensorineural hearing loss has also been noted and a significant proportion of these patients will have a mixed hearing loss (Orvidas et al 1999).

PFEIFFER SYNDROME

Otological manifestations are not as common as in Crouzon syndrome but when they occur they are similar in nature. Ankylosis of the middle ear ossicles, especially stapes fixation and meatal atresia, has been reported (Cremers 1981).

SAETHRE–CHOTZEN SYNDROME

Hearing loss is present in a significant proportion of cases, although the frequency varies in published reports (Pantke et al 1975), and is usually mild to moderate and conductive in nature. Hearing loss may be unilateral or asymmetric reflecting the asymmetry of the craniofacial abnormalities. Mild sensorineural hearing loss has also been seen occasionally.

Diagnosis of hearing loss

As a significant proportion of these children present either at birth or soon after, the diagnosis of any hearing loss can be challenging. Initial otoscopy may fail to detect occasional deep meatal atresia especially in the presence of a normal pinna. Certainly any middle ear defects, especially congenital ossicular fixation, will not be diagnosed by otoscopy but should be borne in mind when assessing these children.

The otoacoustic emissions (OAE) test (transient or distortion product) is currently widely used for neonatal hearing screening. Although the presence of good OAEs is compatible with normal hearing, as the OAE test requires a normally functioning middle ear it will not be useful in children with OME, meatal atresia and congenital ossicular fixation. Further, while the absence of OAEs is indicative of a hearing loss this test alone is not useful in determining the degree of this.

The auditory brainstem response test (ABR) is also widely used in this group of children with a developmental age of less than 6 months, or for those who are uncooperative for behavioural testing, for determining the hearing level. There are a number of methods being used and the commonest is 'click' evoked ABR. The stimulus is a 'click' and the threshold when recorded in optimal conditions is within 10 dB of the behavioural threshold of hearing in the 2–4 kHz frequency range. Tone bursts, filtered clicks and, more recently, steady state evoked potentials have been used for determining frequency-specific auditory thresholds. However, presence of interference, especially background noise when the test is carried out in a non-soundproofed, non-electrically screened environment, and also other factors such as raised intracranial pressure (which is sometimes seen in these children) that may affect conduction of the evoked electrical potential to the surface electrodes on the scalp, will lead to raised thresholds in a child with normal hearing (Edwards et al 1985). Further, although the inner ear is fully formed by the eighth month (of gestation), the auditory pathways up to the brainstem may not be fully matured (myelinated) until 4–6 weeks postnatally. During this early period any raised ABR thresholds must be interpreted carefully. Further, there are some children with delayed auditory maturation and therefore any sensorineural hearing loss diagnosed this early in life must be managed only by experienced audiologists.

Children with a developmental age of 6 months or older can be assessed using behavioural tests. These include visual reinforcement audiometry and distraction tests until the age of 30 months or so, performance and co-operative tests in children from 24 months onwards, and pure tone audiometry using a set of headphones in children who are developmentally over 36 months. Visual reinforcement audiometry, which is being increasingly used in the UK, provides an excellent test to determine ear and frequency specific hearing thresholds, with air and bone conducted stimuli, as young as 6 months of age.

OME and ossicular fixation alone usually produce a mild or moderate hearing loss, while meatal atresia will give rise to a maximum conductive hearing loss (around 60 dBHL). Any hearing loss above this raises the suspicion of a sensorineural hearing loss in addition to the conductive component. Post-grommet hearing assessment is therefore mandatory in order to exclude any residual conductive hearing loss due to ossicular fixation, or sensorineural hearing loss due to cochlear damage.

Tympanometry is usually used to examine the status of the middle ear and can be a very valuable tool when used with the tests described above. In newborn babies it is important to use high frequency tympanometry (Rhodes et al 1999). Conventional frequency tympanometry can be used in babies above 6 months of age with good reliability. In the absence of a tympanic membrane perforation, a flat graph indicates the presence of a middle ear effusion. Significantly higher ear canal volume with a flat graph on tympanometry indicates a tympanic membrane perforation (see below). A normal graph on tympanometry confirms absence of OME but will not exclude ossicular fixation or hypomobility, especially when accompanied by a conductive hearing loss.

Case 1

Mild to moderate conductive hearing loss with flat tympanometry suggesting middle ear effusions. Post-grommet audiogram shows residual low frequency conductive hearing loss due to ossicular hypomobility.

AUDIOGRAM

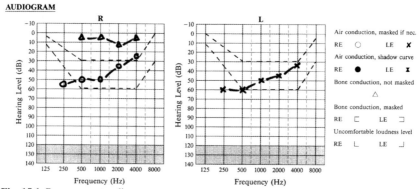

Fig. 15.1 Pre-grommet audiogram.

Fig. 15.2 Flat tympanometry confirming a middle ear effusion.

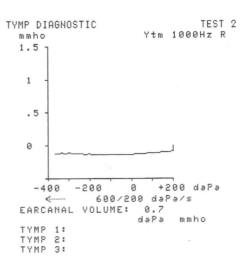

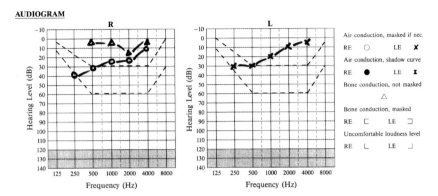

AUDIOGRAM

Fig. 15.3 Post-grommet audiogram – showing residual conductive hearing loss due to ossicular hypomobility.

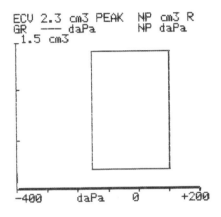

ECV 2.3 cm3 PEAK   NP cm3 R
GR —— daPa   NP daPa
1.5 cm3

-400   daPa   0   +200

Fig. 15.4 Post-grommet tympanogram with large ear canal volume confirming patency of the grommet.

Case 2

A girl with Pfeiffer syndrome with atresia of both external auditory canals and a maximum conductive hearing loss. This girl has excellent aided hearing with a bone-anchored hearing aid (B).

AUDIOGRAM

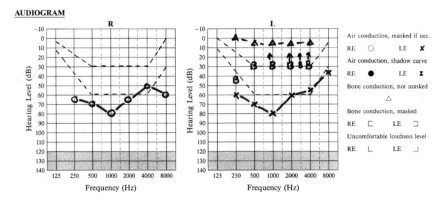

Fig. 15.5 Case 2

Case 3

A child with Pfeiffer syndrome with bilateral sensorineural hearing loss in addition to conductive hearing loss from middle ear effusions.

AUDIOGRAM

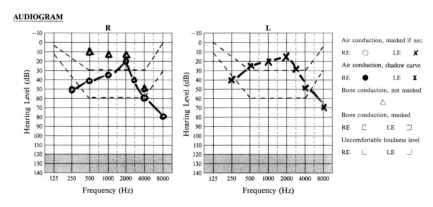

Fig. 15.6 Case 3

Effect of hearing loss on the development of the child

Exposure to sound is essential not only for the development of oral language but also for the normal development of the auditory system. The intensity of speech at normal conversational distance is about 55–60 dBHL, with a range from 35 dBHL to 65 dBHL for different speech sounds (speech spectrum – see below). Phonetic learning, the first stage in the acquisition of oral language, can occur only when there is access to the speech spectrum. Therefore, any child with a hearing loss of more than 70 dBHL is unlikely to hear normal conversational speech and hence will have a significant difficulty in developing normal speech. Further, very loud speech has an average of about 85 dBHL and therefore those with an average hearing loss of more than 90 dBHL will not develop any spoken language without appropriate intervention. Those with a hearing loss between 40 dBHL and 70 dBHL, and thus unable to access the full speech spectrum, may also have a varying degree of difficulty in acquiring normal speech, depending on the severity of hearing loss (Seewald et al 1996). More recently, it has been argued that a hearing level of 15 dBHL (Gelfand 1997) should be used as the upper limit of normal hearing in children.

In addition to the development of speech, development of spoken language is also dependent on hearing. Those children with a profound congenital hearing loss (see Appendix) would not develop spoken language without early auditory intervention but would develop alternative communication skills (Goldin-Meadow 1999). On the other hand, the effects of sound deprivation may not be apparent during the first year of life, even in generally healthy looking infants (Lohle et al 1999). Eillers and Oller (1994) showed that babbling establishes in a normally hearing infant before the age of 11 months and is delayed in a child with severe to profound hearing loss. Bennett et al (2001) showed that deficits in reading ability and interactive behaviour can persist into late childhood in a child with OME with mild to moderate hearing loss. Early detection of significant hearing loss and intervention is essential for better speech and language development (Robinson 1998, Schonweiler et al 1998). Hindley (1997) reviewed 120 publications on psychiatric aspects of hearing impairment and concluded that children with hearing impairment follow many different developmental pathways and are at a greater risk of developing behavioural problems.

Certain craniofacial conditions are associated with a unilateral hearing loss (e.g. in unilateral meatal atresia). Although this is compatible with normal speech and language

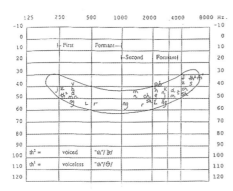

Fig. 15.7 Audiogram showing the intensity of normal conversational speech ('speech banana').

305

development, these children face a number of other problems, which are often ignored. These include:

1. Difficulty in localising a sound source (e.g. directionalising an approaching vehicle when crossing a road).
2. Difficulty in hearing in a noisy environment.
3. Having frequent and prolonged periods of significant hearing loss due to the involvement of normal ear with OME.

About 25 per cent of children with OME, in addition to a small number of craniofacial children who have developmental abnormalities of the vestibular system, do suffer from balance problems (Koyuncu et al 1999), and these children are likely to have delayed physical milestones (e.g. delayed walking).

Some children with resolved OME (or after grommet insertion) may present with hypersensitivity to loud sounds. This is seen usually immediately after resolution of OME (or grommet insertion) and almost always settles without any treatment within a few months.

Evidence for early intervention

Markides (1986) showed that children fitted with hearing aids before the age of 6 months had significantly superior speech intelligibility compared to those fitted with hearing aids later, as rated by teachers on a 7-point scale. Downs (1995) from Colorado showed that a group of infants provided with amplification before the age of 3 months scored 87 per cent of normal on an expressive language test. A similar finding was reported by Yoshinaga-Itano et al (1998) who compared the language abilities of children with hearing loss diagnosed and habilitated before the age of 6 months with those diagnosed after 6 months. There are several other studies showing the benefit of early intervention in hearing loss. These are shown below:

Ramakalawan and Davis (1992)	Early intervention leads to better outcome measures for language
Eillers and Oller (1994)	Children fitted with hearing aids sooner, babbled earlier
Robinshaw and Evans (1995) Robinshaw (1996)	Early intervention leads to normal pattern of speech and language development in some hearing-impaired infants.
Yoshinaga-Itano (1999)	Relationship between the degree of hearing loss and speech and language development (review); the more severe the hearing loss the poorer the speech and language development
Downs and Yoshinaga-Itano (1999)	Effect of early identification and intervention for children with hearing loss (review)

All this recent literature supports early intervention for significant hearing loss.

Management of OME

In children with craniofacial syndromes (especially Apert syndrome) OME is less likely to resolve spontaneously. This is thought to be due to the skull base abnormalities affecting the Eustachian tube function. The disability from OME can be variable, depending on the severity of hearing loss. In addition there is a degree of individual variation of the disability in children, due to a number of other factors such as classroom environment, learning ability and extent of stimulation. Often feedback from teachers and other healthcare professionals (e.g. speech and language therapists, care workers) can be helpful in making a decision, especially in children with mild or mild to moderate hearing loss.

Early intervention is fundamental to the development of spoken language wherever there is a significant hearing loss. However, deciding on the timing of intervention can be difficult, especially when the hearing loss is fluctuating and not so severe. Antibiotics, decongestants, mucolytics, antihistamines and other forms of medical management of OME are not usually useful in children with craniofacial syndromes. Grommets should be considered sooner for significant hearing loss due to OME in these children, although inserting these may be difficult in those children with narrow external ear canals. It is extremely important that hearing is reassessed after grommets are inserted, to exclude rare sensorineural hearing loss or more frequent conductive hearing loss due to ossicular fixation. Providing amplification is an alternative, but fitting hearing aids may not be possible because of pinna abnormalities and narrow ear canals.

Management of bilateral meatal atresia

Bilateral meatal atresia always leads to a significant conductive hearing loss in the region of 50–60 dBHL. In the newborn with this condition, ABR with air and bone conduction stimuli should be carried out to exclude a sensorineural hearing loss. Amplification via a bone conduction hearing aid must be provided as early as possible and will lead to an excellent outcome. Attempts at reconstructing ear canals almost always lead to a disastrous outcome, including possible damage to the facial nerve and chronically discharging ear canals, and are highly unlikely to improve the hearing so that the hearing aids can be discontinued. When the child is about 4 years of age and the skull has reached a minimal thickness, a bone anchored hearing aid could be considered, as these give the child a better quality hearing, especially in noisy situations (Mora Fernandez 2000, Sirimanna 2002).

Sensorineural hearing loss

The occasional child with a sensorineural hearing loss must be managed appropriately. If the hearing loss is mild the child should be followed up regularly to detect any further hearing loss due to OME. The management is similar to the management of OME, requiring grommet insertion or hearing aid fitting, depending on the parental or patient preference. Significant sensorineural hearing loss must be identified early and managed with suitable amplification.

Dealing with the above requires time, expertise in counselling and a multidisciplinary team effort. Greenberg (1983) found that parents who received counselling interacted more positively with their hearing-impaired child than those who did not. Keeping parents informed at all times and discussing management plans will be helpful in getting the parents through this difficult period and shifting the focus to habilitation. Involving parents as part of the team responsible for the habilitation process often helps them feel that they are actively involved in the habilitation of their child. Establishing goals during the process of counselling is extremely helpful and leads to positive participation of the parents (and the rest of the family) (Kample 1989).

Parents will need further information about the condition (hearing loss) as well as introduction to self-help groups and societies dealing with hearing impairment related issues (e.g. National Deaf Children's Society, UK). Exposure to speech and language therapy is unlikely to be useful in the first year of life although involvement of the peripatetic teacher of the deaf will be invaluable especially when the hearing aids are fitted.

Conclusion

Craniofacial syndromes carry a higher than normal incidence of hearing loss, mostly due to OME but occasionally due to other causes such as congenital ossicular fixation with or without meatal atresia and sensorineural hearing loss. Identification of and appropriate intervention in this hearing loss is extremely important in order to optimise the speech and language development and maximise the educational achievement, thus reducing the disability. These children should be managed by experienced audiologists working as part of a team with other professionals involved in the management of the craniofacial problems.

Appendix: Classification of degree of hearing loss

(HL = hearing loss)	Average hearing level over 0.5, 1, 2 and 4 kHz
Normal hearing	≤20 dBHL
Mild HL	20 dBHL ≤40 dBHL
Moderate HL	40 dBHL ≤70 dBHL
Severe HL	70 dBHL ≤95 dBHL
Profound HL	>95 dBHL

Source: *British Journal of Audiology* (1988) 22: 123.

REFERENCES

Bennett KE, Haggard MP, Silva PA, Stewart IA (2001) Behaviour and developmental effects of otitis media with effusion into the teens. *Arch Dis Child* 83: 91–95.
Bergman BM, Beauchaine KL, Gorga MP (1992) Application of the auditory brainstem response in paediatric audiology. *Hear J* 45(9): 19–25.
Bonfils P, Avan P, Francois M, Trotoux J, Narcy P (1992a) Distortion product otoacoustic emissions in the neonates. *Acta Otolaryngol* 112(5): 739–744.
Bonfils P, Francoise M, Avan P, Londero A, Trotoux J, Narcy P (1992b) Spontaneous and evoked otoacoustic emissions in pre-term neonates. *Laryngoscope* 102(2): 182–186.
Bowes M, Smith C, Tan AK, Varette-Cerre P (1999) Screening of high-risk infants using distortion product otoacoustic emissions. *J Otolaryngol* 28(4): 181–184.

Cohen MM, Gorlin RJ (1995) Genetic hearing loss associated with musculo-skeletal disorders. In: Gorlin RJ, Tortello HV, Cohen MM, editors. *Hereditary Hearing Loss and Its Syndromes*. Oxford: Oxford University Press, pp 141–233.

Corey JP, Calderelli DD, Gould HJ (1987) Otopathology in cranial facial dysostosis. *Am J Otol* 8(1): 14–17.

Cremers CW (1981) Hearing loss in Pfeiffer's syndrome. *Int J Paediatr Otolaryngol* 3(4): 343–353.

Dillon H (1996) Compression? Yes, but for low or high frequencies, for low or high intensities, and with what response times? *Ear Hear* 17(4): 287–307.

Downs MP (1995) Universal new-born hearing screening – the Colorado story. *Int J Paediatr Otolaryngol* 32: 257–259.

Downs MP, Yoshinaga-Itano C (1999) The efficacy of early identification and intervention for children with hearing impairment. *Pediatr Clin North Am* 46(1): 79–87. (Review.)

Edwards CG, Durieux-Smith A, Picton TW (1985) Auditory brainstem response audiometry in neonatal hydrocephalus. *J Otolaryngol Suppl* 14: 40–46.

Eillers RE, Oller DK (1994) Infant vocalisation and early diagnosis of childhood hearing impairment. *J Pediatr* 124(2): 199–203.

Engdahl B, Arnesen AR, Mair JW (1994) Otoacoustic emissions in the first year of life. *Scand Audiol* 23(3): 195–200.

Garnham J, Cope Y, Durst B, McCormick B, Mason SM (2000) Assessment of aided ABR thresholds before cochlear implantation. *Br J Audiol* 34: 267–278.

Gelfand SA (1997) *Essentials of Audiology*. New York, NY: Thiem Medical Publishers.

Gliddon ML, Martin AM, Green R (1999) A comparison of some clinical features of visual reinforcement audiometry and the distraction test. *Br J Audiol* 33(6): 355–365.

Goldin-Meadow S (1999) What children contribute to language learning? (Review). *Sci Progress* 82(pt 1): 89–102.

Gould HJ, Calderelli DD (1982) Hearing and otopathology in Apert syndrome. *Arch Otolaryngol* 108: 347–349.

Greenberg M (1983) Family stress and child competence: the effects of early intervention for families with deaf infants. *Am Ann Deaf* 128: 407–417.

Hayes D (1994) Hearing loss in infants with craniofacial abnormalities. *Otolaryngol Head Neck Surg* 110: 30–35.

Hayes D, Northern JL (1996) *Infants and Hearing*. San Diego, CA: Singular Publishing Group.

Hindley P (1997) Psychiatric aspects of hearing impairments. *J Child Psychol Psychiatry* 38(1):101–117.

Kample C (1989) Parental reaction to a child's hearing impairment. *Am Ann Deaf* 134: 255–259.

Koyuncu M, Saka MM, Tanyeri Y, Sesen T, Unal R, Tekat A, Yilmaz F (1999) Effects of otitis media with effusion on the vestibular system in children. *Otolaryngol Head Neck Surg* 120(1): 117-121.

Kreiborg S (1981) Crouzon syndrome. *Scand J Plast Reconstr Surg Suppl* 18: 1–198.

Liden G, Kankkunen A (1969) Visual reinforcement audiometry. *Acta Otolaryngol* 67: 281–292.

Lindsay JR, Black FO, Donnelly WH Jr (1975) Acrocephalosyndactyly (Apert syndrome): temporal bone findings. *Ann Otol Rhinol Laryngol* 84(2 pt 1): 174–178.

Lohle E, Holm M, Lehnhardt E (1999) Preconditions of language development in deaf children. *Int J Pediatr Otolaryngol* 47(2): 171–175.

Markides A (1986) Age of fitting of hearing aids and speech intelligibility. *Br J Audiol* 20: 165–167.

Meadow-Orlans K (1995) Sources of stress for mothers and fathers of deaf and hard of hearing infants. *Am Ann Deaf* 140: 352–357.

Møller K, Blegvad B (1976) Brainstem response in patients with sensorineural hearing loss. *Scand Audiol* 5: 115–127.

Moore JM, Wilson WR, Thompson G (1977) Visual reinforcement of head-turn responses in infants under 12 months of age. *J Speech Hear Dis* 42: 328–334.

Mora Fernandez J (2000) Parental questionnaire on BAHA in children. MSc thesis, Institute of Laryngology and Otology, University College London, London

Oller DK, Eilers RE (1988) The role of audition in infant babbling. *Child Dev* 59(2): 441–449

Orvidas LJ, Lee B, Fabry LB, Diacova S, Thomas J, McDonald TJ (1999) Hearing and otopathology in Crouzon syndrome. *Laryngoscope* 109(9): 1372–1375.

Pantke OA, Cohen MM Jr, Witkop CJ Jr, Feingold M, Schaumann B, Pantke HC, Gorlin RJ (1975) The Saethre–Chotzen syndrome. *Birth Defects Orig Artic Ser* 11(2): 190–225.

Paradise J, Smith C, Bluestone C (1976) Tympanometric detection of middle ear effusion in infants and young children. *Pediatrics* 58: 198–210.

Ramakalawan TW, Davis AC (1992) The effects of hearing loss and the age of intervention on some language metrics in young hearing impaired children. *Br J Audiol* 26: 97–107.

Renier D, Lajeunie E, Arnaud E, Marchac D (2000) Management of craniosynostosis. *Childs Nerv Syst* 16(10–11): 645–658. (Review.)

Robinshaw HM (1995) Early intervention of hearing impairment: differences in the timing of communicative and linguistic development. *Br J Audiol* 29(6): 315–334.

Robinshaw H (1996) The pattern of development from non-communicative behaviour to language by hearing impaired children. *Br J Audiol* 30: 177–198.

Robinshaw H, Evans R (1995) *Assessing the Acquisition of Auditory, Communicative and Linguistic Skills of a Congenitally Deaf Infant Pre- and Post-Cochlear Implantation*. London: British Association of Teachers of the Deaf.

Robinson K (1998) Implications of developmental plasticity for the language acquisition of deaf children with cochlear implants. *Int J Pediatr Otolaryngol* 46(1–2): 71–80.

Rhodes MC, Margolis RH, Hirsch JE, Napp MA (1999) Hearing screening in the newborn intensive care nursery: comparison of methods. *Otolaryngol Head Neck Surg* 120(6): 799–808.

Ruben RJ (1997) A time frame of critical/sensitive periods of language development. *Acta Otolaryngol (Stockh)* 117: 202–205.

Schonweiler R, Ptok M, Radu HJ (1998) A cross-sectional study of speech and language abilities of children with normal hearing, mild fluctuating conductive hearing loss, or moderate to profound sensorineural hearing loss. *Int J Pediatr Otolaryngol* 44(3): 251–258.

Seewald RC, Ramji KV, Sinclair ST, Moodie KS, Jamieson DG (1993) *Computer-assisted Implementation of the Desired Sensation Level Method for Electroacoustic Selection and Fitting in Children. User Manual.* London, Ont: University of Western Ontario.

Seewald RC, Moodie KS, Sinclair ST, Cornelisse LE (1996) Traditional and theoretical approaches to selecting amplification for infants and young children. In: Bess FH, Gravel JS, Tharpe A, editors. *Amplification for Children with Auditory Deficits.* Nashville, TN: Bill Wilkerson Press, pp 161–192.

Seewald RC, Cornelisse LE, Ramji KV, Sinclair ST, Moodie KS, Jamieson DG (1997) DSL v 4.1 for Windows: A software implementation of the Desired Sensation Level (DSL) Method for fitting linear gain and wide dynamic range compressions hearing instruments. Hearing Healthcare Research Unit, University of Western Ontario, Canada.

Sirimanna T, Tungland P (2002) *Speech in Noise with Bone Anchored Hearing Aid, Proceedings of the International Society of Audiology Conference*, Melbourne, Australia.

Sulik KK, Cotanche DA (1995) Embryology of the ear. In: Gorlin RJ, Tortello HV, Cohen MM, editors. *Hereditary Hearing Loss and Its Syndromes.* Oxford: Oxford University Press, pp 22–42.

Tucker SM, Battacharya J (1992) Screening of hearing impairment in the new-born using the auditory response cradle. *Arch Dis Child* 67(7): 911–919.

Werner L (1996) The development of auditory behaviour. *Ear Hear* 17: 438–446.

Westwood GFS, Bamford JM (1995) Probe-tube microphone measures with very young infants: real ear to coupler differences and longitudinal changes in real ear unaided response. *Ear Hear* 16(3): 263–273.

Wilson WR, Thompson G (1984) Behavioural audiometry. In: Jerger J, editor. *Pediatric Audiology.* San Diego, CA: College Hill Press, pp 1–44.

Yoshinaga-Itano C (1999) Benefits of early intervention for children with hearing loss. *Otolaryngol Clin North Am* 32(6): 1089–1092. (Review.)

Yoshinaga-Itano C, Sedey AL, Coulter DK, Mehl AL (1998) Language with early and late identified children with hearing loss. *Pediatrics* 102(5): 1161–1171.

16
FEEDING PROBLEMS IN SYNDROMIC CRANIOSYNOSTOSIS

Valerie Pereira

Introduction

Feeding patterns in children with craniosynostosis are poorly described in the literature and remain relatively ill-defined. Hence, the prevalence of feeding difficulties in this population remains unknown and much of our current knowledge of the specific relationships between feeding and craniosynostosis is based on clinical experience and local evidence. With such a complex array of functional problems and a significantly altered oral-facial anatomy, the potential for feeding difficulties that are not only wide-ranging in nature but also extend across the whole spectrum of feeding development is always present.

This chapter discusses the predisposing risk factors for feeding difficulties in syndromic craniosynostosis and describes the nature of these difficulties throughout the main stages of feeding development from bottle-feeding to biting and chewing. It also addresses the potential effects of midface advancement on swallowing. Assessment issues are covered, with a focus on useful assessment tools including standardised feeding assessments as well as the more usual diagnostic tests and procedures. Clinical studies and case histories based on our own extensive experience will also be presented in order to illustrate the complexity of feeding difficulties in syndromic craniosynostosis and the range of management strategies required for this group.

To put feeding difficulties in syndromic craniosynostosis in context, the chapter begins with a brief background to the development of feeding skills in infants, describing the normal and abnormal swallow.

The development of feeding skills

'Feeding' is a term that is widely used in the general paediatric literature to refer not only to the act of swallowing but also sucking, biting and chewing. The term 'dysphagia' refers to any difficulty in any phase of the swallowing process including difficulties with the oral preparation of fluid or food.

The development of feeding skills is associated with the types of liquids and solids taken and how these are presented, e.g. via a bottle or spoon. Table 16.1 summarises the normal progression of feeding skills according to the type of liquid or food given at specific ages and the manner of presentation. Age levels shown are only approximate, and development

TABLE 16.1
The development of feeding skills according to type of food given and manner of presentation

Manner of presentation	Age in months	Liquid/food	Milestone
Bottle/breast-feeding	0–6	Liquids, e.g. milk/juice	Suckling/sucking
Cup-feeding introduced Spoon-feeding introduced	4–6	Liquids Smooth puree, e.g. commercially available 4-month jar baby foods, liquidised semi-solids	Forward-backward tongue movements when spoon is introduced Sucking from spoon
Finger/self-feeding introduced	6–12	Mashed food Finger foods	Upper lip begins to be active in removing food from spoon nearer 9–12 months With finger foods, biting down on food begins/'munch' emerges
Weaning off bottle/breast	12–18	Firmer table food is chopped	Chewing emerges with rotary jaw movements Biting on cup to stabilise jaw
	18–24	Foods requiring chewing	Rotary jaw movements whilst chewing Internal jaw stability present for biting down and breaking off biscuit Internal jaw stability developing for cup drinking

Source: Adapted from Morris and Klein (1987: 61–82) and Winstock (1994: 6–11).

of feeding skills varies from one child to the next. For a detailed discussion of the normal development of feeding skills, the reader is referred to Morris and Klein (1987).

The normal swallow

Swallowing can be described according to the following phases: oral-preparatory, oral, triggering pharyngeal, pharyngeal and oesophageal (see Fig. 16.1).

Oral-preparatory phase: The oral-preparatory phase involves events which are associated with reception of food or liquid into the oral cavity, and the formation of a bolus when the food or liquid mixes with saliva. When food or liquid enters the oral cavity, a labial seal is required to ensure that there is no leakage of food or fluid from the mouth. During this phase, the larynx and pharynx are at rest, the airway is open and nasal breathing continues (Logemann 1998). The oral-preparatory phase is voluntary and its duration depends on physical properties of the food or fluid, including bolus volume and food texture.

Oral phase: Following the formation of the bolus, the tongue then propels the bolus posteriorly within the oral cavity. As the bolus enters the pharynx, the nasopharynx is sealed off as the soft palate elevates against the posterior pharyngeal wall (Tuchman 1994, Arvedson and Lefton-Greif 1998). As cited in Arvedson and Lefton-Greif (1998), the oral phase lasts for about 0.5 seconds (Dodds et al 1990) and does not vary with texture.

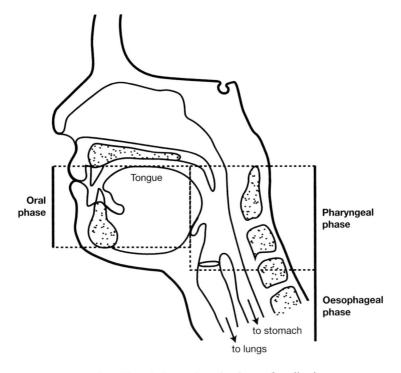

Fig. 16.1 Schematic drawing of lateral view to show the phases of swallowing.

Triggering pharyngeal phase: The triggering of the pharyngeal phase occurs when 'the bolus head passes any point between the anterior faucal arches and the point where the tongue base crosses the lower rim of the mandible' (Logemann 1998: 29). In infants, this swallow trigger can occur only when the bolus accumulates in the valleculae (Arvedson and Lefton-Greif 1998). If the swallow has not been triggered by this time, the swallow is said to be delayed.

Pharyngeal phase: Once the swallow reflex is activated, the soft palate or velum elevates to close off the nasopharynx and the posterior pharyngeal wall constricts. The larynx closes and elevates and the epiglottis folds down to cover the open airway. The true and false vocal cords also approximate to provide more airway protection. Respiration ceases during this time to allow the bolus to move through the pharynx by the combined action of pharyngeal peristalsis and changing pressure gradients towards the relaxed upper oesophageal sphincter.

Oesophageal phase: This phase begins with the opening of the upper oesophageal sphincter. The oesophageal phase consists of peristaltic wavelike movements which carry the bolus to the stomach.

The abnormal swallow

Swallowing difficulties can occur in any of the four phases. In the oral phase, the infant may have a weak or inefficient suck resulting in inadequate expression of milk from the teat or nipple. The infant may also have difficulties maintaining lip closure or seal around the teat, resulting in fluid loss and inadequate intake. Difficulties in this phase also include poor chewing skills to effectively manage firmer foods. Oral stage difficulties can have an adverse impact on the pharyngeal stage of swallowing.

Two significant symptoms of swallowing difficulties are laryngeal penetration or aspiration. Laryngeal penetration occurs when fluid or food penetrates to the inferior surface of the epiglottis or the part of the laryngeal vestibule that is still above the level of the true vocal cords. Aspiration on the other hand occurs when fluid or food enters the trachea below the level of the true vocal cords (see Fig. 16.2). Aspiration may be associated with an observable behaviour, e.g. a cough, or may sometimes be asymptomatic or 'silent'. This reflexive coughing is one of the primary protective functions of the larynx and acts as a 'backup protection when the primary airway protective mechanisms during swallowing fail to function adequately' (Arvedson and Lefton-Greif 1998: 27). With aspiration, there is a potential risk of bacterial pneumonia, pneumonitis and bronchitis (Arvedson and Brodsky 1993).

Swallowing difficulties can also be classified according to the timing of occurrence of laryngeal penetration or aspiration. Aspiration before the swallow is usually caused by oral stage difficulties which can cause premature spillage of the liquid/food into the pharynx. If it occurs during a swallow, it can be caused by reduced or insufficient laryngeal elevation and closure (Wolf and Glass 1992) or pharyngeal/respiratory incoordination (Arvedson and Lefton-Greif 1998). Aspiration after the swallow is caused by a variety of reasons including reduced laryngeal elevation or nasopharyngeal reflux (Arvedson and Lefton-Greif 1998).

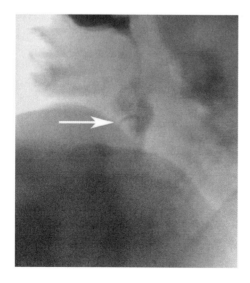

Fig 16.2 Lateral view of videofluoroscopic evaluation using barium. Laryngeal penetration is indicated by the arrow.

314

Predisposing risk factors for feeding difficulties in syndromic craniosynostosis

The complexity of the oral-facial and cranial morphology of syndromic craniosynostosis can often result in raised intracranial pressure, upper airway difficulties, sleep apnoea and ophthalmologic problems. Abnormalities of the central nervous system have also been reported in Apert, Crouzon and Pfeiffer syndromes (Cohen and Kreiborg 1993b, Slaney et al 1996, Cohen and MacLean 2000, Peterson-Falzone et al 2001) and in Saethre–Chotzen syndrome (Elia et al 1996). Additionally, both cardiovascular and respiratory anomalies have been found in children with Apert, Crouzon and Pfeiffer syndrome (Cohen et al 1993, Cohen and MacLean 2000). Gastrointestinal anomalies have also been documented in both Apert and Pfeiffer syndromes (Cohen and MacLean 2000). These are all risk factors that predispose the infant or child with syndromic craniosynostosis to feeding difficulties (see Table 16.2)

ABNORMAL ORAL-FACIAL ANATOMY

Abnormalities of the oral-facial anatomy of varying degrees and types occur in all four syndromic craniosynostosis groups. Maxillary hypoplasia results in a typical class III jaw occlusion and an anterior open bite. Delayed dental development and dental overcrowding are also common. The hard palate is high and arched, and in Apert syndrome, 'the palatal vault is characterised by progressive accumulation of the soft tissue along the palatine shelves' (Peterson-Falzone et al 2001: 51). A median furrow is also characteristic and was identified in 94 per cent of cases reviewed by Kreiborg and Cohen (1992). Clefts of the palate or submucous clefts in Apert syndrome occur in about 30 per cent of cases (Ferraro 1991), although Kreiborg and Cohen (1992) reported that clefts of the soft palate or bifid uvula occur in approximately 75 per cent of cases. Slaney et al (1996) found that the overall prevalence rate for clefts of the soft palate including bifid uvula was 57.6 per cent of their cases. With such a complex and altered oral-facial anatomy, the potential for oral-motor difficulties affecting feeding is clearly present.

The impact of oral-motor dysfunction on feeding cannot be overemphasised. There is increasing evidence in the literature to suggest that there is an association between oral-motor deficits and poor nutritional intake and failure to thrive (Gisel and Patrick 1988, Mathisen et al 1989, Alper and Manno 1996, Reilly et al 1999). The hypoplastic maxilla can adversely affect lip seal around a teat during bottle-feeding, resulting in liquid loss. A

TABLE 16.2
Predisposing risk factors for feeding difficulties in syndromic craniosynostosis

Abnormal oral-facial anatomy
Upper airway obstruction
Visual impairment
Motor difficulties/delayed development
Malformations of the central nervous system
Cardiovascular and respiratory anomalies
Gastrointestinal anomalies

TABLE 16.3
Common oral-motor deficits in syndromic craniosynostosis
and clinical manifestations of feeding difficulties

Oral-motor deficit	Clinical symptom
Hypoplastic maxilla (retropositioned and retruded)	Poor lip seal around teat/nipple during nipple-feeding leading to potential liquid loss
High arched palate	Poor/inefficient suck leading to inadequate expression of milk from teat/nipple (may also affect success of breast-feeding) Food may get stuck on hard palate causing distress or putting the child at risk for later choking
Cleft palate	Poor/inefficient suck leading to inadequate expression of milk from teat/nipple (may also affect success of breast-feeding) May result in nasal regurgitation
Class III malocclusion	Limited/no rotary jaw movements leading to minimal intake of firmer foods or prolonged mealtimes

cleft of the soft palate may affect the infant's ability to develop adequate negative intraoral pressure for effective sucking. Interestingly, clinically this is not always the case with infants with Apert syndrome with diagnosed unrepaired clefts of the palate. One possible reason for this is the existing diminished nasopharyngeal space which makes creating negative intraoral pressure easier. Nasal regurgitation is reported in only some cases of Apert infants with a diagnosed cleft palate. In Apert syndrome, the high arched palate and median groove may cause food to get stuck within this midline furrow. Some children become distressed as they are unable to remove this food with their tongue. If the food is left in the median groove, it potentially places the child at risk for later choking. Poor chewing is also often seen in syndromic craniosynostosis and a plausible cause for this is the characteristic class III malocclusion. This is discussed in detail in later sections of this chapter. The common oral-motor deficits seen in syndromic craniosynostosis and the clinical manifestations of the associated feeding difficulties are illustrated in Table 16.3.

UPPER AIRWAY OBSTRUCTION

Upper airway obstruction in syndromic craniosynostosis is well reported in the literature (Lauritzen et al 1986, Moore 1993, Perkins et al 1997, Sculerati et al 1998, Lo and Chen 1999). The nasal cavity is narrow and the height is decreased anteriorly and there is diminished nasopharyngeal space (Cohen and Kreiborg 1996). In addition, the palate is long, soft and floppy and there are widespread cartilaginous abnormalities (Moore 1993). The severity of upper airway obstruction in syndromic craniosynostosis ranges from nasal obstruction and increased work of breathing to severe obstructive sleep apnoea and respiratory distress. Possible consequences of airway obstruction include 'developmental delay, suboptimal neurologic development and failure to thrive' (Sculerati et al 1998: 1806).

The relationship between airway and swallowing is well documented in the paediatric dysphagia literature (Stevenson and Allaire 1991, Wolf and Glass 1992, Arvedson and Brodsky 1993, Tuchman and Walter 1994, Brodsky 1997). For a safe and effective swallow to occur, not only must the pharyngeal and laryngeal musculature co-ordinate precisely, but the airway has to be patent for breathing and protected for swallowing (Brodsky 1997). In early feeding, the acts of sucking, swallowing and breathing have to co-ordinate accurately and effectively with each other for safe bottle-feeding to occur. The suck and swallow pattern is usually in a 1:1 ratio and at a rate of one suck per second, with respiration occurring between swallows, at birth and during the neonatal period. As the infant grows and matures, this increases to about two to three sucks per second. The co-ordination of sucking, swallowing and breathing is described in great detail in Wolf and Glass (1992), with a focus on the specific impact of swallowing on breathing, breathing on sucking and sucking on swallowing.

The adverse effects of airway difficulties on bottle-feeding in children with midface hypoplasia have been documented in the literature (Thompson et al 1994, Tuchman and Walter 1994, Posnick 1996, Brodsky 1997, Perkins et al 1997). As a result of decreased narrow nasal airways and, in some cases, choanal atresia, the suck–swallow–breathe co-ordination is adversely affected. This inadvertently puts the infant with syndromic craniosynostosis at risk of aspiration while bottle-feeding. This is discussed in detail in the section on 'Bottle-feeding'.

VISUAL IMPAIRMENT
Ophthalmologic problems in syndromic craniosynostosis can include infection, corneal ulceration, recurrent prolapse of the orbital contents as well as progressive visual deteri-oration (Thompson et al 1994). From birth, vision plays an important part in feeding and visual impairment can affect both the development of self-feeding and the social interaction between the child and the feeder. There are special issues to consider when feeding the child with a visual impairment. These include modifications of the environment and position during feeding, encouraging the use of smell and tactile aspects, and a carefully planned system of communication. These issues are discussed and described in detail in Winstock (1994) and Klein and Delaney (1994). Feeding development in a child with visual impair-ment should be seen in light of their other developmental milestones.

MOTOR DIFFICULTIES/DELAYED DEVELOPMENT
Motor development plays a crucial role in the acquisition of feeding skills – for example, head control and trunk stability. Oral-motor movements which are important for the development of feeding occur 'after the head and trunk have achieved stability, symmetry and alignment' (Stevenson and Allaire 1996: 19). Motor development in syndromic craniosynostosis may also be delayed as part of an overall developmental delay. The prevalence rates of developmental delay in syndromic craniosynostosis continue to be ill-defined in the literature.

Additionally, as a result of syndactyly of the hands, the development of fine motor skills is at major risk in infants with Apert syndrome. Limitations of elbow extensions and rotation may also occur in Apert syndrome (Cohen and Kreiborg 1993b), and in Pfeiffer syndrome, ankylosis or synostosis of the elbows has been reported (Peterson-Falzone et al 2001). These difficulties may have an adverse impact on self-feeding. In such cases, an assessment by an occupational therapist is necessary to determine the need for and type of adaptive feeding equipment (e.g. angled spoon) required.

MALFORMATIONS OF THE CENTRAL NERVOUS SYSTEM

Feeding difficulties may also be associated with malformations of the central nervous system. The prevalence rates of these malformations and anomalies are not as yet defined, as infants and children with syndromic craniosynostosis are not routinely investigated for these. Malformations of the central nervous system have been reported in Crouzon, Pfeiffer and Apert syndromes (Cohen and Kreiborg 1993b, Slaney et al 1996, Cohen and MacLean 2000, Peterson-Falzone et al 2001) and in Saethre–Chotzen syndrome (Elia et al 1996). In a review of 136 cases of Apert syndrome, Cohen and Kreiborg (1993b) identified CNS abnormalities including malformations of the corpus callosum, the limbic structures or both. In a review of 70 cases with Apert syndrome, Slaney et al (1996) found similar malformations of the CNS including posterior fossa abnormalities in 20.8 per cent of cases, although they did also state that this might be an overestimate. The exact nature of and relationship between such malformations of the central nervous system and feeding development in syndromic craniosynostosis remains unknown.

CARDIOVASCULAR AND RESPIRATORY ANOMALIES

Infants and children with Apert syndrome are also at risk of feeding difficulties associated with cardiovascular and respiratory anomalies. From a review of 136 cases with Apert syndrome, Cohen and Kreiborg (1993c) found cardiovascular anomalies in 10 per cent of cases. Cardiovascular anomalies including ventricular septal defect and patent ductus arteriosus have been documented in Pfeiffer syndrome (Cohen and MacLean 2000). Additionally, anomalies of the respiratory system were found in 1.5 per cent of the same Apert cohort (Cohen and Kreiborg 1993c). Cases with complete or partial cartilage sleeve abnormalities have been documented in Apert, Crouzon and Pfeiffer syndromes (Cohen and MacLean 2000). A solid cartilaginous trachea may result in respiratory inefficiency or an inability to clear secretions (Cohen and MacLean 2000).

Cardiopulmonary disorders can adversely affect bottle-feeding in infants and children. Infants and children with such difficulties present with fatigue effects with bottle-feeding. Such infants usually start off well with fairly good suck–swallow–breathe co-ordination but deteriorate as the feed progresses. In many cases, the infant stops feeding and is unable to complete the feed, resulting in inadequate intake and subsequent failure to thrive.

GASTROINTESTINAL ANOMALIES

Gastrointestinal anomalies have also been documented in both Apert and Pfeiffer syndromes. Cohen and Kreiborg (1993c) documented that such anomalies occurred in about 1.5 per cent of their cohort. They reported two cases with oesophageal atresia. Other gastrointestinal anomalies including pyloric stenosis and intestinal malrotation have been identified in Pfeiffer syndrome (Cohen and MacLean 2000). Long-term complications of oesophageal atresia include oesophageal dysmotility which can contribute to gastroesophageal reflux. Disordered motility can also lead to intraesophageal reflux which can result in aspiration or interfere in swallowing (Wolf and Glass 1992). Gastroesophageal reflux can contribute negatively to dysphagia, and not only can it result in insufficient nutritional intake and consequently failure to thrive, but it may also lead to an aversion or even refusal to feed (Hyman 1994, Mathisen et al 1989). According to Hyman (1994: S104), 'the frustration arising from conflict between the drive to eat and the drive to escape pain may contribute to irritability and fussiness'.

The nature of feeding difficulties in syndromic craniosynostosis

BOTTLE-FEEDING

Bottle-feeding difficulties in syndromic craniosynostosis have been documented in the literature and are attributed to airway difficulties (Thompson et al 1994, Tuchman and Walter 1994, Posnick 1996, Brodsky 1997). Infants tend to be obligatory nasal breathers often up to the age of 3 months. When normal nasal breathing is not possible, as is often the case in syndromic craniosynostosis, these infants are immediately at risk of bottle-feeding difficulties. Bottle-feeding in syndromic craniosynostosis can therefore not only be prolonged, with an increase in noisy breathing as the feed progresses, but an uncoordinated suck–swallow–breathe pattern is also often seen (Thompson et al 1994, Posnick 1996). As a result, many of these infants cough and even 'choke' during feeding (Tuchman and Walter 1994). Such feeding difficulties, if not resolved or managed, may result in inadequate calorie intake and, in more severe cases, failure to thrive.

In a study looking at airway management in children with midface hypoplasia including syndromic craniosynostosis (Perkins et al 1997), the authors reported feeding difficulties in a third (n=45) of this cohort. However, no details as to the nature of these difficulties were given.

Clinically, we have made similar observations of bottle-feeding difficulties especially in infants and children with Apert, Crouzon and Pfeiffer syndromes. The most obvious cause usually appears to be airway and/or cardiac difficulties. However, other factors are indicated in some cases.

Although bottle-feeding difficulties are clearly indicated in this group of infants and children and fairly well documented in the literature, there has yet to be an objective study looking at feeding difficulties in syndromic craniosynostosis. To establish the extent of bottle-feeding difficulties in syndromic craniosynostosis and to better understand the nature of these difficulties, a clinical audit was undertaken on all infants and children with Apert syndrome seen by the unit over a three-year period (Pereira et al 2002–, work in progress).

Thirteen infants with Apert syndrome were seen for a bottle-feeding assessment out of a total of 17 new referrals to the craniofacial unit. Three of the infants had already been weaned off the bottle and the other was 'nil by mouth' and fed via a gastrostomy. All 13

319

infants received a bedside clinical evaluation of their bottle-feeding and a nutritional assessment. A subset of this cohort (n=7) underwent videofluoroscopy swallow evaluations because of clinical indicators of aspiration, including coughing and choking during feeding, recurrent chest infections and slow weight gain and/or failure to thrive.

The results of the clinical audit showed that all the infants assessed had bottle-feeding difficulties and presented with incoordinated suck–swallow–breath patterns as evidenced by nasal flaring and increased noisy breathing as the feed progressed. It is therefore not surprising that, with liquid loss and increased work during breathing, 10 out of the 13 infants were at a less than 0.4th percentile for weight and required long-term nutritional supplements including Infatrini, Duocal, Maxijul and Calogen (Pereira et al 2002–, work in progress).

As a result of airway difficulties, the infant with syndromic craniosynostosis has to work even harder to breathe during bottle-feeding. With increased energy expenditure, calories are consumed or lost and this contributes to the resultant weight loss and, in more severe cases, failure to thrive. Additionally, excess sweating is often reported in Apert syndrome and this may lead to elevated temperatures (Cohen and Kreiborg 1993b).

Videofluoroscopic swallow evaluations (n=7) showed delayed swallow onset, pooling and post-swallow residue in the valleculae and/or pyriform sinuses for all cases. More than half of this cohort of infants (n=4) showed laryngeal penetration or aspiration. In all four cases, this occurred *during* the swallow as opposed to either before or after the swallow. Laryngeal penetration or aspiration during a swallow is associated with either reduced laryngeal closure or elevation and/or pharyngeal or respiratory incoordination. Another interesting observation was that none of the children made any response to this laryngeal penetration or aspiration, e.g. by coughing, and none made any attempt to clear the airway. In such cases, possible causes include receptor dysfunction or a neurologic indication.

SPOON-FEEDING

Infants and children with syndromic craniosynostosis can present with feeding difficulties at this stage. The infant or child may have difficulty using their upper lip to remove the food from the spoon. Parents may consequently resort to tilting the spoon upwards and scraping the food off the spoon onto the child's upper teeth or gums before removing the spoon from the child's mouth. The child may also have difficulty accepting lumps and may remain on a smooth puree consistency for an extended period of time. There may also be difficulties with managing mixed textures (e.g. gravy mixed with peas) which may put the child at risk of aspiration. With such foods, the child has to be able to swallow the softer consistency (the gravy), while retaining the harder food (the peas) within the oral cavity for further oral manipulation.

A fairly common parental report is that food tends to get stuck on the child's hard palate, especially in cases where there is a deep median groove. The older child may be seen removing the stuck food with their own fingers or may get parents to do so. With a younger child, who may not be able to do this independently and who is not yet cognitively able to inform parents, the food may remain on the hard palate between the palatine shelves for a period of time. In such cases, there may be a risk of choking if the food then falls posteriorly in the oral cavity.

BITING AND CHEWING

Clinically, parents of children with syndromic craniosynostosis often report that they have to chop up firmer foods into smaller pieces or that mealtimes can be stretched as the child takes a long time to 'chew' his/her food properly. Alternatively, the child who is unable to break the piece of food down into smaller and more manageable pieces for swallowing may attempt to swallow the pieces whole. Clinical indicators of this include an 'effortful' swallow attempt manifested by facial grimacing or the use of concomitant head movements to aid in the swallow. Some children may eventually spit the food out.

Most children with syndromic craniosynostosis also tend to chew with their mouths open or have intermittent lip closure while chewing. Children with syndromic craniosynostosis often rely on mouth breathing because of their narrow nasal airways or, in some cases, atresia. As such, it is difficult for them to maintain complete and consistent lip closure when chewing, especially with firmer foods that require a longer chewing time. Clinical manifestations of this include leakage of food and dribbling of saliva.

Children with syndromic craniosynostosis generally present with good or functional vertical jaw movements but appear to have either very limited or no rotary jaw movements, which results in poor chewing. Interestingly, teenagers who have undergone their final major midfacial advancement surgery, of which improved dental-occlusal relationships are one result, often report improved chewing abilities.

There is currently no literature that reports on biting and/or chewing in syndromic craniosynostosis. There is however research that has looked at chewing in adults with a class III malocclusion. Deguchi et al (1995) compared the chewing abilities of 20 adults with a class III malocclusion and 20 adults with a normal jaw alignment, using a method called DL-EMG or differential lissajous electromyography, which 'describes the co-ordinated electromyographic activity of the bilateral masseter and temporal muscles during chewing' (Deguchi et al 1995: 151). They reported that the electromyographic activity of the masseter and temporal muscles was not only less, but that there was also a lower percentage of clockwise rotation and irregular co-ordination of the activity in the four muscles in the adults with the class III malocclusion. Zhou and Fu (1995) reported that the masticatory efficiency in adults with a class III malocclusion was only 60 per cent of that for adults with normal jaw alignment. Similarly, Eckardt et al (1997) attributed weak muscle activity to this group of adults.

It is however important to stress that the results of these studies should be interpreted with caution, for two main reasons. First, the studies are based on the adult population and, apart from having a class III malocclusion, no other medical diagnoses are reported. Second, at present, we do not yet know the exact nature of the motor unit physiology and character in syndromic craniosynostosis and such electromyographic studies on 'normal' or non-syndromic adults may not be relevant. However, such studies are a starting point in helping us to understand the nature of chewing difficulties in individuals with syndromic craniosynostosis.

MIDFACIAL ADVANCEMENT AND SWALLOWING

Midfacial advancement in syndromic craniosynostosis is undertaken for various reasons. Functional reasons include raised intracranial pressure, ocular proptosis and airway obstruction. Psychosocial reasons are also often indicated both in children and in teenagers. Midfacial advancement is conventionally treated by midfacial osteotomies. One of the main limitations of conventional osteotomies however is that the degree of advancement is limited. Additionally, the use of bone grafts is required. Distraction osteogenesis of the midfacial skeleton which involves the use of internal or external distractors not only allows a bigger forward advancement but does not involve the use of bone grafts (Dunaway 2002).

There is currently no literature that has commented on the direct relationship between midfacial advancement and any phase of the swallowing process in syndromic craniosynostosis.

Clinically, however, we have had cases who have presented with significant swallow difficulties post distraction osteogenesis, resulting in the need for alternative methods of feeding, at least in the short term. Interestingly, these tend to be cases with long-term and continuing swallow difficulties, but with no objective evidence of laryngeal penetration or aspiration prior to distraction. Videofluoroscopy swallow evaluations provide objective evidence of laryngeal penetration or aspiration post distraction osteogenesis (see Fig. 16.3). The case is described in Case study 4.

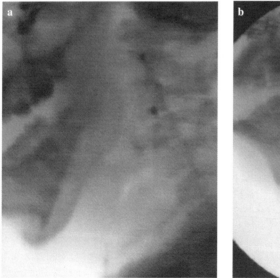 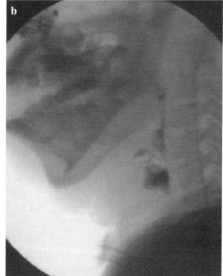

Fig. 16.3 Videofluoroscopy swallow evaluations in lateral view of a teenager with Crouzon syndrome. (a) View prior to distraction. No laryngeal penetration or aspiration evident. Note there is very slight pharyngeal residue post-swallow. (b) View post-distraction. Note the laryngeal penetration and significant pharyngeal residue especially in the pyriform.

With midfacial advancements, the forward movement is accompanied by a differential downward displacement of the palate in relation to the posterior pharyngeal wall. As the hard palate moves further away from the pharyngeal wall, 'the need for a modified, if not greater, effort' of the velum occurs (Scheuerle and Habal 2001: 69). In swallowing, the soft palate to posterior pharyngeal wall contact forms a seal between the nasopharynx and the oropharynx. A strong seal not only helps prevent nasopharyngeal reflux, but also helps 'maintain the propulsive forces necessary to transport the bolus through the hypopharynx, upper oesophageal sphincter and into the oesophagus' (Tuchman 1994: 11). It is therefore important to consider the effects of the large advancements possible with distraction osteogenesis on the swallowing status of a child or teenager, especially in cases where there are known swallowing difficulties at the presurgery stage.

The nature of feeding difficulties seen in syndromic craniosynostosis is summarised in Table 16.4. The behavioural and psychosocial consequences of some of these feeding difficulties cannot be overemphasised. Behavioural feeding problems may arise not only from gastroesophageal reflux or long-term tube-feeding but also from early or initial 'skill deficits' such as 'an inability to chew, swallow or consume an age-appropriate texture' (Babbitt et al 1994: 77). These problems can then become motivationally based, as the child whose *skills* increase or improve over time continues to choose the easier to manage or softer food texture. If not treated early, this can continue on into adolescence and can result in acute malnutrition, rendering supplementary or alternative tube-feedings essential.

TABLE 16.4
The nature of feeding difficulties seen in syndromic craniosynostosis

Bottle-feeding	poor lip seal around teat poor/ineffective suck poor ability to co-ordinate suck–swallow–breathe patterns inability to maintain sucking bursts fatigue effects resulting in inadequate nutritional intake
Spoon-feeding	poor upper lip movement to remove food from spoon difficulty accepting lumps delayed transition to more difficult textures difficulty managing mixed textures potential for food to get stuck on hard palate within median groove
Biting/chewing	firmer foods have to be chopped up into smaller pieces, e.g. pizza limited or poor rotary jaw movements potential for swallowing pieces of firmer foods whole, putting child at risk of choking. This may sometimes be manifested as an 'effortful swallow' or 'gulpy' swallow sounds can be heard may chew with only intermittent lip closure due to a dependency on mouth breathing, which may result in leakage of food bolus and/or dribbling preference for softer foods even as older children or teenagers social consequences
Midfacial advancement using distraction osteogenesis	swallowing difficulties may be exacerbated with bigger midfacial advancements alternative methods of feeding may be required in the short term

TABLE 16.5
Professions that are essential to the feeding assessment process: the GOSH CFU experience

Craniofacial team members	Other professions
Speech and language therapy	Dietetics/nutrition
Otolaryngology/ENT	Gastroenterology
Nurse specialists (craniofacial, respiratory)	Cardiology
Craniofacial surgeon	Neurology
Orthodontics	Radiology
Neurosurgery	Physiotherapy
Nursing	Occupational therapy
Ophthalmology	Feeding team (Department of psychological medicine)

Feeding difficulties can very often also have social consequences. The older child who is unable to manage firmer foods and is on a soft food diet may withdraw from group mealtimes at school or other social situations as they feel embarrassed. Younger children may not understand why they cannot have what their friends are having and may have to be supervised both at home and at school. Mealtimes at home may be prolonged and stressful for both the child and the parent. In certain cases, families may refrain from eating out in public and may restrict mealtimes to within the home environment.

Assessment of feeding in syndromic craniosynostosis
Due to the complex array of problems present in syndromic craniosynostosis, assessment of feeding in this population should not only be multifactorial in approach but multi-disciplinary in nature. The knowledge base that each profession brings to the team is essential not only in the accurate and holistic assessment of the nature of the child's feeding difficulties but also in the effectiveness of the management of these difficulties. Table 16.5 lists the professions that should be involved in the assessment and management of feeding difficulties in craniosynostosis. Some of these professions are already core members of the existing craniofacial unit at Great Ormond Street Hospital for Children.

THE FEEDING ASSESSMENT
Assessment of feeding in syndromic craniosynostosis involves taking a full medical, developmental and feeding history (Table 16.6), evaluating the child's readiness to feed orally, observing the child feeding (bottle-feeding/spoon-feeding/biting and chewing, wherever appropriate) and performing special investigations, e.g. videofluoroscopy swallow investigations, pH probe studies, as required.

As infants and children with syndromic craniosynostosis present with such a complex array of problems that may have an adverse impact on feeding, it is important that all aspects of predisposing factors that can have an adverse impact on feeding and swallowing are known or investigated. Additional information can be gathered from the child's medical/case notes and from further investigations by various relevant members of the feeding team. The information gained will also determine the rest of the assessment process and the need for additional or special investigations.

TABLE 16.6
Past and current medical, developmental and feeding and nutrition information
needed when assessing feeding in a child with syndromic craniosynostosis

Medical	Syndrome
	Other medical diagnoses, e.g. laryngeal cleft
	Sensory impairments, e.g. vision
	Significant events, e.g. hypoxic event at birth, seizures
	Medications
	Cardiopulmonary, respiratory status including any trouble breathing during feeds/increased noisy breathing
	Malformations of the central nervous system
	Gastrointestinal problems
	Airway status, e.g. mouth breathing, sleep apnoea
	Active airway intervention, e.g. nasopharyngeal prong, tracheostomy
	Medical tests, e.g. pH probe studies looking at reflux
	Surgical interventions, e.g. major cardiac surgery, major midface advancement
Development	Overall cognitive levels
	Acquisition of gross and fine motor milestones
	Acquisition of speech and language milestones
Feeding and nutrition	Tube-feeding: if yes, when? How long? Why? Type? Schedule? How much? Position?
	Any oral-facial defensiveness?
	Utensils, e.g. bottle, cup, spoon
	Types of food/liquid: food textures
	Diet per day
	Food allergies/intolerance
	Duration of meals and intervals
	Feeding position
	Main feeder(s)/self-feeding
	Preferred foods
	'Difficult' foods: reaction/response to such foods
	Signs of distress during feeding, e.g. turning head away, crying
	Coughing/choking during or after feeds
	Gurgly voice quality during/after feeds
	Vomiting or rumination
	Oro-motor feeding skills

When evaluating the child's readiness to feed, it is important to ascertain the child's body posture and positioning needs and to note if special equipment is required, e.g. seating, supplementary oxygen. Note also the general state of alertness of the infant, breathing patterns and the child's responses to touch to the face and mouth. Aversive reactions to this may be indicative of underlying gastrointestinal problems like reflux. A pre-feeding assessment of the infant's or child's oral-motor structure and function is essential. This normally includes an assessment of the lips, tongue and palate. With infant feeding, an assessment of reflexes such as the rooting reflex and a non-nutritive feeding assessment using the adult's gloved fifth finger or a dummy/pacifier are also essential. It is important that the infant or child receives a nutritional assessment which includes measuring the child's weight and length. Observe also the quality and nature of the interaction between the infant or child and the parent. Oral-motor and feeding assessment in infants and children is described in great detail by Wolf and Glass (1992), Arvedson and Brodsky (1993) and Morris and Klein (2000).

SOME USEFUL ASSESSMENT TOOLS TO ASSESS FEEDING IN SYNDROMIC
CRANIOSYNOSTOSIS

When assessing the child's feeding, feeding assessment tools, including both the use of standardised feeding assessments such as the Schedule for Oral-Motor Assessment (SOMA) (Reilly et al 1995) and the Neonatal Oral-Motor Assessment Scale (NOMAS) (Braun and Palmer 1985/6) as well as more diagnostic tests and procedures such as cervical auscultation, pulse oximetry and videofluoroscopic swallow studies, can be used. These are described briefly below.

Neonatal Oral-Motor Assessment Scale (NOMAS) (Braun and Palmer 1985/6)
The NOMAS assesses infant bottle-feeding and gives a diagnosis of 'normal', 'disorganised' or 'dysfunctional' feeder, where *disorganised* refers to 'a lack of rhythm of total sucking activity' or a lack of rhythm of the suck–swallow–breathe pattern, and *dysfunction* refers to 'the interruption of the feeding process by abnormal movements of the tongue and jaw' (Palmer et al 1993: 29). It also assesses non-nutritive sucking in infants. Reliability studies have been undertaken with the NOMAS (Palmer et al 1993). The NOMAS can also aid in the planning of appropriate treatment strategies and can be used as a pre- and post-test measure of progress. No special or additional equipment is required.

Schedule for Oral-Motor Assessment (SOMA) (Reilly et al 1995)
The SOMA was developed to rate and 'record oral-motor skills objectively in infants between the ages of 8 and 24 months', and aims to 'identify areas of dysfunction that could contribute to feeding difficulties' (Reilly et al 1995: 177). In the published version, the oral-motor challenge categories assessed include *liquids* presented via a bottle or trainer cup, *puree* (e.g. fromage frais), *semi-solids* (e.g. baked beans) and *solids* (e.g. fruit cocktail) all via spoon-feeding, and *cracker* (e.g. digestive biscuits) via finger-feeding. Each of these oral-motor challenge categories is described on three levels: *functional areas*, which refers to the muscle group or structure being investigated, e.g. head and trunk control, lip function, tongue function and jaw function; *functional units*, which includes refusals (unwillingness to accept food) and reactivity (reactions to food presented); and *discrete oral-motor behaviours*, which refers to the individual oral-motor movements (Reilly et al 1995). For each oral-motor challenge category, a score is given and this determines if the child has an oral-motor dysfunction for that particular food type. Specific equipment and food types have to be used as described in the administration manual. Video recording of the assessment for later scoring is highly recommended.

Non-standardised feeding assessments are also available and can be used as part of the clinical evaluation process. These include the 'Clinical Feeding Evaluation of Infants' by Wolf and Glass (1992), the 'Developmental Pre-Feeding Checklist' by Morris and Klein (1987/2000) and the 'Oral-Motor and Feeding Evaluation Checklist' by Arvedson and Brodsky (1993).

Cervical auscultation

A stethoscope or a microphone is used to 'detect changes in the upper aero digestive tract sounds that occur during breathing, swallowing and bolus passage' (Arvedson and Lefton-Greif 1998: 6). It allows the trained user to detect acoustic changes in swallow sounds associated with the occurrence and the timing of penetration or aspiration of the liquid or food bolus (Wolf and Glass 1992). Although debate continues over the best type of acoustic detector unit to use for detecting swallow sounds, there is agreement over the optimal placement sites (Takahashi and Groher 1994, Cichero and Murdoch 2002).

Pulse oximetry

Pulse oximetry can be used to measure changes in pulse rate and oxygen saturation levels prior to the start of the bottle-feed, during and after feeding. Infants generally have an oxygen saturation level of 95 per cent and above, and if this dips down to below 90 per cent, hypoxia may be indicated (Wolf and Glass 1992). The use of pulse oximetry can also inform with regard to the need and effectiveness of oxygen therapy in helping with bottle-feeding.

Videofluoroscopy swallow study

The videofluoroscopy swallow study not only defines anatomy and physiology of the swallowing mechanism during feeding, but also identifies bolus and positioning variables and feeding strategies that enhance the safety of swallowing (Arvedson and Lefton-Greif 1998, Logemann 1998). It also defines the 'reason' for the swallowing dysfunction and detects laryngeal penetration and/or aspiration (Arvedson and Lefton-Greif 1998: 5). Clinical indicators of swallowing dysfunction and aspiration may arise from the information gathered during the clinical evaluation of the infant's or child's feeding, such as a history of frequent upper respiratory infections or pneumonias, frequent low-grade fevers, coughing and choking during feeding, a gurgly voice quality after individual swallows, or increased noisy breathing over the course of feeding.

Management strategies

The main aims of any feeding management programme should include maintenance of adequate nutrition and hydration intake, maximising the swallow safety of the child and ensuring that feeding time is a positive experience for both the parent and the child. The management plan should be based on the results of a comprehensive multidisciplinary assessment and will depend greatly on many factors, including the oral-facial anatomy, the severity of the airway difficulty and the type of airway intervention, the presence of other co-occurring factors such as cardiac and gastrointestinal anomalies, neurologic impairment, as well as any impending craniofacial or other surgical intervention. The decisions made around the feeding management plan should also consider not only parental concerns but whether parents understand and accept the feeding management plan, as they will usually be the persons who will have to carry out the recommendations made.

The wide-ranging nature of feeding difficulties in syndromic craniosynostosis lends itself to a whole host of management strategies. The next section describes general management strategies that can be used to help the infant or child with feeding difficulties and is followed by case studies to illustrate how some of these strategies have been used in managing feeding difficulties in syndromic craniosynostosis.

POSITIONING AND POSTURE CHANGES

- Positioning the infant or child such that there is a 'base of central stability with good body alignment' with good head and neck control or external support (Arvedson 1998: 456). Some children benefit from being fed in a tumbleform chair. Infants with an unrepaired cleft of the palate benefit from being in an upright position to prevent nasopharyngeal reflux. If positioning or posture is a significant concern, the child needs to be assessed by an occupational therapist or a physiotherapist.

CHANGING/ALTERING THE ROUTE OF NUTRITION AND HYDRATION

- Using a non-oral tube-feeding method (naso/oro-gastric/gastrostomy) where the infant's swallow is assessed to be unsafe for oral feeding or the infant is refusing to feed orally.
- Using supplementary tube-feeding when the infant starts to show aspiration with fatigue while bottle-feeding or when nutritional intake via oral means is inadequate.

NUTRITIONAL GUIDELINES

- Increasing the caloric density of the milk formula by prescribing nutritional supple-ments, e.g. Infatrini and Duocal, where the infant is losing calories with increased respiratory effort and fatigue or where there is failure to thrive. These are usually prescribed by the child's paediatrician or paediatric dietician.

ALTERATIONS IN BOLUS SIZE AND CONSISTENCY

- Using a slower flow teat to reduce the bolus size to improve swallow safety.
- Thickening the milk formula to 'create' a more cohesive bolus to provide the infant/child with more sensory information. Milk formula can be thickened by using a prescribed thickening agent.
- Thickening the base consistency of puree to 'hide' tiny soft lumps which are of similar texture to this base consistency. This is a good way to gradually introduce the child to lumps. Lumps which are of distinct texture from the base consistency (e.g. hard peas in runny gravy) can be difficult for a child to manage as he/she has to deal with two very distinct textures.
- Eradicating firmer foods from the oral diet of a child who presents with oral-motor deficits and is assessed to be unable to manage such foods safely.

- **Bottles**: There is a wide variety of bottles available and what may suit some infants may not be suitable for others.

  Soft plastic squeezy bottles with teats: e.g. Mead-Johnson cleft palate nurser (Evansville, IN), Softplas bottle with teat (see Fig. 16.4(a)).

  Medela Haberman feeder: there is a one-way valve in the mouthpiece which allows easy flow of the liquid forward. The slit-valve opening also closes in between sucks thereby preventing too fast a flow. Parents can also control the flow rate of the milk or other liquid by using one of three flow rates that are indicated by line markings on the nipple itself (see Fig. 16.4(b)).

  These bottles were developed to help the infant with a cleft of the palate. However, some of our parents have found them useful for use with their infant with syndromic craniosynostosis.

- **Teats**: As with bottles, there is a wide variety of teats available. Parents have found the wide orthodontic teat shape to be useful in helping their infant with retruded maxilla achieve better lip closure around the teat and thus preventing liquid loss. Teats also come with varying flow rates, i.e. slow, medium and fast. It is important that the appropriate flow rate is used. A faster flow rate gives the infant less time to co-ordinate the suck–swallow–breathe pattern.

- **Spoons**: Using a flatter-bowled spoon can help prevent food getting stuck on the child's hard palate or within the median groove. An angled spoon can help the child with hand/elbow anomalies self-feed better.

CHANGES IN FEEDING SCHEDULE AND EXTERNAL PACING

- Limiting the length of the feeding session to just 10 to 15 minutes, for example. This works well for the infant who shows decreased endurance after that time period.

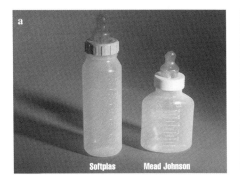
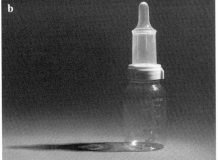

Fig. 16.4 Soft plastic squeezy bottles with teats. (a) Mead-Johnson cleft palate nurser (Evansville, IN) and the Softplas bottle with teat. (b) Medela Haberman feeder. Note the line markings on the nipple, indicating three different flow rates.

Pushing the infant to feed further may result in loss of calories with increased effort.

- Reducing the time interval between feeds, which results in the infant having to take a smaller volume at each feed.
- Using external pacing. Here, the aim is to help the infant by removing the teat from the infant's mouth after a fixed number of sucks, e.g. two to three sucks, and allowing the infant to 'catch his breath'.

PROVIDING SUPPLEMENTAL OXYGEN

- Providing additional respiratory support by using supplemental oxygen during feeding if the need has been determined with pulse oximetry.

ORAL-MOTOR TREATMENT

- Placing food in between upper and lower molars on each side alternately to encourage biting. It is important to use food textures that are assessed to be safe for the child. Close supervision is maintained to ensure that the child is not at risk of choking.
- Specific exercises to improve and encourage tongue lateralisation for chewing.

CARDIOPULMONARY RESUSCITATION (CPR) TRAINING

- Formal CPR training for parents/carer or other professionals involved in the feeding management of a child, especially in cases where there is a known history risk of choking with solids.

Follow-up and monitoring of the child's feeding abilities by the speech and language therapist trained in feeding is important, as these may change with time. It is important that once the child is out of hospital and is home with the parent/carer, other professionals such as the community nurse and the health visitor are aware of the feeding needs of the child. This also includes the child's schoolteachers, special needs teachers/co-ordinators, learning support assistants or helpers, when the child starts to attend school with continuing feeding difficulties and needs. Such two-way liaison is necessary and should be on a regular basis.

Case study 1

Jake is a little boy with Apert syndrome and was referred at the age of 2 months. He had mild to moderate upper airway obstruction and was having significant difficulties feeding. To manage his airway obstruction, Jake had a tracheostomy placed when a nasopharyngeal prong was assessed to be inadequate to resolve his airway difficulties.

Following this, a videofluoroscopy swallow study was carried out to determine swallow safety and to aid in a feeding management plan. The results showed persistent trace aspiration and silent aspiration with thin liquids as the feed progressed, indicative of fatigue aspiration. No aspiration was seen with thickened liquids. Nasopharyngeal reflux was also evident, which could be attributable to notching of the soft palate. Jake was seen by a dietician and was assessed as having poor nutritional status and was prescribed a high-calorie milk formula. The dietician also prescribed a thickening agent as he was found to be 'safe' with small amounts of thickened milk. With this feeding profile, Jake went on to have a maximum of 10 mls of thickened milk formula via a bottle with external pacing and received the remainder of his nutritional requirements via a nasogastric tube. To prevent nasopharyngeal reflux, he was also fed in a more upright feeding position. Jake was consequently discharged to his local hospital which continued to review and manage his feeding. During this time, Jake was gradually taking more milk orally and was also putting on weight. A few months later, a repeat videofluoroscopy swallow study, to reassess his swallow function and safety with liquids and puree, showed that he was now safe to manage even thin liquids and could move on to smooth puree.

Comment
This is an important example highlighting that even when airway difficulties are managed, in this case with a tracheostomy, feeding may not necessarily improve. The presence of a tracheostomy may in itself have its own adverse impact on swallowing and therefore any assumptions of swallow safety following active airway intervention should not be made without objective assessment. This case also shows the importance and necessity of continued and close monitoring, as the infant's swallowing status can change and thus feeding management must likewise be altered. Specific feeding management strategies used in this case include:

- Positioning
- Changing and altering the route of nutrition
- Changing nutritional guidelines
- Alterations in bolus consistency
- External pacing

Case study 2

Lisa has Crouzon syndrome with a history of and current obstructive sleep apnoea. She was referred for a feeding assessment at the age of 3 as there were parental concerns of poor chewing as well as choking episodes requiring parental intervention in the form of informal CPR. There were also parental concerns about how to manage feeding at nursery. From clinical evaluation of her oral-motor skills during eating, Lisa managed solid textures such as puree, mash and easy to bite and dissolvable solids, e.g. Wotsits/Skips, but was unable to manage firmer and more chewy textures, e.g. pizza. Lisa was unable to break these firmer foods down and was swallowing such foods whole, thereby putting herself at risk of aspiration and choking. Additionally, Lisa was unable to manage mixed textures, e.g. peas and gravy. Because of this, firmer foods and more chewy textures were removed from Lisa's daily intake oral diet. Lisa was also not given mixed textures. If she wanted peas and gravy, the peas were mashed down and given with a thicker consistency of gravy. Lisa was also seen by a dietician who provided her parents with a list of different types of puree and mash foods, as well as a list of foods that could be added to these to increase her calorie intake. Additionally, her parents were given formal CPR training on the ward in the event of possible future choking episodes. At nursery, she was closely supervised at all mealtimes by a member of staff who was CPR trained. Her meals were also brought from home. No further reports of choking have since been reported.

Comment

This case highlights the significant risks and consequences that can arise from chewing difficulties and the importance of a detailed oro-motor feeding assessment. There are varying levels of difficulty in managing different types of solids and it is important that an assessment of which types of solids a child can and cannot manage safely is undertaken. This case also shows the importance of liaison with the child's school when mealtimes are part of the child's daily routine there. In such cases, it is necessary to ensure that all persons involved in monitoring and supervising the child at mealtimes, including parents, are trained in CPR. Specific feeding management strategies used in this case include:

- Nutritional guidelines
- Alterations in bolus consistency/texture
- CPR training

Case study 3

Neil has Pfeiffer syndrome and was first seen at the age of 15. He had a tracheostomy placed when he was younger but had since been decannulated. Neil was not referred specifically for a feeding assessment but parental concerns about his feeding, nutritional status and growth were raised during the speech and language therapy assessment. It was reported that Neil had episodes of vomiting when young as well as a history of and continuing chest infections. His parents also reported that he had feeding difficulties as a baby.

Neil's current intake of food was not only limited in terms of the amount/volume taken but was also significantly restricted and specific in terms of range. A typical day's diet was orange juice for breakfast, a packet of crisps for lunch, chips for tea and either crisps or Milky Way chocolate bars for dinner. Neil reported that he was having about 50 Milky Way bars and 60 litres of orange juice a week. Additionally, Neil felt that his feeding difficulties were affecting his social life in that he felt embarrassed to eat in public. His parents also reported inconsistent choking with different food textures, e.g. crisps or ice-cream. From videofluoroscopy swallow evaluation, there was no evidence of laryngeal penetration or aspiration with different food textures, although his swallow function presented as 'abnormal'.

An assessment by a dietician showed his dietary intake to be grossly inadequate and, although nutritional supplements were offered, Neil had little appetite and refused to co-operate with this. It was also recommended that Neil be seen within a behaviour feeding clinic to help him extend his range of tastes and, again, Neil was not receptive to this approach. Additionally, as it was further assessed that food supplements were not going to be adequate and thus a useful means to correct his malnutrition, supplementary tube-feeding in the form of a gastrostomy with overnight feeds was recommended and implemented.

Neil is reported to be very happy with how this is going, not only because he is now putting on weight and growing in terms of height, but also because the focus and the pressure of taking more foods orally, which he still finds difficult, have decreased. He continues not to be keen on the idea of a behavioural feeding clinic to help him extend his range of tastes and foods, and has chosen to decide on this after his upcoming major midfacial advancement surgery. Neil continues to be monitored by his local team including his speech and language therapist and dietician.

Comment

This case highlights how early feeding difficulties, if not managed effectively, can persist and develop into very significant problems even into adolescence, resulting in malnourishment, poor growth and behavioural feeding difficulties. As a consequence, the need for long-term supplementary tube-feeding to improve nourishment and growth was clearly indicated. The psychosocial consequences of Neil's feeding difficulties are also apparent. As with any medical intervention with older children and teenagers, it is vital to engage individuals in their treatment. The role of the dietician is clearly shown. Specific feeding management strategies include:

- Changing the route of nutrition
- Nutritional guidelines

Case study 4

Jane is 15 years of age and has Crouzon syndrome. She had cyanotic episodes at birth and severe respiratory problems in the neonatal period resulting in a tracheostomy at 4 months of age. She was also diagnosed with a laryngeal cleft, which was repaired at 18 months, and has since had repeated failed trials of decannulation. Jane has a history of long-term nasogastric tube-feeding as well as aspiration on thin liquids. She also developed aversive feeding behaviours as a child and was then seen in the feeding programme under the Department of Psychological Medicine.

At 14 years of age, Jane underwent distraction osteogenesis, for airway as well as aesthetic/cosmetic reasons. Preoperatively, videofluoroscopic evaluation of her swallow function showed no laryngeal penetration or aspiration with liquids or solids, puree or mash. Her swallow function was assessed to be only at a functional level and was characterised by reduced airway closure with liquids and poor movement of the bolus through her pharynx with the solids. Postoperatively, food-stained secretions were noted on suctioning from her tracheostomy site and the immediate postoperative videofluoroscopy swallow study revealed laryngeal penetration with liquids and puree. Jane then went on to receive all her nutritional requirements via supplementary nasogastric tube-feeding.

A repeat videofluoroscopy swallow study two months post-surgery showed laryngeal penetration only with thin liquids. Jane started having purees and mash orally, as well as thickened liquids, e.g. milkshakes or liquids with a prescribed thickening agent.

Comment

This case serves to highlight the importance of monitoring cases with a borderline swallowing status prior to midfacial advancement for potential swallowing difficulties following surgery. In such cases, where there is a known history of feeding difficulties and/or a borderline swallowing status presurgery, postsurgery swallow assessment, in the form of a clinical bedside evaluation as well as a more objective swallow assessment using videofluoroscopy swallow evaluation, should be undertaken to inform management. As this case illustrates, regular monitoring for adapted function over time is emphasised. Specific feeding management strategies include:

- Changing the route of nutrition
- Alterations in bolus consistency

334

Summary and conclusions

Infants, children and teenagers with syndromic craniosynostosis present with a wide range of feeding difficulties that can arise at any one or all of the main stages of feeding development. The complex nature of the syndromes sets the foundation for feeding difficulties in this population. Assessment and management of these feeding difficulties has to be both holistic and interdisciplinary in nature, involving not only the core members of the craniofacial team but also other relevant professions, as well as parents and the child or teenager. Regular monitoring of the child's feeding difficulties is important as these may change over time. With discharge from the acute setting, close liaison with relevant professionals involved in the care of the child locally is vital. Objective and systematic research in this field is clearly indicated and warranted.

REFERENCES

Alper B, Manno CJ (1996) Dysphagia in infants and children with oral-motor deficits: assessment and management. *Semin Speech Lang* 17(4): 283–310.

Arvedson J (1992) Infant oral-motor function and feeding. In: Brodsky L, Holt L, Ritter-Schmidt P, editors. *Craniofacial Anomalies: An Interdisciplinary Approach*. St Louis: Mosby.

Arvedson J (1998) Management of pediatric dysphagia. *Otolaryngol Clin North Am* 31(3): 453–476. Review.

Arvedson J, Brodsky L, editors (1993) *Paediatric Swallowing and Feeding: Assessment and Management*. San Diego, CA: Singular Publishing Group.

Arvedson J, Lefton-Greif MA (1998) *Paediatric Videofluoroscopic Swallow Studies: A Professional Manual with Caregiver Guidelines*. San Antonio, TX: Communication Skill Builders.

Arvedson J, Rogers B, Buck G, Smart P, Msall M (1994) Silent aspiration prominent in children with dysphagia. *Int J Paediatr Otorhinolaryngol* 28: 173–181.

Babbitt RL, Theodore AH, Coe DA (1994) Behavioural feeding disorders. In: Tuchman DN, Walter RS, editors. *Disorders of Feeding and Swallowing in Infants and Children. Pathophysiology, Diagnosis and Treatment*. San Diego, CA: Singular Publishing Group.

Biron Campis L (1991) Children with Apert syndrome: developmental and psychologic considerations. *Clin Plast Surg* 18(2): 409–416.

Braun MA, Palmer MM (1985/6) A pilot study of oral-motor dysfunction in at-risk infants. *Phys Occup Ther Paediatr* 5(4): 13–25.

Brodsky L (1993) Drooling in children. In: Arvedson J, Brodsky L, editors. *Paediatric Swallowing and Feeding*. San Diego, CA: Singular Publishing Group, pp 395–398.

Brodsky L (1997) Dysphagia with respiratory/pulmonary presentation: assessment and management. *Sem Speech Lang* 18(1).

Cichero JA, Murdoch BM (2002) Detection of swallowing sounds: methodology revisited. *Dysphagia* 17: 40–49.

Cohen MM Jr (1986) Perspectives on craniosynostosis. In: Cohen MM Jr. *Craniosynostosis: Diagnosis, Evaluation and Management*. New York: Raven Press.

Cohen MM Jr (1990) Selected clinical research involving the central nervous system. *J Craniofac Genet Dev Biol* 10: 215–238.

Cohen MM Jr, Kreiborg S (1990) The central nervous system in the Apert syndrome. *Am J Med Genet* 35: 36–45.

Cohen MM Jr, Kreiborg S (1993a) Growth pattern in the Apert syndrome. *Am J Med Genet* 47: 617–623.

Cohen MM Jr, Kreiborg S (1993b) An updated pediatric perspective on the Apert syndrome. *Am J Dis Child* 147: 989–993

Cohen MM Jr, Kreiborg S (1993c) Visceral anomalies in the Apert syndrome. *Am J Med Genet* 45: 758–760.

Cohen MM Jr, Kreiborg S (1994) Cranial size and configuration in the Apert syndrome. *J Craniofac Genet Dev Biol* 14: 153–162.

Cohen MM Jr, Kreiborg S (1996) A clinical study of the craniofacial features in Apert syndrome. *Oral Maxillofac Surg* 25: 45–53.

Cohen MM Jr, MacLean RE, editors (2000) *Craniosynostosis: Diagnosis, Evaluation and Management*. 2nd edn. New York and Oxford: Oxford University Press.

Cohen MM Jr, Russell J, Kreiborg S (1992) Upper and lower airway compromise in the Apert syndrome. *Am J Med Genet* 44(1): 90–93.

Deguchi T, Garetto LP, Sato Y, Potter RH, Roberts WE (1995) Statistical analysis of differential lissajous EMG form normal occlusion and class III malocclusion. *Angle Orthod* 65(2): 151–160.

Dikeman K, Kazandjian M (1995) *Communication and Swallowing: Management of Tracheostomized and Ventilator-Dependent Adults*. San Diego, CA and London: Singular Publishing Group.

Dodds WJ, Logemann JA, Stewart ET (1990) Radiological assessment of abnormal oral and pharyngeal phases of swallowing. *Am J Roentgenol* 154: 965–974. (Review article.)

Dunaway D (2002) Mid-facial distraction osteogenesis. *ENT News* 11(1).

Eckardt L, Harzer W, Schneevoigt R (1997) Comparative study of excitation patterns in the masseter muscle before and after orthognathic surgery. *J Craniomaxillofac Surg* 25: 344–352.

Elia M, Musumeci SA, Ferri R, Del Gracco S, Stefanini MC (1996) Saethre–Chotzen syndrome: a clinical, EEG and neuroradiological study. *Childs Nerv Syst* 12(11): 699–704.

Ellis E III, Throckmorton G, Sinn DP (1996) Functional characteristics of patients with anterior open bite before and after surgical correction. *Int J Adult Orthod Orthognathic Surg* 11(3): 211–223.

Fehlow P (1993) Craniosynotosis as a risk factor. *Childs Nerv Syst* 9: 325–327.

Ferraro NF (1991) Dental, orthodontic, and oral/maxillofacial evaluation and treatment in Apert syndrome. *Clin Plast Surg* 18(2): 291–307.

Fucile S, Wright PM, Chan I, Yee S, Langlais M, Gisel EG (1998) Functional oral-motor skills: do they change with age? *Dysphagia* 13: 195–201.

Gisel EG (1988) Chewing cycles in 2- to 8-year-old normal children: a developmental profile. *Am J Occup Ther* 42(1): 40–46.

Gisel E, Patrick J (1988) Identification of children unable to maintain a normal nutritional state. *Lancet* I: 283–286.

Gisel EG, Birnbaum R, Schwarta S (1998) Feeding impairments in children: diagnosis and effective intervention. *Int J Orofac Myol* 24: 27–33. (Review.)

Howlett C, Stavropoulos MF, Steinberg B (1999) Feeding complications in a six-week-old infant secondary to distraction osteogenesis for airway obstruction: a case report. *J Oral Maxillofac Surg* 57: 1465–1468.

Hyman PE (1994) Gastroesophageal reflux: one reason why baby won't eat. *J Pediatr* 125(6 pt 2): S103–109. (Review.)

Jarund M, Lauritzen C (1996) Craniofacial dysostosis: airway obstruction and craniofacial surgery. *Scand J Plast Reconstr Surg Hand Surg* 30(4): 275–279.

Kaloust S, Ishii K, Vargervik K (1997) Dental development in Apert syndrome. *Cleft Palate Craniofac J* 34(2): 117–121.

Kaplan LC (1991) Clinical assessment and multispeciality management of Apert syndrome. *Clin Plast Surg* 18(2): 217–225.

Klein MD, Delaney TA (1994) *Feeding and Nutrition for the Child with Special Needs: Handouts for Parents*. Tucson, AZ: Therapy Skill Builders.

Kreiborg S, Cohen MM Jr (1992) The oral manifestations of Apert syndrome. *J Craniofac Genet Dev Biol* 12: 41–48.

Kreiborg S, Aduss H, Cohen J, Russell MM (1999) Cephalometric study of the Apert syndrome in adolescence and adulthood. *J Craniofac Genet Dev Biol* 19(1): 1–11.

Lauritzen DC, Lilja J, Jarlstedt J (1986) Airway obstruction and sleep apnoea in children with craniofacial anomalies. *Plast Reconstr Surg* 77: 1–5.

Lee S, Seto M, Sie K, Cunningham M (2002) A child with Saethre-Chotzen syndrome, sensorineural hearing loss, and a TWIST mutation. *Cleft Palate Craniofac J* 39(1): 110–114.

Lo LJ, Chen YR (1999) Airway obstruction in severe syndromic craniosynostosis. *Ann Plast Surg* 43(3): 258–264.

Logemann J (1998) *Evaluation and Treatment of Swallowing Disorders*, 2nd edn. Austin, TX: Pro-Ed.

McGill T (1991) Otolaryngological aspects of Apert syndrome. *Clin Plast Surg* 18: 309–313.

Marsh JL, Galic M, Vannier MW (1991a) The craniofacial anatomy of Apert syndrome. *Clin Plast Surg* 18(2): 237–249.

Marsh JL, Galic M, Vannier MW (1991b) Surgical correction of the craniofacial dysmorphology of Apert syndrome. *Clin Plast Surg* 18(2): 251–275.

336

Mathisen B, Skuse D, Wolke D, Reilly S (1989) Oral-motor dysfunction and failure to thrive among inner-city infants. *Dev Med Child Neurol* 31: 293–302.

Miller AJ (1999) *Neuroscientific Principles of Swallowing and Dysphagia*. San Diego, CA and London: Singular Publishing Group.

Moore MH (1993) Upper airway obstruction in the syndromal craniosynostoses. *Br J Plast Surg* 46: 355–362.

Moore MH, Cantrell SB, Trott JA, David DJ (1995) Pfeiffer syndrome: a clinical review. *Cleft Palate Craniofac J* 32(1): 62–70.

Morris SE, Klein MD (1987) *Pre-Feeding Skills. A Comprehensive Resource for Feeding Development*. Tuscon, AZ: Tuscon Therapy Skill Builders.

Palmer MM, Crawley K, Blanco IA (1993) Neonatal Oral-Motor Assessment Scale: a reliability study. *J Perinatol* 13(1): 28–35.

Pereira V, Sacher P, Ryan M, Hayward (2002–) Dysphagia and nutrition in Apert syndrome. Work in progress.

Perkins JA, Sie KCY, Milczuk H, Richardson MA (1997) Airway management in children with craniofacial anomalies. *Cleft Palate Craniofac J* 34(2): 135–140.

Peterson-Falzone SJ, Pruzansky S, Parris PJ, Laffer JL (1981) Nasopharyngeal dysmorphology in the syndromes of Apert and Crouzon. *Cleft Palate J* 18(4): 237–250.

Peterson-Falzone S, Hardin-Jones M, Karnell M (2001) *Cleft Palate Speech*. 3rd edn. London: Mosby.

Posnick JC (1996) Craniofacial dysostosis syndromes: a staged reconstructive approach. In: Turvey TA, Vig KW, Fonseca RJ, editors (1996) *Facial Clefts and Craniosynostosis: Principles and Management*. London: WB Saunders.

Reilly S, Skuse D, Mathisen B, Woke D (1995) The objective rating of oral-motor functions during feeding. *Dysphagia* 10: 177–191.

Reilly SM, Skuse DH, Wolke D, Stevenson J (1999) Oral-motor dysfunction in children who fail to thrive: organic or non-organic? *Dev Med Child Neurol* 41: 115–122.

Rynearson RD (2000) Case report: orthodontic and dentofacial orthopedic considerations in Apert's syndrome. *Angle Orthod* 70(3): 247–252.

Scheuerle J, Habal MB (2001) Functional impact of distraction osteogenesis of the midface on expressive language development. *J Craniofac Surg* 12(1): 69–73.

Sculerati N, Gottlieb MD, Zimbler MS, Chibbaro PD, McCarthy JG (1998) Airway management in children with major craniofacial anomalies. *Laryngoscope* 108(12): 1806–1812.

Sidhu SS, Deshmukh RN (1989) Oro-dental anomalies in Apert's syndrome. *Indian Pediatr* 26: 501–504.

Skuse D, Stevenson J, Reilly S, Mathisen B (1995) Schedule for Oral-Motor Assessment (SOMA): methods of validation. *Dysphagia* 10: 192–202.

Slaney SF, Oldridge M, Hurst JA, Morriss-Kay GM, Hall CM, Poole MD, Wilkie AOM (1996) Differential effects of FGFR2 mutations on syndactyly and cleft palate in Apert syndrome. *Am J Hum Genet* 58: 923–932.

Southall A, Schwartz A, editors (2000) *Feeding Problems in Children: A Practical Guide*. Oxford: Radcliffe Medical Press.

Stevenson RD, Allaire JH (1991) The development of normal feeding and swallowing. *Pediatr Clin North Am* 38(6): 1439–1453.

Stevenson RD, Allaire JH (1996) The development of eating skills in infants and young children. In: Sullivan P, Rosenbloom L, editors (1996) *Feeding the Disabled Child*. Cambridge: Cambridge University Press.

Takahashi K, Groher ME (1994) Methodology for detecting swallowing sounds. *Dysphagia* 9: 54–62.

Thompson D, Jones B, Hayward R, Harkness W (1994) Assessment and treatment of craniosynostosis. *Acta Neurochir (Wien)* 120: 123–125.

Tuchman DN (1988) Dysfunctional swallowing in the pediatric population. *Dysphagia* 2: 203–208.

Tuchman DN (1994) Physiology of the swallowing apparatus. In: Tuchman DN, Walter RS, editors (1994) *Disorders of Feeding and Swallowing in Infants and Children. Pathophysiology, Diagnosis and Treatment*. San Diego, CA: Singular Publishing Group.

Tuchman DN, Walter RS, editors (1994) *Disorders of Feeding and Swallowing in Infants and Children. Pathophysiology, Diagnosis and Treatment*. San Diego, CA: Singular Publishing Group.

Turvey TA, Vig KW, Fonseca RJ, editors (1996) *Facial Clefts and Craniosynostosis: Principles and Management*. London: WB Saunders.

Walker JW (1985) Case report: the case of craniofacial dysostosis syndrome of Apert. *Br Orthop J* 42: 72–79.

Winstock A (1994) *The Practical Management of Eating and Drinking Difficulties in Children*. Bicester: Winslow Press.

Wolf LS, Glass RP (1992) *Feeding and Swallowing Disorders in Infancy. Assessment and Management*. San Antonio, TX: Therapy Skill Builders.

Wolf LS, Glass RP (1996) The therapeutic approach to the child with feeding difficulty. In: Sullivan P, Rosenbloom L, editors. *Feeding the Disabled Child*. Cambridge: Cambridge University Press.

Zhou Y, Fu M (1995) Masticatory efficiency in skeletal class III malocclusion. *Chung Hua Kou Chiang Hsueh Tsa Chih* 30(2): 72–74.

17
THE ROLE OF THE CLINICAL NURSE SPECIALIST

Andrea White

There have been many changes over recent years in the delivery of healthcare. As a result of these health reforms, nursing is changing its boundaries. A generation of 'expert practitioners' is emerging. The Royal College of Nursing in the United Kingdom issued a document in 1988 that reflected its ethos on the clinical nurse specialist (CNS) – 'Specialist practice involves a clinical and consultative role, teaching, management, research and the application of relevant nursing research. Only if a nurse is involved in all these is he or she a specialist' (cited in Hansa 2002).

This chapter will describe the role undertaken by the CNS within the craniofacial team in terms of the CNS's relationship and partnership with the children and their families, and the local community teams, as well as the CNS's relationship with and responsibilities to the craniofacial team itself.

The chapter will describe what has been set up in the craniofacial unit at Great Ormond Street Hospital for Children NHS Trust to facilitate and improve the care and treatment these children receive, and what is being looked at in the future to promote quality care.

The clinical nurse specialist

SOME GENERAL OBSERVATIONS.
The CNS is a relatively new concept, involving a multifaceted role that now incorporates elements of clinical practice exposed by the reduction of junior doctors' hours.

In 1982, Castledine (cited in Hansa 2002) emphasised that the clinical nurse specialist should be someone who has practised and should continue to practise nursing. Indeed, it is essential that practical nursing skills are not lost, not only for the sake of the child and his or her family but also for the nurse. Combining practical and theoretical knowledge, clinical experience and expertise enables a holistic approach to be undertaken to the management of the children – and this can be described as the essence of the CNS role.

With clinical developments in areas of relative rarity (like those congenital craniofacial disorders that include craniosynostosis), a need for 'expert practitioners' has emerged. The CNS as just such an 'expert practitioner' is in a position to influence patient care by utilising advanced knowledge, leadership and expertise in a multidisciplinary environment (Bousfield 1997, cited in Cattini and Knowles 1999) in which a single profession or individual can no longer deliver a complete service (Gillam and Irvine 2000, cited in Kenny

2002). The craniofacial service thus becomes a prime example of a multidisciplinary approach to delivering continuity of care, and the CNS has the pivotal role in ensuring that this continuity is ongoing.

It is becoming increasingly recognised that patients and their families are becoming more knowledgeable about their health. They are using the internet to search for the 'best' in treatment and medical and nursing care. The demand for appropriate and effective healthcare is increasing exponentially. A most important role of the CNS must therefore be to encourage the handing over of knowledge and decision making to the patient and/or the family (Pearson 2002) – a role that should be shared with and supported by the other members of the multidisciplinary craniofacial team. This process will enable the child and/or family to use the complex information they acquire appropriately and safely.

The CNS's core competencies can be defined as shown in Table 17.1.

The core components of the CNS's role are clinical, educational, research and communicative (or consultative) (Jones 2002, cited in Hansa 2002).

CLINICAL ROLE
The clinical role involves maintaining and updating nursing skills, and being involved in all levels of healthcare for the child. This provides a standard of excellence in nursing practice to pass on to ward staff and nurses involved in the child's care both in the specialist unit and in the local community.

EDUCATION
With this responsibility comes the role of educator to fellow team members, to ward staff, to local services and most importantly to the children and their families. Providing information is essential to quality care and the knowledge that the CNS and other members of the multidisciplinary team possess must be shared. This is an integral part of the CNS's role.

TABLE 17.1
Core competencies of the CNS

Key roles	Key statements	Standard of competency	Mode of achievement
To be the acknowledged nurse expert in a specified subject within the Trust	Contributes to the effective delivery of care	Care given is of a quality that is auditable according to agreed guidelines	Standards agreed by the CNS with the multidisciplinary team
To be a major resource in the Trust of current research-based practice in their specific subject	Monitors the delivery of care to maintain best clinical practice	Uses a variety of methods to ensure that knowledge and usage of CNS role are maximised	Standards developed and agreed by CNS and reviewed and audited
To provide professional support to staff, children and families in the clinical field	Provides up-to-date advice and education	Is available and contactable	Staff and patients aware of the position and role of the CNS

Source: Cattini and Knowles (1999).

340

The education of other team members about the patient's family – its attitudes, how it functions, its concerns about the child's health (both mental and physical) – is also essential. Equally important, if not of paramount importance, is the education of the family – and particularly the parents/carers – so that issues concerning development, behaviour and health that may appear throughout the childhood and adolescence of a patient with craniofacial anomalies can be addressed (Warschausky et al 2002).

RESEARCH

To back up these core components, the CNS must engage in both audit and research in order to provide evidence-based practice and improve current concepts of care. The acquisition of additional knowledge and skills enhances the CNS's role within the multidisciplinary team and provides improved care and treatment for the children (Department of Health 2001).

COMMUNICATION

Improving practice and increasing communication between the CNS and the many people he or she interacts with on a day-to-day basis is a further key component of the CNS role (Lethem 2000).

The CNS is thus in the best position to adopt a leadership role in children's nursing, and patients (and their families) place an increasing responsibility on them to do this. The CNS is in an ideal position to recognise the children's needs, and promote a specialist service just for them (Khair and Madge 2002). Flexibility in care provision, especially in this group of patients, is essential.

The clinical nurse specialist and the craniofacial service

Strauss (1999) described craniofacial care as being optimally delivered by organised teams. He stated that the benefits of working in teams included their ability to co-ordinate a complex service, to meet the psychological and social needs of these children and families, and to give evaluations that were multifaceted. The children with craniosynostosis, especially those with conditions such as Crouzon and Apert syndromes, have complex needs that involve all members of the team and require a systematic approach. When a variety of specialists and disciplines are providing care and assessment, there is a risk of dehumanising both child and family, and so it is essential that a personal touch is given. The CNS's role is to co-ordinate assessments and treatments (surgical and non-surgical) to enable the children to receive a high standard of personal care. This involves meeting the family on their arrival at the hospital, and being available on a day-to-day basis to answer questions, as well as to support and be there for the children and their families. For outpatients the personal touch can be maintained by telephone calls to keep the family informed of what to expect and when.

The responsibilities of a CNS working within the multidisciplinary craniofacial team are centred around interlinking roles that have been described well by Long (2002):

1   Assessment
2   Co-ordination and communication
3   Technical and physical care
4   Therapy integration
5   Emotional support
6   Involving the family

The *assessment* ensures that actual and potential problems are addressed. From this process referrals to other teams and community services are made.

Co-ordination and communication is an intricate responsibility that involves delegation of aspects of care to other team members, including ward staff, and requesting input from other team members. If the gathering, synthesising, and dissemination of information is central to the role of the CNS, then it is liaison, referral, negotiation and discharge planning, within and without the craniofacial unit, that makes up the largest part of that role.

Emotional support for the families is essential. It involves following up, and going through, what has been said by the team members in clinic sessions and on the ward rounds, helping in the continuation of care, and ensuring that the families have taken in and understood what has been said to them. By being there the CNS provides a reassuring and familiar presence.

Providing the rest of the craniofacial team with an insight into the family dynamics, their coping strategies, and degrees of understanding, is often something that only the CNS can do. This enables the team to plan their care and treatment strategies more appropriately.

These roles and responsibilities also apply to the community teams involved in the child's ongoing care. The CNS can provide them with essential and up-to-date information on the child's progress. Some families come from far reaches of the country – some from overseas – and in such cases it is essential to have someone to liaise with locally so that they can offer support and care on a personal level close to home.

There are obvious problems for families in having a child who does not look as they expected. There is the difficulty of balancing normal family life and parenting with prolonged and often unexpected treatments, as well as the additional physical duties, if the child has airway difficulties, a tracheostomy or nasal prong, for example. This can make bonding even more difficult. Crittenden and Ainsworth (1989 cited in May 2001) found that babies who had a facial disfigurement were at a higher risk of developing insecure attachments. At around 2 days of age babies who were considered less attractive were given less physical contact and held less close than those babies considered to be attractive (Langois and Swain 1981). Parents in this situation need support from specialists who understand the complexity of their child's condition and can provide the information the parents need. Pain (1999) looked at the function of information for parents of children with disabilities and concluded that it was a vital requirement for parents in understanding the practical implications of their child's condition, and in facilitating their adjustment to it. Not surprisingly, problems associated with attachment will be exacerbated in proportion to the impairment of the child either in facial appearance or development (Endriga and Kapp-Simon 1999).

As parents/carers are the centre-point of the physical and emotional well-being of the family, the extent to which they adapt to living with a child with a craniofacial condition will, ultimately, have an impact on the physiological and psychological health of that child, and also that of his or her siblings (Fisher 2001). The CNS as part of the multidisciplinary team therefore has an important role to play from the moment of initial contact onwards – a role that is ongoing and long-term, guided by the CNS's growing relationship with the family.

Children across all cultures depend on adult care for their survival, though the extent and nature of an individual child's needs will obviously differ (Thorne 2002). Children with a severe facial disfigurement soon start to form their own opinions on how they look, how others see them and their role within the healthcare system they have grown up in. Giving them a choice in their own care as they grow helps them to see their place in society, because this is something that the family can sometimes overlook in their desire to protect their child. This should be encouraged and supported by the CNS along with the other members of the craniofacial team. Part of the CNS's responsibility is to focus on the children's developmental needs, by using play and education while emphasising the importance of their family, and their own place within it. Included also is the need to liaise with local schools, social services, and local medical and nursing teams, to ensure that these children receive the specialist help and education they are entitled to.

The CNS's role in advocacy/leadership is to act for both the child and the family, for the rights of the child within the family as an individual and within the craniofacial care team. The children have a right to knowledge about their condition, to express their views and make their own decisions (Flatman 2002). These are issues raised by the Bristol enquiry as part of the challenge of decision making in clinical medicine. As these children grow and mature, so their needs change. They become increasingly involved in their own care and the CNS's role changes too – with increasing emphasis on acting as an advocate for them in planning their care and treatment, allowing them choices and listening to their voice.

The CNS as a key worker with the family has to be seen as approachable, and the information that he or she provides must be tailored to the children and their families' particular needs. It is important for the CNS to retain the personal touch and not become someone who just hands out paper information – or, as one of our families put it, 'There is no substitute for real people.' They found that the really important information came from people in face-to-face conversations, and that although written information was good to take away and digest, it was not enough. Pain (1999) identified three themes that emerged from a study of how such information was used by families. These were: to enhance the management of their child, to help the parents/carers cope emotionally, and to enable them to access benefits and services.

The role the CNS undertakes can, for convenience, be divided into two, although the two are not totally separate. One concerns the care and co-ordination of services for the non-syndromic (usually single suture synostosis) child, and the other concerns the complex, syndromic child. These roles differ just as the children's and their families' needs differ.

343

The child with non-syndromic craniosynostosis
A care pathway has recently been developed by our unit to look at the route the child and family with a non-syndromic condition take through our service (see Fig. 17.1).

The children with simple suture conditions have relatively few functional problems, although some require ophthalmological and others speech and language or psychological services, depending on their age. Essentially their surgery is for cosmetic reasons. Their conditions are associated with a low incidence of problems such as developmental delay or visual loss, and treatment is discussed by the surgeon in terms of improving present appearance and the prevention of further deformity as the child grows and develops (Moos and Hide 1993). This lack of functional problems should not lead to any underestimation of the effect that the child's appearance may have both on the child and his or her family. The children in this group are usually aged 6 months to around 2 years and too young to make a choice themselves. Parental choice therefore leads the decision-making process.

Making a decision to have – or not to have – surgery in a situation in which the surgeon has essentially ruled out the treatment of functional problems can be extremely difficult for the family. On the one hand they have worries about what their child will have to put up with in terms of teasing and bullying if they do not go ahead with an operation. On the other hand, if they decide to have the surgery, there are natural concerns about the safety of the operation and its outcome. The CNS's role is not to make up their minds for them but to provide them with all the information available. This includes 'before and after' pictures, and putting them in touch with other families who have been through similar experiences, in order to enable them to make a more informed decision. The CNS often sees the family separately from the surgeon – outside the clinic room, or in the CNS's office, for example – for informal chats to help them to make that decision.

At Great Ormond Street Hospital, the child with single suture synostosis is seen first in a craniofacial clinic by the plastic surgeon or neurosurgeon to whom the referral was originally made. But before this, the consultant and the CNS review the referral letter and assess the urgency of the appointment. For example, if the child has sagittal synostosis and is coming up to 6 months old, it is essential to speed up the process to ensure that they do not miss the opportunity of being offered surgery at the optimum age (see Chapter 19). In the clinic the diagnosis is made – or confirmed – predominantly on clinical findings. The family then discuss with the consultant the implications of the diagnosis and the management options, including the outlook both with and without surgery. After the consultation the CNS sees new families in order to follow up on any questions they may have, give them some written information and discuss the next steps should they decide to have surgery.

Children with single suture synostosis are listed for surgery according to their age and diagnosis (see Chapter 19). The CNS calls the family at home to let them know the planned date usually about six weeks in advance. The CNS liaises with the craniofacial administrator about any other appointments, such as ophthalmology, they may require, and also arranges for three-dimensional CT if this is required for surgical planning.

The children come to the ward for a preoperative assessment during the week before their surgery. Here they have blood taken, and are seen by the registrar, to go once again through the details of the procedure and the risks associated with it. The CNS also sees

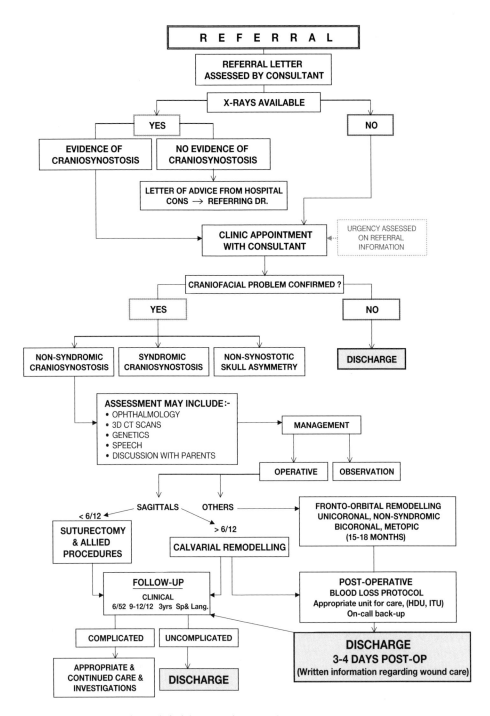

Fig. 17.1 Non-syndromic craniofacial synostosis care pathway.

them and goes through with the families again the details of the pre- and postoperative care.

Following their surgery, the children are usually in hospital for three to five days, at the most. Postoperative care is in a neurosurgical high dependency unit for the first night, and they return to the plastics/craniofacial ward the following day. Part of the CNS's clinical role is to work on the unit for the postoperative period, not only to care for the children but also to provide education for the ward nurses on how to manage the children after their surgery. The children are finally discharged home with an advice sheet on the care of the wound, hair washing, school and other activities.

Follow-up is in a craniofacial clinic around six weeks later. Between discharge and review, the family have the CNS as a contact, for any queries or worries they may encounter once at home.

The child with complex/syndromic craniosynostosis

The child with a craniofacial syndrome has a variety of complex needs not all of which are directly related to their facial appearance and structure, and a care pathway has been developed for these children too (see Fig. 17.2). This is a simplified way of guiding the clinician through the difficulties of this group of children's care. The children are likely to remain under the care of the craniofacial service for many years, often until early adulthood when their final reconstructions are carried out. Building up a relationship with the family and children based on trust and shared responsibilities is essential to their ongoing care and treatment.

The diagnosis for these children can be made at any time from birth onwards, but ideally they should be referred to a craniofacial centre as soon after they are born as possible, so that the specialist and multidisciplinary care and treatment they require can be started as early on as possible. Many families tell us how they found that before being referred to such a specialist service they did not receive the necessary level of support and were confronted with an uncertain future on discharge from the obstetric unit – a view supported by Kerr and McIntosh (2000) who described how parents could feel abandoned in this situation. The problem of course is that local hospitals cannot always be expected to have the specialist knowledge necessary when dealing with conditions of such complexity and rarity that each appears unique.

The pathway through the craniofacial service for the child with complex craniosynostosis commences on referral. The referral letter is assessed by one of the 'lead' consultants and the CNS as to its urgency. Usually, the CNS will call the family at home or, if the patient is a newborn, visit them either at home or in hospital in order to introduce them to the craniofacial unit, provide them with some preliminary information and give them some idea of what to expect in terms of care and treatment. The child is then brought into our hospital for a period of formal assessment. This consists of a Monday to Thursday stay during which the child and family will meet all the various specialists within the craniofacial team. The details of the initial and subsequent assessments are given in Table 17.2.

In order to streamline the assessment process, at our unit we have set up a parent-held dictaphone system. The dictaphones are given to the families when they arrive on the ward

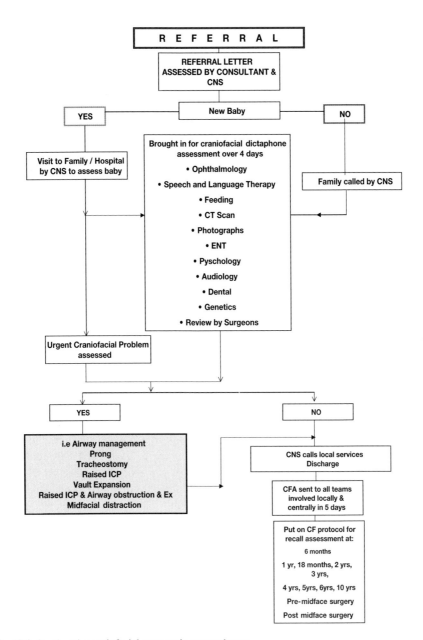

Fig. 17.2 Syndromic craniofacial synostosis care pathway.

TABLE 17.2
Follow-up protocol for syndromic craniofacial patients

Age at appointment	Speciality opinions required
Presentation	Audiology Dental ENT Genetics Ophthalmology/Orthoptics Speech & Language Sleep study 3D CT scan MRI (usually for the children with complex craniofacial conditions, i.e. Pfeiffer syndrome)
6 months	Audiology Ophthalmology/Orthoptics Psychology Photography Sleep study performed if problems shown up on sleep study at presentation/to check follow-up from presentation
9 months	Ophthalmology/Orthoptics Photography Sleep study if parental concerns about noisy breathing or follow-up if airway intervention was required previously, i.e. nasal prong
12 months	Dental ENT Ophthalmology/Orthoptics Pyschology Photography Speech & Language Sleep study as per previous statements
18 months	Audiology Ophthalmology/Orthoptics Psychology Photography Speech & Language
2 years	Opthalmology/Orthoptics Photography
3 years	Audiology Dental ENT Ophthalmology/Orthoptics Psychology Photography Speech & Language Sleep study if previous concerns
4 years	Audiology ENT Ophthalmology/Orthoptics Psychology Photography Speech & Language

6 years	ENT
	Ophthalmology/Orthoptics
	Psychology
	Photography
	Speech & Language
10 years	Dental
	Psychology
	Photography
	Speech & Language
Pre-midfacial surgery	Dental
	ENT
	Ophthalmology/Orthoptics
	Psychology
	Photography
	Speech & Language
	VPI studies and palatal screening
	3D CT scan
	Sleep study whether there have been previous problems or not
Post-midfacial surgery	Dental
	ENT
	Ophthalmology/Orthoptics
	Psychology
	Photography
	Speech & Language
	VPI studies and palatal screening
	3D CT scan
	Sleep study

and they keep them until discharge. As the child and family see each specialist a summary of his or her findings and recommendations is dictated onto the tape. The results are reviewed at a weekly team meeting, during which the details of the patients being operated on over the next two weeks are also reviewed and any other outstanding problems addressed.

These weekly meetings are attended by:

- Consultant neurosurgeon
- Consultant craniofacial/plastic surgeons
- Orthodontic surgeon
- Craniofacial registrar
- Plastic surgery registrar
- Hand specialist registrar
- The CNS
- Neurosurgical and maxillo-facial registrars

A summary of the recent assessment is made at this meeting and then the completed recording is typed up and sent out to local services by the following week. It is now accessible on the computer for the unit's various teams to review; it can also be e-mailed externally and the parents receive a copy too. It has proved, so far, to be an excellent way of information sharing. The information is now much more detailed and accurate than a conventional discharge summary. It has been prepared directly by each specialty and goes a long way towards providing the detailed information that has become – rightly – an important goal of contemporary medicine and nursing.

As children with complex craniosynostosis undergo intensive, long-term treatment by many different members of the team, we have adopted the use of shared care records along the lines already used by other specialties such as oncology. The aim of the shared care folder is to provide the family with printed information about their child's condition. All assessments are put into the records as well as details of their various tests, surgical procedures, airway management and ophthalmological findings. In this way families will eventually build up a comprehensive overview of how their child is progressing.

These records are also useful for local support services, who can photocopy and distribute the information they contain. They provide them with comprehensive documentation about each child's condition of the sort that does not always get sent out to them. The information is regularly updated on each visit to the craniofacial unit and copies of letters are also sent to families for them to incorporate in the records. At the moment, these shared care records are being provided for each new family referred to us, but the aim eventually will be to give them to all families currently within the service and backdate them to include their child's progress to date. This will help us achieve our goal of providing a quality service that administers to the needs of the child and family as well as the needs of those caring for them. 'The provision of quality is measured in terms of prompt access, good relationships and efficient administration' (The NHS Confederation 1999: 6).

What happens after the initial assessment depends upon the condition of the child. Early surgical intervention may be required, but if not the child will continue to be reviewed on a regular basis. Children with Apert, Crouzon, Pffeifer and Saethre–Chotzen syndrome are followed up on the basis of the assessment protocol (Table 17.2) and are therefore recalled for regular review as dictated by that protocol. Other children experiencing continuing problems and those requiring more frequent assessments than had previously been predicted will also be reviewed according to this protocol.

Children with syndromic craniosynostosis or other complex problems are also seen in the joint craniofacial clinics (CRANF) that take place once a month. These are attended by craniofacial/plastic surgeons, neurosurgeon, orthodontic surgeon, ENT surgeon, craniofacial registrar, speech and language therapist, psychologist and CNS. The children and their parents will see the different members of the team and be able to ask questions about ongoing issues; surgery can be discussed in detail and more concrete plans for further treatment and care can be put into action. I personally bring children into this clinic (where the consultation times are longer than our other clinics). I see my role there as ensuring that the child and their family have understood what has been discussed and that they have been able to get their views across.

Some children will be having 'early' surgery because of raised ICP, airway difficulties, and/or problems with eye protection (see appropriate chapters). This surgery can sometimes be required urgently and the child may be quite young. The play specialist and the CNS will discuss how play might aid their preparation. Different types of play can help the child to make sense of their environment and what is happening to them. Non-directive play provides a warm and friendly relationship with the children, showing them total acceptance and allowing freedom for them to express their feelings openly. We use multidimensional play as this allows us to choose the boundaries and level of interpretation to suit the child. It allows us to be as creative as the child, and incorporates such qualities as acceptance and trust. It also acknowledges that the use of simple behavioural interpretations will enable the children to make sense of their world (Holyoake 1998).

Adolescents provide additional challenges when they are approaching major surgery, and their preparation is complex. They are old enough to join the medical decision-making process along with their parents/carers and the craniofacial team (Endriga and Kapp-Simon 1999). It is important that they feel able to voice their opinions and make informed choices about their care and treatment.

As the (usually) older child or adolescent approaches such complex surgery as monobloc, Le Fort III or midfacial bipartition, the CNS commences a timetable of prepa-ration. Because the operation is planned some months in advance, there is time for a treatment plan to be devised. This involves the child being reviewed by the different teams as part of an assessment one month before the surgery, as well as three months afterwards in order for the team to review what physiological and psychological changes have occurred as a result.

Another equally important aspect of surgery is the emotional preparation of both the child and the family. I like to discuss with the parents/carers how they wish to approach this preparation and then work with them. A clinical psychologist will also be involved in assessing how the children view what is going to happen to them, their expectations and their ability to understand all the issues involved.

Such preoperative preparation involves visits to the hospital. The CNS has pre- and postsurgery pictures so that the children can see how their facial appearance might be changed. They can also see what vascular lines, dressings and attachments they will have for monitoring in the high dependency unit, and how these are gradually reduced during the recovery period. During this process the CNS works closely with the play specialist who will be helping to support the children once they are in the hospital.

Some of the children of course already know the ward and its staff well, having been under the care of the craniofacial service for many years, and this helps them in preparing for the surgery ahead.

The children who undergo midface or monobloc distraction using an external distraction frame experience great anxiety at the thought of having the frame attached to their head and the implications this has. In preparing this group of children I have a frame they can see and touch, and they can put it up to their faces and view themselves in the mirror to see how it will look. They can play with it and place it on a doll's head to enact what may happen to them. The adolescents are often interested in the practicalities of distraction and they can perform the distraction manoeuvres on the show frame. After their surgery these children go home with their frame on. Preparation of both the child and the family for this stage is essential and should be started as early as possible. Once the child is back at home the CNS contacts local services, and the GP, to ensure that they have adequate information and understanding to care for the child in the community. The CNS will also visit the child at home to provide reassurance, to check on their progress and to report back to the craniofacial team.

Schools will often be reluctant to have the child back full-time while the frame is on, because of safety issues. They should then provide home tuition, and this will usually have been arranged in advance as part of the preparation the CNS undertakes. If the child wishes to visit the school while the frame is still on, the CNS will go with them, to provide the nursing care and to help them to face their class. The CNS will also prepare their teachers, with the use of pictures and literature describing what their pupil has experienced and how they are progressing. The CNS will speak to the other children, either in the class or in school assembly, with the aim of trying to allay some of their fears about what has happened to their friend/classmate. We have also encouraged school friends to come on a visit to the hospital to see their friend. In this way they can see the environment, the play and the activities available, and de-mask some of the negative anticipation they may have about the whole process.

The future
Looking to the future, there are several projects – some proposed, some already being undertaken – that I would like to describe. The aim of them all is to enhance patient care and to improve their journey through the service.

In 2003 we will be setting up a preoperative assessment clinic for children with (predominantly) single suture synostosis and those with syndromes who require fronto-orbital remodelling and/or vault expansion. This clinic will involve bringing in all the children to be electively operated on during that month to an outpatient appointment about one month before the planned surgery date. The aim will be for the senior house officer (SHO) to pre-clerk the children and assess them. Blood will be taken for preoperative checks and cross-matching. The family will also receive the consent form and accompanying written and verbal information regarding consent, in line with current Commission for Health Improvement (CHI) recommendations. The family will be able to take the form home with them so that they can peruse it and any other information they have received about the planned operation, its aims and the risks involved.

This clinic will also provide them with a chance to meet other parents, and for their children to meet other children. It has been suggested that it can be of great benefit in terms of stress reduction when parents are able to share and compare their experiences with other parents in similar circumstances (Kerr and McIntosh 2000).

There will be a play specialist at this clinic to help with the preparation of the children by playing games, telling stories and answering questions. The families will have a chance to talk about the surgery with the CNS and ask questions about what to expect pre- and postoperatively. There will be 'before and after' pictures, as well as pictures of children from the day of surgery through to the day of discharge, so that they can see how a child progresses. The day of assessment and preparation will finish with a visit to the ward to meet the staff and familiarise themselves with the environment. 'Pre-op' clinics, particularly in the ENT field, have been shown to be an efficient way of physically preparing the child for the surgery and making it all a more positive experience for them. It also provides the

352

parents/carers with information to help them with talking with their child at home about coming into hospital for an operation.

Another ambition is to improve the transition of care from child to adult services. The children with complex problems are under the care of the craniofacial unit until all major reconstructive surgery has been completed, which means that some will stay with the service until they are in their early twenties. Our vision for the future is to be able to provide a smooth transition from paediatric to adult services, should these be required. Such a transition needs to be made over a period of time to enable the child and family to adjust to the new teams involved in their care.

Healthcare management is complex, and trying to involve separate hospitals and other institutions in one goal means operating across domains. This makes it important to find out from the children and their families what their expectations of transferring care are – and when they think the time is right for this. The CNS must be involved in helping the transition to go smoothly and ensuring that the family does not feel cut off abruptly. Saying goodbye is important for both the adolescent and the parent/carer. Clinics held jointly between paediatric and adult services would ease the transition and I would aim to visit a new hospital with them for the first few occasions to ensure that there is a comprehensive multidisciplinary handover.

Care pathways for children with syndromic and non-syndromic craniosynostosis have been developed, as already shown. From these we would like to progress to the production of an even more detailed integrated pathway that would provide a comprehensive guide to the assessment, and pre- and postoperative care of patients undergoing craniofacial surgery. This document would provide an overview of the child's care, and would complement existing documentation. It would form part of the notes on discharge of the patient and, we hope, would tighten up all the documentation involved in our multidisciplinary approach while ensuring that all the paperwork associated with the child's care is in one pack.

As one of four supraregionally funded craniofacial units in England it is important for us to stay in touch with each of the other centres. Such contacts help us to compare and contrast experiences and share new ideas and treatments. We have set up a nursing benchmarking group with the other units that allows us to compare practices and identify opportunities for improvement. Such benchmarking activity can be an effective way to identify the scope for improving a service. Its ultimate goal is to eliminate areas of practice that are not working and to identify best practice – what Grout (Grout et al 2001) describes as the benchmarking cycle, the overall result of which is to improve patient care.

Conclusion

The CNS's role, as can be seen, is a multifaceted one but essentially it is to communicate and to co-ordinate the delivery of care. Entwined in this are the many individual roles and responsibilities to the craniofacial team, to the community services and ultimately to the children and their families. These responsibilities ensure augmentation of care delivery to the child and their family. It is important to remember that, whatever roles are undertaken, extended or considered by a professional dealing with the child and his or her family, at the centre of everything are the best interests and rights of that child and that family. It is their right to have access to appropriate and up-to-date specialist healthcare, and it is our duty to give them the information, education, care and treatment they need in an experienced, professional and supportive environment. In this the CNS has a pivotal role.

Despite numerous challenges and problems, many children with craniofacial conditions become productive, contributing, and happy individuals. It is important to remember that most will live healthy, satisfying and full lives (Strauss 2001) and that it is our task to ensure that each and every one of them grows up to develop to the full potential of which they are capable.

REFERENCES

Cattini P, Knowles V (1999) Core competencies for clinical nurse specialists: a usable framework. *J Clin Nurs* 8: 508–509.

Department of Health (2001) Strengthening the nursing, midwifery and HV contribution to health and health care. *Making a Difference*. London: Department of Health.

Endriga MC, Kapp-Simon KA (1999) Psychological issues in craniofacial care: state of the art. *Cleft Palate Craniofac J* 36(1): 5.

Flatman D (2002) Consulting children: are we listening? *Paediatr Nurs* 14(7): 28–30.

Grout PA et al (2001) *Benchmarking and Incentives in the NHS*. London: Department of Health.

Hansa RJ (2002) Role boundaries – research nurse or clinical nurse specialist? A literature review. *J Clin Nurs* 11(4): 13–15.

Holyoake D (1998) Reflections on the process of play interaction. *Paediatr Nurs* 10(2): 15.

Kenny G (2002) Children's nursing and interprofessional collaboration: challenges and opportunities. *J Clin Nurs* 11: 307.

Kerr SM, McIntosh JB (2000) Coping when a child has a disability: exploring the impact of parent-to-parent support. *Child Care Health Dev* 26(4): 2.

Khair K, Madge S (2002) The leadership and advocacy roles of the paediatric nurse specialist. *Prof Nurse* 17(5): 289.

Langois JH, Swain DB (1981) Infant physical attractiveness as an elicitor of parenting behaviour. Paper presented at the Society for Research in Child Development, Boston.

Lethem W (2000) Education and the novice clinical nurse specialist. *Nurs Times* 96(8): 43.

Long AF (2002) The role of the nurse within the multi-professional rehabilitation team. *J Adv Nurs* 37(1): 5.

May L (2001) *Craniosynostosis, Paediatric Neurosurgery: A Handbook for the Multidisciplinary Team*. London: Whurr, p 164.

Moos FM, Hide R (1993) Craniofacial surgery – surgical correction of congenital deformities. *Surgery* (The Medicine Group (journals) Ltd), p 458.

The NHS Confederation and The Nuffield Trust (1999) Consultation: the modern values of leadership and management in the NHS.

Pain H (1999) Coping with a child with disabilities from the parents' perspective: the function of information. *Child Care Health Dev* 25(4): 9.

Pearson A (2002) Just what does the patient want? *Int J Nurs Practice* 8(2): 67. (Letter.)

Strauss RP (1999) The organization and delivery of craniofacial health services: the state of the art. *Cleft Palate Craniofac J* 36(3): 189.

Strauss RP (2001) 'Only skin deep': health, resilience, and craniofacial care. *Cleft Palate Craniofac J* 38(3): 226–227.

Thorne B (2002) From silence to voice: bringing children more fully into knowledge. In: *Childhood*. London: Sage, p 254.

Warschausky S et al (2002) Health-related quality of life in children with craniofacial anomalies. *Plast Reconstr Surg* 110: 7.

18
ANAESTHESIA FOR CRANIOSYNOSTOSIS SURGERY

S. Mallory and R. Bingham

The history of anaesthesia for corrective surgery on infants and children with disfiguring conditions can be traced back to the introduction of anaesthesia. Since then it has been employed to facilitate improved and increasingly complex surgical techniques. The patients requiring craniosynostosis surgery broadly fall into two groups: otherwise normal children with a single suture craniosynostosis undergoing cosmetic procedures, or syndromic individuals with multiple abnormalities and multiple suture synostoses. In both groups the anaesthetist plays a vital role in ensuring the risk/benefit ratio is acceptable for the proposed surgery. The care of these often highly complex patients requires meticulous planning and preparation prior to anaesthesia.

Despite its elective nature, the surgical correction of craniofacial abnormality carries a high risk of extensive blood loss and other serious intra-operative and postoperative complications. Craniofacial surgery may be indicated for functional and/or cosmetic reasons. Functional indications include raised intracranial pressure, compromised respiratory function (with central and airway components), feeding difficulties, proptosis and visual deterioration. Cosmetic correction is of central importance, particularly in the older child, because of the psychological issues involved.

The development of multidisciplinary and interdisciplinary teams to co-ordinate services has been central in the management of these patients. Because each discipline may see the patient's problems and needs from a different viewpoint, co-operation between specialists is felt to enhance patient care. In addition, there have been significant advances in imaging, allowing precise surgical planning (Thompson et al 1994) and objective assessment of surgical outcome. Anaesthetists are involved in the preoperative assessment and optimisation of the patient as well as their perioperative care, as part of the inter-disciplinary craniofacial team.

Our experience at Great Ormond Street Hospital is based on approximately 125 cases annually. In 2001, for example, we anaesthetised for 11 facial bipartition/monobloc procedures (with or without distraction), 56 fronto-orbital reconstructions and vault expansions, 18 ICP monitoring probe insertions and 72 related procedures. The figures for 2002 show an increase in the number of major procedures – particularly those involving the use of distraction. Of these, approximately 2–3 per cent were monobloc osteotomies, 2–3 per cent were facial bipartitions, 1–2 per cent were Le Fort III, 20 per cent were fronto-orbital remodelling, and 5–6 per cent sagittal and calvarial remodelling.

Craniofacial syndromes and anaesthesia

THE AIRWAY

Craniofacial abnormalities can result in a wide spectrum of airway problems, which may present perioperative challenges to the anaesthetist. Between 20 and 37 per cent of patients undergoing major craniofacial surgery have airway problems (Palmisano and Rusy 2002). In the subset of patients with craniofacial synostosis, approximately 50 per cent of patients have problems with airway management (Handler et al 1979). There may be shortening of the oropharyngeal and nasopharyngeal airways as a result of a truncated cranial base (Shprintzen 1982, Kreiborg et al 1999), and the mandible may be hypoplastic (Shprintzen 1992), with the tongue placed posteriorly. Maxillary hypoplasia may result in reduced nasal and postnasal spaces. Additional anomalies peculiar to a given syndrome, such as choanal atresia, can also compromise the airway. Anatomical abnormalities may be further compounded by neurological dysfunction, which can produce pharyngeal hypotonia and incoordination (Sher 1992).

OBSTRUCTIVE SLEEP APNOEA

Patients with this condition often have noisy breathing and snoring. They may be tired during the day with detrimental effects on schoolwork and behaviour. Right heart failure and pulmonary hypertension may exist at the extreme end of the spectrum. The occurrence of obstructive sleep apnoea in craniofacial patients is well documented (Lauritzen et al 1986, Argamaso 1992), and we routinely perform sleep studies as part of the preoperative work-up if this condition is suspected. These often demonstrate prolonged and profound oxygen desaturation when sleeping.

The mechanism of obstruction has been shown to result from a number of factors, in addition to the already anatomically reduced upper airway. Abnormal tongue movement against the posterior pharyngeal wall and medial movement of the lateral pharyngeal walls, along with pharyngeal constriction, can all produce airway obstruction during sleep (Sher et al 1986). The mechanism of obstruction may also exhibit a central component in individuals with herniation of the hindbrain through the foramen magnum. Airway optimisation in children with obstructive sleep apnoea may require nasal stenting, nasal continuous positive airway pressure (CPAP), or choanal dilatation. In some individuals tracheostomy may be indicated, and in others soft tissue procedures may be performed (Moore 1993). This is fully addressed in Chapter 9 in this book.

INTRACRANIAL PRESSURES AND THE EFFECT OF ANAESTHESIA

Intracranial pressure may be increased by variations in tissue, blood or cerebrospinal fluid (CSF) pressure. In patients at risk of intracranial hypertension, these fluctuations are monitored preoperatively. Any rise in intracranial pressure affects cerebral perfusion pressure and in turn cerebral blood flow. This may manifest initially as headaches, nausea and altered behaviour. As the skull is essentially a rigid box, once compensatory mechanisms have been exhausted, intracranial pressure rises rapidly. If allowed to progress, the Cushing response may become apparent (a fall in heart rate with a concomitant rise in blood pressure).

356

This may be followed by herniation of the brainstem through the foramen magnum ('coning'), resulting in coma and death.

While mean arterial pressure remains within a given range, cerebral perfusion is controlled by auto-regulatory mechanisms. If excessive hypo- or hypertension occurs, then these mechanisms fail. This failure to auto-regulate also becomes apparent under other circumstances, for example during periods of hypoxia, hypercarbia and cerebral ischaemia. In addition, volatile anaesthetic agents themselves are responsible for inhibiting auto-regulation via a dose-dependent cerebral vasodilation.

Cerebral perfusion pressure is a product of a number of factors:

$$CPP = MAP - (ICP + CVP)$$

CPP, cerebral perfusion pressure
MAP, mean arterial pressure
ICP, intracranial pressure
CVP, central venous pressure

All these aspects of patient physiology may be affected by surgery and anaesthesia. It is therefore important that 'balanced' anaesthesia is delivered, with the intention of minimising any such changes. This starts with avoidance of opioids or excessively sedative premedication, as respiratory depression may result in hypercarbia. Cerebral excitatory drugs are avoided at induction of anaesthesia and a volatile agent with minimal vasodilatory action is used. Isoflurane is currently our volatile agent of choice. Surges in arterial pressure are avoided, both at laryngoscopy and intra-operatively, by using generous doses of fentanyl. Cerebral venous obstruction is avoided by careful patient positioning prior to surgery and the use of 'head-up' tilt. Neuromuscular blockade is monitored continuously in order to prevent coughing leading to intracranial pressure surges.

Mild hyperventilation intra-operatively to a minimum $PaCO_2$ of 3.5 kPa will reduce cerebral blood volume via vasoconstriction. However, cerebral ischaemia has been described if the CO_2 is allowed to fall too low. We avoid hypotensive agents such as sodium nitroprusside, as they may cause increased ICP via vasodilation and impair auto-regulatory compensation. Acute rises in ICP are usually managed with moderate hyperventilation and mannitol administration.

ASSOCIATED ABNORMALITIES
Over 100 syndromes associated with craniosynostosis have been described, although many are extremely rare (Elmslie and Reardon 1998). Crouzon syndrome is the most common of the syndromic synostoses. However, any syndrome can present a wide number of abnormalities which may challenge the anaesthetist. Speech difficulties, optic atrophy, conductive hearing loss and delayed intellectual development can make preoperative communication difficult for patient and doctor. Venous access may be difficult or limited due to limb abnormalities such as syndactyly. Upper airway obstruction may not be the only difficulty encountered at induction. Laryngocopy may be difficult due to limited mouth opening, and

cervical vertebral abnormalities may result in restricted neck movement, which limits extension for the 'sniffing the morning air' position preferred for intubation. In addition, choanal stenosis or atresia, tracheal stenosis or abnormal tracheal cartilage may further compromise the airway and limit tube position, with nasal intubation being impossible.

Patient positioning, often prone, may be problematic in those at risk of skeletal fractures (Antley–Bixler syndrome) or those with joint contractures. Protecting proptotic eyes is particularly difficult in the prone position.

Other abnormalities that may require modification of anaesthesia, analgesia and post-operative care include renal or urogenital abnormalities such as polycystic kidneys and hydronephrosis, cardiac anomalies such as atrial septal defect (ASD), ventricular septal defect (VSD), pulmonary stenosis and overriding aorta (10 per cent incidence in Apert syndrome) and pulmonary aplasia.

Preoperative preparation

Facial deformity has wide-ranging effects on a child's psychological development. Bullying at school and other negative social experiences may lead to varying degrees of behavioural problems. These aspects must not be overlooked in children presenting for surgery, and psychological assessment forms an integral part of the preoperative work-up. Surgery will alter cosmetic appearance, and patients and parents need the necessary support. This may be especially relevant when the indication for such a major procedure and all its inherent risks may not be an identifiable physical function but improved self-image alone.

A recent series at Great Ormond Street Hospital looked at satisfaction following facial bipartition procedures for improved cosmesis in 22 patients. This series, completed in 2002, reported a high level of both patient and parent satisfaction. Improved self-image has been shown previously to decrease behavioural problems for these patients (Lefebvre and Barclay 1982). This information is helpful to the anaesthetist seeking to reassure the anxious child and parents fearing alteration in appearance. However, these are major procedures, with an associated morbidity and mortality. Patients with complex problems, such as difficult or compromised airways, are at particular risk (Whitaker et al 1979), and for each individual the risk/benefit ratio, including that of anaesthesia, needs to be assessed and explained. In a study of 126 children undergoing craniofacial surgery, 20 per cent required transfusion in excess of their circulating volume, 29 per cent required postoperative ventilation and 3 per cent received intra-operative epinephrine and/or cardio-pulmonary resuscitation following complications (Moylan et al 1993). Mortality with craniosynostosis repair from massive haemorrhage also remains a possibility (Meyer et al 1993).

INVESTIGATIONS

Numerous preoperative investigations are required. At Great Ormond Street Hospital, admission for any major craniofacial procedure occurs a week preoperatively and the patient's pathway through the hospital is carefully mapped out with a multidisciplinary approach (Fig. 18.1). The anaesthetist will make their preoperative visit during this time in order to be able to answer a patient's or family's questions, request any specific investigations, and plan their anaesthesia.

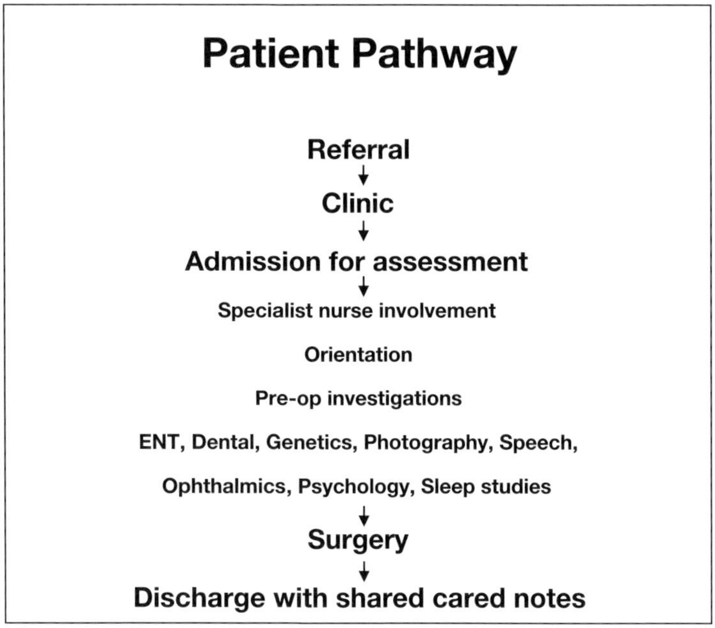

Patient Pathway

Referral
↓
Clinic
↓
Admission for assessment
↓
Specialist nurse involvement

Orientation

Pre-op investigations

ENT, Dental, Genetics, Photography, Speech,

Ophthalmics, Psychology, Sleep studies
↓
Surgery
↓
Discharge with shared cared notes

Fig. 18.1 Craniofacial patient pathway

The preoperative investigations are tailored to fit the needs of the individual patient. Those of particular relevance to anaesthesia will include sleep studies, intracranial pressure measurement, otolaryngological review, a check of current haematological and biochemical parameters, cross-matching of packed red blood cells, and cardiology review, if appropriate. The intra-operative death of a child with cloverleaf skull syndrome has led to selected complex patients having cerebral venous imaging as part of their preoperative investigations. In the aforementioned case, pre-existing obstruction of intracranial venous drainage due to abnormal bone development led to the development of extracranial collaterals. Intra-operatively this network of collaterals was disrupted and fatal venous hypertension ensued (Thompson et al 1995). Venous imaging may be helpful in identifying other patients with anomalous venous drainage for whom such surgery could be catastrophic (Anderson et al 1997).

PREMEDICATION

Premedication is usually used for one of three reasons: to facilitate pain-free cannulation, as an anxiolytic, or as an antisialagogue. Local anaesthetic creams, such as eutectic mixture of local anaesthetic (EMLA) or Ametop, are applied to likely cannulation sites preoperatively. This may facilitate the siting of a venous cannula that can be used to administer anaesthesia. Limb abnormalities and recurrent cannulation can be problematic and this should be borne in mind.

In the anxious patient, a sedative premedication may, along with psychological preparation, make the experience less distressing and induction smoother. The commonly employed agents are benzodiazepines, midazolam for infants and young children (0.5 mg/kg; max. 15 mg), and temazepam for older children (0.5 mg/kg; max. 20 mg). However, sedative premedication should be used with great caution in patients with airway compromise or raised ICP.

Finally, in children where secretions may prove hazardous to the airway, such as the very young and/or those with anticipated difficult intubation, atropine may be given orally (40 mcg/kg; max. 500 mcg).

Intra-operative techniques and agents

AIRWAY MANAGEMENT

Laryngoscopy
Difficulty at laryngscopy in this group of patients may be encountered for a number of reasons, usually in combination. Respiratory reserve may be poor, with rapid desaturation occurring once mask ventilation is halted to perform laryngoscopy. When positioning the patient, cervical abnormalities, such as synostosis, may limit neck extension, preventing optimal positioning. Mouth opening can be restricted by trismus or temporomandibular joint synostosis. Once the mouth is opened, oral crowding secondary to maxillary hypoplasia and macroglossia can hinder the introduction of the laryngoscope. Mandibular hypoplasia, presenting the larynx as anterior, can restrict the view of the vocal cords.

We have found that the physical appearance of individuals is not always an accurate guide to difficulty with laryngoscopy (Fig. 18.2). In particular, those with maxillary hypoplasia look abnormal but do not usually present a problem. Children who have undergone corrective surgery may look normal, but often laryngoscopy is more difficult due to maxillary advancement and temporomandibular joint limitation. This finding has been reported by other centres, and previously uneventful anaesthesia may be falsely reassuring, especially in relation to specific procedures such as removal of maxillary distraction devices (Roche et al 2002).

Difficult laryngoscopy is associated with numerous risks; there may be hypoxia, aspiration of gastric contents leading to lung injury, trauma causing airway oedema, and hypertensive responses leading to raised ICP. Some centres advocate the use of elective fibreoptic intubation as reliable and safe where some degree of difficulty with endotracheal intubation is anticipated (Blanco et al 2001, Roche et al 2002). The use of the fibreoptic bronchoscope requires training and experience. However, even in experienced hands failure of the technique is possible (Gallagher et al 1980). We do not use awake fibreoptic intubation as we regard it as too distressing for the child. Instead we introduce the fibreoptic bronchoscope through a laryngeal mask airway which has the dual effect of controlling the airway and simplifying visualisation of the larynx.

Indications for tracheostomy
A minority of individuals may require a tracheostomy preoperatively. Some cases of severe respiratory obstruction may not improve with age and may actually deteriorate over time

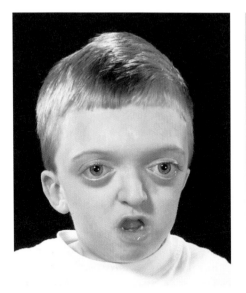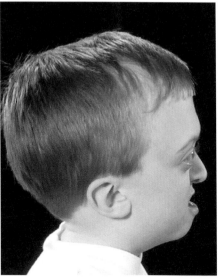

Fig. 18.2 Maxillary hypoplasia, an appearance that does not predict a difficult laryngoscopy. However, corrective surgery may result in a more problematic airway.

(Mixter et al 1990, McGill 1991). In these circumstances, if preoperative optimisation by other measures is not possible or effective, a tracheostomy needs to be sited preoperatively, as early surgery on the airway may not be in the interest of the patient. A tracheostomy will provide time for the required growth prior to a procedure and prevent the potentially serious long-term sequelae of chronic airway obstruction. Elective tracheostomy is sometimes performed where extensive facial osteotomies are to be undertaken, or where reintubation would be impossible were it to be required intra-operatively or postoperatively. The complications of the surgical airway are well known, but in addition there is an increased risk of meningeal infection after cranial reconstruction in children with a pre-existing tracheostomy (Jones et al 1992).

INDUCTION OF ANAESTHESIA

Induction may be with an intravenous or inhalational agent. In our practice inhalational induction is more common, with just 9.5 per cent of patients receiving intravenous inductions (Moylan et al 1993). This is for a number of reasons. Venous access may be difficult in the awake infant with limb abnormalities and where multiple cannulations have occurred in the past. Inhalational induction may be preferable where a difficult airway is anticipated. Cautious gaseous induction is unlikely to result in apnoea, and the maintenance of spontaneous ventilation initially allows time to confirm the ability to deliver controlled ventilation, prior to administration of a muscle relaxant. This confers an additional degree of safety. The gaseous agent of choice is currently sevoflurane, although halothane was commonly used, to good effect, in the past. Intravenous induction may still be preferred in the older child and where the ability to ventilate is predictable. The agent most commonly employed in the past was thiopentone, but currently propofol is preferred.

Even at this early stage of anaesthesia, problems may be encountered. Ill-fitting face-masks due to facial asymmetry or maxillary hypoplasia make establishing a seal difficult. The presence of exophthalmos may also cause difficulty with mask ventilation. Soft-seal facemasks with highly deformable rims make this problem less likely. Where leaks around the facemask persist, high gas flows may be required to permit adequate bag and mask ventilation.

In many patients with midface hypoplasia, airway obstruction may become apparent and problematic, even at light levels of anaesthesia. This may create a problem, as patients are not sufficiently anaesthetised to tolerate an oropharyngeal airway. This can usually be overcome by employing distending pressure, via the mask, until an airway is accepted.

Muscle relaxation is administered only after the ability to ventilate manually with a bag and mask has been confirmed. Agents commonly used include atracurium or vecuronium. The choice of airway for the procedure depends on the proposed surgery. For intraoral procedures and where intermaxillary fixation (IMF) is to occur, the nasal route is commonly requested although, in most children, IMF can be achieved with an oral tube routed posterior to the molar teeth. In midfacial surgery, reinforced orotracheal tubes are usually employed as they are more likely to resist crushing or kinking during the procedure and they can be secured by means of a circum-mandibular wire. Since the neck is usually extended to avoid any obstruction of the cervical veins, the tube position is optimised by first confirming endobronchial intubation and then withdrawing the tube until breath sounds are heard bilaterally. In older children (>6 years) a cuffed tube is preferred. Along with a throat pack, a cuff prevents blood and debris entering the respiratory tract and also assists in stabilising the tube's position, thus helping to prevent intra-operative displacement. The tube's stability once secured is vital, as the airway and the surgical field are largely shared. The list of complications involving the endotracheal tube in craniofacial surgery is extensive. Despite extreme caution, it remains a possibility that accidental surgical displacement or puncture of the tube or its pilot balloon may occur intra-operatively. In the event of tube displacement occurring while facial bones are mobile and access is limited during midface advancement, a laryngeal mask has been successfully employed in our institution, its insertion in the interim allowing continued oxygenation and anaesthesia, prior to formal reintubation

For cranial vault surgery a pre-formed south-facing oro-tracheal tube is satisfactory for procedures in the supine position, and armoured tubes with complete facial strapping are used if the child is to be placed prone. Two large bore venous lines are established, as massive transfusion is a possibility and adequate access for this eventuality is essential. One is a large bore peripheral line (usually in the long saphenous vein) and in most cases the second line is inserted via the femoral vein, also allowing for central venous pressure monitoring. Antibiotic prophylaxis including anaerobe cover is usual on induction.

INTRA-OPERATIVE ANAESTHESIA
Anaesthesia may be maintained using a balanced technique involving fentanyl (up to 10 mcg/kg) for analgesia and a gaseous anaesthetic agent, such as isoflurane, carried in either

nitrous oxide/oxygen or air/oxygen mixtures. Alternatively, total intravenous anaesthesia (TIVA) may be used. However, the use of TIVA in this group of patients is unusual as the infusion requires a separate dedicated intravenous line and the pharmacokinetics of propofol (the usual agent) have not been fully described for children. Moreover, the use of propofol in small children or infants has led to increased mortality in the intensive care setting (Parke et al 1992). The potent and very short-acting analgesic agent remifentanil may be delivered by continuous intravenous infusion as an alternative to boluses of fentanyl.

MONITORING AND PATIENT POSITIONING
Monitoring of oxygen saturation, end-tidal carbon dioxide, ECG, invasive blood pressure, central venous pressure, rectal temperature and peripheral nerve function is standard for all patients. Invasive monitoring is employed primarily to allow close monitoring of blood loss, as direct measurement is difficult. It has been suggested that there may be inaccuracies in the above parameters (Wolf et al 1986), but the alternatives, such as pulmonary artery catheters, present their own difficulties in the child. These devices are invasive and not without considerable risk. Experience and availability of the non-invasive alternative, transoesophageal echocardiography, are limited in the paediatric population (Reich et al 1993), and its manipulation restricted in this instance by the surgical access required. One study into non-invasive monitoring of aortic blood flow measurement in infants undergoing craniofacial surgery has been promising (Orliaguet et al 1998). This study utilised a paediatric oesophageal probe, inserted at induction of anaesthesia, to provide a continuous Doppler measurement of aortic blood flow. The study showed that not only was such monitoring feasible for such procedures but the technique also provided reliable data.

The temperature of the patient is monitored rectally and the aim is to maintain normothermia. With the large volumes of fluid transfused intra-operatively, fluid warming devices are essential and we use a co-axial counter-current device, which warms the fluid right up to the point it enters the patient. In addition, a forced air-warming blanket is used for the duration of the procedure. In a recent audit of 20 major craniofacial cases at our institution, only one had documented intra-operative hypothermia

Positioning of the patient has to be exercised with attention to detail. The airway will be in the surgical field, and all connections to the endotracheal tube need to be securely fixed with adequate slack to tolerate surgical movement intra-operatively. Many bony abnormalities, contractures and synostoses may make positioning difficult, particularly when the modified prone position is required (Fig. 18.3). Once all pressure points are protected and the abdomen is free, allowing for diaphragmatic movement with ventilation, the chest is auscultated to confirm that endotracheal tube position is still satisfactory.

Intra-operative complications have included bronchial intubation during surgical flexion of the neck (Moylan et al 1993) and this can be minimised by following the above manoeuvres. Cerebral venous congestion must also be avoided. The patient is usually in a slightly 'head-up' position and therefore there is the potential risk of venous air embolism (VAE). We have found end-tidal carbon dioxide measurement to be satisfactory for the monitoring of VAE, provided the alarm parameters are closely set. The greatest risk of VAE is in those patients who are hypotensive and undergoing complex vault and sagittal procedures

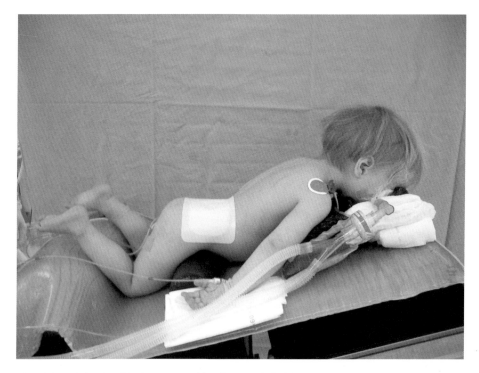

Fig. 18.3 A child placed in the prone position for a craniofacial procedure such as a posterior vault expansion (see Chapter 19). Note that the padding under the pelvis ensures that the abdomen is free of any compression and also that the eyes have been well protected. For operations involving access to the entire calvarium (vault reconstructions for the older child with scaphocephaly, for example) the neck can be extended by increasing the padding under the chin.

(Faberowski et al 1999), although, in our practice, it is an extremely rare event, in the order of 0.8 per cent (Moylan et al 1993).

Acute bradycardia due the oculocardiac reflex is another well-documented risk. This sudden fall in heart rate of >30 beats/min can occur with manipulation around the orbits and its occurrence in our experience is of the order of 10–15 per cent. In the majority of cases, this complication responds to cessation of the stimulus or vagolysis with atropine or glycopyrolate. However, one patient did not respond to standard treatment, became asystolic, and required adrenaline and external cardiac massage. Recovery in this instance was complete (Moylan et al 1993).

Postoperative care

INDICATIONS FOR INTENSIVE CARE

Improvements in anaesthetic and surgical techniques have led to a reduction in admission rate to our intensive care unit, from 64 per cent in 1986, to 6.5 per cent in 1989 (Moylan et al 1993). In more recent years, the percentage of craniofacial patients being admitted to intensive care postoperatively has continued to be less than 10 per cent. Improving expertise and confidence has meant that, despite the increasingly complex procedures being undertaken, the majority of children can be extubated at the end of the procedure. Postoperative care is performed by specialist medical and nursing staff on a neurosurgical high dependency unit, with the continued use of invasive monitoring allowing uninterrupted haemodynamic assessment.

At the end of the procedure, tissue swelling may be so great that it influences the decision to extubate or ventilate. Where airway swelling presents the potential for postoperative upper airway obstruction, such as where maxillary surgery has been undertaken, the insertion of bilateral nasopharyngeal airways has considerably reduced the need for prolonged intubation. These may be left *in situ* for up to seven days (in the case of facial bipartition surgery) or until the oedema has resolved.

Continued oedema and/or haematoma formation in the initial 48 hours is reduced by nursing these patients 'head-up'. When extensive facial surgery has been performed, 'frost sutures' may be necessary in order to temporarily close the palpebral fissures, to protect the cornea from the sequelae of postoperative swelling.

Previous studies at Great Ormond Street Hospital found that the indications for postoperative ventilation included body temperature <35°C, major intra-operative complications, or excessive length of surgery (Moylan et al 1993). We have recently found, in a series of patients undergoing facial bipartition surgery, that age is also an important factor determining the likelihood of a patient requiring intensive care treatment postoperatively. Patients under 14 months old had a higher risk of both major haemorrhage and the requirement for postoperative ventilation. In addition, in this age group, the difficulties of estimating and accurately replacing blood loss were also found to be greater.

FLUID MANAGEMENT

Large fluid losses continue into the immediate postoperative period, necessitating continuous careful monitoring of clinical parameters. It is not only accurate assessment of losses from surgical drains, haematoma formation and cerebrospinal fluid that needs to be monitored; some of these individuals may also be at risk of developing diabetes insipidus, which is thought to be related to the retraction of the frontal lobes required in some procedures (Poole 1988). As well as correcting any remaining fluid deficit, we aim to maintain a haematocrit of >25 per cent and a haemoglobin concentration of >8 g/dl. Problems associated with large volume replacement with crystalloid mixtures, such as hyponatraemia, have been reported, with patients becoming symptomatic in some instances (Wilkinson et al 1992). However, this should be avoidable by the use of isotonic solutions, and hypovolaemia remains the most common problem for these patients. A number of different perioperative regimens have been adopted at different centres. Our protocol (Appendix) has proved effective in our unit and a recent audit revealed no clinically shocked patients in recovery or on arrival in the high dependency unit or paediatric intensive care unit.

Postoperative fluid replacement consists of 50 per cent of calculated maintenance fluids using dextrose 4 per cent and saline 0.18 per cent for 24 hours, and replacement of ongoing losses with colloid solutions (colloidal gelatin). We try to minimise recipient exposure by

365

avoiding transfusion unless haemoglobin falls to less than 8 g/dl, and when blood transfusion is required we maximise the use of the unit even if it results in a raised haematocrit, in order to reduce the need for another transfusion in the postoperative period. Correction of coagulopathy is also essential to reduce haematoma formation postoperatively. Clotting screens are repeated after 80 ml/kg of volume replacement. Fresh frozen plasma, 10 ml/kg, is considered after rapid infusion of one circulating volume, and platelets, 5 ml/kg, depending on the platelet count. In a recent series of 20 cases where major craniofacial procedures were undertaken, we found that one or more clotting indices in postoperative blood specimens were outside the normal range in all the patients. Prothrombin time was the most frequently affected. Where two patients in this series received massive blood transfusions during procedures lasting in excess of 10 hours, an aprotonin infusion was also used postoperatively to aid haemostasis.

PAIN MANAGEMENT

Intra-operative analgesia is achieved in infants using fentanyl in doses of 5–10 µg/kg. This provides adequate analgesia for procedures during which surgical stimulus is extremely varied. Prior to emergence from anaesthesia, paracetamol, 30 mg/kg, and codeine suppositories, 1–1.5 mg/kg, are given. Diclofenac is also used, 1mg/kg, if not contraindicated by coagulopathy. Despite the extensive nature of the surgery, adequate analgesia is usually achieved via these means.

In older children, particularly if remifentanil has been used intra-operatively, a small bolus of intravenous morphine may be given at the end of the procedure, along with paracetamol and diclofenac suppositories. In a few instances, where older children have undergone major procedures, patient-controlled analgesia with morphine has been used, but this approach is not routinely required. In those who require postoperative ventilation, morphine infusions are instituted at the end of the procedure.

When bone grafts (such as iliac crest or rib grafts) have been taken, patients may require more analgesia than would be expected for the cranial aspect of the procedure alone. In these children, we use a bupivacaine infusion, 0.125 per cent at 0–3 ml/hr, direct to the donor site, via a fine bore catheter. This augments the additional systemic analgesia postoperatively.

Management of blood loss

Corrective surgery for many craniosynostosis patients is performed early. In primary craniosynostosis repair, the factor presenting greatest risk to the infant is blood loss and major transfusion, with patients frequently requiring transfusion of more than one circulating volume. Over a five-year period, in one centre, packed red cell transfusion was required in 96.3 per cent of patients. From 20 to 50 per cent of circulating volume can be lost over a 30-minute period in some instances (Meyer et al 1993). This degree of blood loss may be deemed by some as presenting a disproportionate risk where the indication for surgery is cosmesis alone.

Aside from the possibility of errors in cross-matching, the main immediate risks of transfusion include coagulopathy, hypocalcaemia, acidosis and hyperkalaemia. One study demonstrated significantly elevated potassium levels in 10/11 children undergoing craniofacial surgery (Brown et al 1990). The presence of hyperkalaemia has been associated with cardiac arrest in this group of patients (Buntain and Pabari 1999). The risk from hyperkalaemia is probably increased as a result of the coexisting metabolic acidosis and hypocalcaemia that may be present in these circumstances. The inadvertent infusion of high concentrations of potassium with massive blood transfusion has been avoided in some centres by routinely washing banked blood (Board 2000).

Other complications of massive transfusion include haemoglobinuria lasting for 24 hours, and skin rashes (Moylan et al 1993). It is not only these immediate risks that are of concern. The increasing awareness of the risks of transfusion-transmitted infections, amongst both the medical profession and the public, has led to concerns that unnecessary transfusion should be avoided wherever possible.

Assessment of blood loss in craniofacial surgery is particularly difficult because of the copious volumes of irrigation fluid used for the surgical power tools and the blood loss onto the surgical drapes. The methods normally employed, such as suction canister volumes and swab weights, are inaccurate in this setting. A variety of other suggestions have been advanced in the literature. These have included analysis of arterial waveforms, differential pressure, peripheral pulse waves, urinary output (Scholtes et al 1985) and preoperative and postoperative haematocrit measurements (Kearney et al 1989). Anaesthetists tend to underestimate blood loss (Faberowski et al 1999) but the risks of over-transfusion may also cause problems. The age of the patient was a strong predictor of over-transfusion of red cells in our recent series of 20 cases, with all three patients with excessive haematocrits being under 14 months old. This is similar to findings in other major craniofacial surgery series where slight over-transfusion occurred in 32 per cent (Meyer et al 1993).

Our patients are transfused according to vital signs including capillary refill, invasive-monitoring parameters (particularly arterial pressure waveform) and regular blood gas measurements (which provide base excess, haematocrit and haemoglobin concentration). We aim for a haemoglobin concentration of >8 g/dl at the conclusion of surgery. Significant blood loss is usually encountered as the scalp-flap is raised by the surgeon. Errors are still possible as large, rapid blood loss may require replacement over a short time to maintain patient stability.

VOLUME REPLACEMENT FLUIDS

Blood loss may be replaced with a number of different fluids, each of which has its own risks and benefits. Whole blood is the source of all blood products, but it is infrequently issued by blood banks and, despite containing clotting factors and platelets, these become inactive following one week of storage. Packed red cells are the most commonly issued blood product. These have been reduced by plasma removal and are leucocyte depleted to reduce incompatibility problems. Packed cell units have a haematocrit of 0.6–0.7.

As mentioned earlier, massive blood transfusion has a potential for numerous complications. Many of these can be reduced by meticulous documentation and checking prior to transfusion, and effective warming of the blood before it enters the patient. Initially the haemoglobin in transfused blood carries oxygen poorly, due to depleted 2, 3 diphosphoglycerate (DPG); it is 24 hours before 2, 3 DPG stores are replaced and the transfused blood functions optimally.

Crystalloid and colloid solutions are also transfused, either if red cells are not required, or to adjust the haematocrit to normal levels. Amongst the crystalloids available, dextrose-containing solutions should not be used unless there is a measured hypoglycaemia, as they can cause hyponatraemia and may increase the cerebral insult on reperfusion after spells of ischaemia. Balanced salt solutions (e.g. Hartmann's solution or 0.9 per cent saline) are the preferred crystalloid fluids. These solutions expand the extracellular fluid and move into interstitial and plasma spaces in varying amounts, depending on their osmolarity. Colloidal solutions contain molecules which are retained in the intravascular space, and produce a greater initial expansion of this compartment. There is constant debate as to which fluid is most effective in given circumstances. Theoretically, colloid should be the natural choice to replace blood loss, as it remains in the vascular space in greater volumes and for a longer duration. However, given in sufficient volume crystalloid should have the same effect and, since in acute haemorrhage the extracellular space may be depleted by fluid moving into the vascular compartment, crystalloid may prevent depletion of extracellular fluid more effectively than colloid. Other issues may be important for particular individuals, for example colloids have the potential to trigger an allergic reaction in some instances.

AVOIDANCE OF TRANSFUSION

In recent years the concern of infection risk relating to blood transfusion has increased, and a number of suggestions have been put forward in an attempt to reduce transfusion requirement. First, preoperative measures can be taken, including erythropoietin stimulation to raise haemoglobin concentration and autologous blood donation.

Erythropoietin has been used in the past for the treatment of anaemia and for stimulating red cell production prior to autologous donation. Preoperative erythropoietin has been used in a number of major procedures including scoliosis surgery. In craniofacial surgery it has been shown to have a place in certain situations. It has formed part of protocols in some centres for older Jehovah's Witness children in whom transfusion is unacceptable (Polley et al 1994). Given three times a week, beginning three weeks prior to surgery, in otherwise healthy children, it acts to increase haematocrit and reduces the requirement for transfusion (Helfaer et al 1998). It has also been suggested that the increased viscosity directly reduces blood loss. In this study, however, 64 per cent of those receiving erythropoietin also received blood, making cost-effectiveness an issue.

Preoperative autologous blood donation may be employed along with erythropoietin treatment, but presents a number of problems. First, small children (<30 kg) cannot donate blood, as their small circulating volume does not permit loss of a clinically useful amount of blood. Second, the blood donated only remains available for 28 days, making the scheduling of surgery difficult; and lastly, the resulting administrative changes may increase the cost prohibitively. In addition, blood loss needs to be anticipated in order for prior donation to be cost-effective, but, in reality, blood loss is often unpredictable. Autologous blood donation does not avoid all the risks of blood transfusion. Infection from bacterial contamination, non-haemolytic reactions or a mishap with labelling are still possible.

However, possible protocols for preoperative and intra-operative donation have been explored in 11 infants undergoing craniofacial surgery (Longatti et al 1991), and it remains a possibility for the future.

Intra-operative measures to reduce the need for transfusion include induced hypotension, scalp infiltration, acute normovolaemic haemodilution and intra-operative blood-salvage techniques (Tatum 1999), as well as meticulous attention to haemostasis by the surgeon.

Hypotension may be used to limit blood loss and present a clearer surgical field for the procedure. Practice is varied, as hypotension presents significant risks, and opinion as to its effectiveness varies. It is only employed in the absence of any contraindicating disease, such as a coexisting cardiac anomaly. It requires careful monitoring of intravascular volume to avoid any spells of hypovolaemia leading to poor organ perfusion. Cerebral ischaemia is a potential risk with hypotensive techniques, so excessive hyperventilation is avoided and tissue perfusion is monitored with frequent arterial blood gas analyses. We do not employ controlled hypotension in infants undergoing synostosis repair, beyond that caused by anaesthesia and 'head-up' tilt. The role of formal induced hypotension in craniosynostosis repair is unclear (Diaz and Lockhart 1979). It could compromise cerebral perfusion where intracranial pressure is unpredictable

In the older child undergoing major midfacial procedures we do induce a moderate degree of hypotension, using a combination of clonidine and remifentanyl infusions. However, in the past, other centres have used a variety of agents, including nitroglycerin, propranolol, labetalol, pentolinium or sodium nitroprusside.

Scalp infiltration is frequently employed and has been shown to reduce bleeding; however the majority of surgical blood loss is from the bone and periosteum (Eaton et al 1995). We routinely employ surgical infiltration of the subcutaneous tissue with a combination of bupivacaine, lidocaine, hyalase and adrenaline (Neil-Dwyer et al 2001).

Acute normovolaemic haemodilution has not been shown to reduce either the incidence of blood transfusion or the volume of other fluids required in patients undergoing surgical correction of craniosynostosis (Hans et al 2000). It has been successfully used for other procedures, such as infant liver resection, with a degree of success (Schaller et al 1984). However, its use is limited by the small circulating volume and relatively low preoperative haematocrit in the majority of patients.

Intra-operative blood-salvage techniques have been limited in the past by unfamiliarity with the technique and concerns regarding re-infusing thromboplastic material from brain tissue (Velardi et al 1999). Recently, interest has increased, as more sophisticated blood-salvage systems have become available. Blood-salvage is unable to cope with the rapid and massive volume replacement requirements of infants undergoing craniofacial surgery (Meyer et al 1993). However, there may be a role for blood-salvage in older children, and we are increasingly employing this technique; and with the increasing cost of blood it is cost-effective if the transfusion of one unit of blood is avoided.

While these techniques may reduce transfusion requirements in certain patient groups, they have not been effective in reliably reducing the incidence or volume of transfusion required.

Patients do fall into 'risk groups' for transfusion despite normal haematological parameters preoperatively. Transfusion requirements have been shown to differ between surgeons and anaesthetists. This may be expected as surgical technique, dexterity and speed may affect blood loss. However, in one study, the factor most likely to determine the magnitude of any intra-operative transfusion was not primarily the surgeon or the suture involved, but the anaesthetist (Eaton et al 1995). Age is also a risk factor for large volume blood loss (Meyer et al 1993). In our recent series of facial bipartition patients, replacement with blood volumes greater than circulating volumes was required in four patients (20 per cent). All of these patients were less than 14 months old.

MANAGEMENT OF COAGULOPATHY

Massive transfusion is associated with coagulopathy. A prescriptive view of coagulation factor replacement has suggested that coagulation profiles should be checked after a transfusion of 40 ml/kg, and fresh frozen plasma should be given depending on coagulation results (Wilkinson et al 1992). This study also suggested that a blood loss in excess of 40 ml/kg would lead to difficulties in achieving haemostasis. Others believe that loss of as little as 30 per cent of estimated blood volume should prompt the administration of fresh frozen plasma (Imberti et al 1990). However, some authors suggest the empirical transfusion of 20 ml/kg of fresh frozen plasma only once a whole blood volume has been lost (Orliaguet et al 1998). Indeed, a previous audit of our practice demonstrated that, provided tissue perfusion is maintained, coagulopathy is not a major problem until at least one circulating volume has been lost. This is also the experience of other centres (Eaton et al 1995).

Summary and conclusions

Craniofacial patients, with their complex airway and associated anomalies, present anaesthetists with a number of challenges. These require meticulous preoperative assessment and planning by the anaesthetist as part of an interdisciplinary team. The physical risks and psychological aspects of surgery that is sometimes for cosmesis alone must not be forgotten. The surgical procedures themselves pose specific intra-operative problems for airway management and may result in large volume blood loss that is difficult to assess accurately, especially in the infant. The increasing awareness of the risks of blood transfusion means that, in the future, techniques such as intra-operative blood-salvage may be increasingly utilised. Where blood loss is large and rapid, metabolic disturbances and coagulopathy may further complicate the situation. While improvements in anaesthesia have reduced the demand for postoperative intensive care, these patients still require specialist care on a neurosurgical high dependency ward for continued assessment and treatment following surgery.

Appendix: Craniofacial unit protocol for postoperative fluid replacement

Aim:

- Maintain normal circulating blood volume by continuous assessment and reassessment of fluid balance:
  - Give maintenance fluid
  - Replace fluid losses:
    - **Blood:** drain losses, haematoma
    - Urine: losses may be excessive with diabetes insipidus
    - CSF

Maintenance fluid:

- 4% dextrose 0.18% dextrose. **Give 50% of full maintenance for the first 24 hours**

Moderate blood loss <10 ml/kg/hr

- Measure losses at **half-hourly** intervals and replace at the appropriate **hourly** rate (if 25 ml blood lost in first half hour, replace at a rate of 50 ml/hr). Monitor hourly fluid balance to avoid over/under-transfusion.
- Measure haematocrit after each 20ml/kg of infusion.
- **Replace with blood or colloid to maintain haemoglobin >8 g/dl (haematocrit >24).**
- 4 ml/kg packed cells raises Hb by approximately 1g/dl (hct by approx 3). Minimise donor exposure when blood is used (if used, make full use of a pack of blood – transfuse to Hb approx 12g/dl, avoid opening a new pack unless necessary).

Massive blood losses >10ml/kg/hr

Occasionally, massive postoperative blood loss may occur. It is important to keep up with transfusion to maintain the circulating blood volume and haematocrit.

Use plasma reduced blood (hct approx 60%) +/or colloid (Gelofusine).

- **If Hb 10–12 g/dl**   give blood:colloid 1:1

i.e. if blood loss 100 ml, give 50 ml blood, 50 ml colloid

- **If Hb >12 g/dl**   give blood:colloid approx 1:2

i.e. if blood loss 100 ml, give 30 ml blood, 70 ml colloid

- **If Hb <10 g/dl**   give blood:colloid approx 2:1

i.e. if blood loss 100 ml, give 70 ml blood, 30 ml colloid

- **Measure clotting** after each 80 ml/kg of infusion (i.e. after infusion of estimated blood volume, EBV).
- FFP 10 ml/kg is usually required after rapid transfusion of 1 EBV.
- Platelets 5 ml/kg usually required after transfusion of 2 EBV.

Hypovolaemia is the most common problem after craniofacial surgery

Signs:	Tachycardia
	Delayed capillary refill (>2 seconds)
	Cool, mottled peripheries
	Hypotension – this is a late sign
Immediate treatment:	**Give an immediate fluid bolus of 10 ml/kg**
	Reassess and repeat as necessary

REFERENCES

Anderson PJ, Harkness WJ, Taylor W, Jones BM, Hayward RD (1997) Anomalous venous drainage in a case of non-syndromic craniosynostosis. *Childs Nerv Syst* 13: 97–100.

Argamaso RV (1992) Glossopexy for upper airway obstruction in Robin sequence. *Cleft Palate Craniofac J* 29: 232–238.

Blanco G, Melman E, Cuairan V, Moyao D, Ortiz-Monasterio F (2001) Fibreoptic nasal intubation in children with anticipated and unanticipated difficult intubation. *Paediatr Anaesth* 11: 49–53.

Board J (2000) Hyperkalaemia and massive transfusion. *Anaesth Intensive Care* 28: 111 (Letter.)

Brown KA, Bissonnette B, MacDonald M, Poon AO (1990) Hyperkalaemia during massive blood transfusion in paediatric craniofacial surgery. *Can J Anaesth* 37: 401–408.

Buntain SG, Pabari M (1999) Massive transfusion and hyperkalaemic cardiac arrest in craniofacial surgery in a child. *Anaesth Intensive Care* 27: 530–533.

Diaz JH, Lockhart CH (1979) Hypotensive anaesthesia for craniectomy in infancy. *Br J Anaesth* 51: 233–235.

Eaton AC, Marsh JL, Pilgram TK (1995) Transfusion requirements for craniosynostosis surgery in infants. *Plast Reconstr Surg* 95: 277–283.

Elmslie FV, Reardon W (1998) Craniofacial developmental abnormalities. *Curr Opin Neurol* 11: 103–108.

Faberowski LW, Black S, Mickle JP (1999) Blood loss and transfusion practice in the perioperative management of craniosynostosis repair. *J Neurosurg Anesthesiol* 11: 167–172.

Gallagher DM, Hyler RL, Epker BN (1980) Hemifacial microsomia: an anesthetic airway problem. *Oral Surg Oral Med Oral Pathol* 49: 2–4.

Handler SD, Beaugard ME, Whitaker LA, Potsic WP (1979) Airway management in the repair of craniofacial defects. *Cleft Palate J* 16: 16–23.

Hans P, Collin V, Bonhomme V, Damas F, Born JD, Lamy M (2000) Evaluation of acute normovolemic hemodilution for surgical repair of craniosynostosis. *J Neurosurg Anesthesiol* 12: 33–36.

Helfaer MA, Carson BS, James CS, Gates J, Della-Lana D, Vander Kolk C (1998) Increased hematocrit and decreased transfusion requirements in children given erythropoietin before undergoing craniofacial surgery. *J Neurosurg* 88: 704–708.

Imberti R, Locatelli D, Fanzio M, Bonfanti N, Preseglio I (1990) Intra- and postoperative management of craniosynostosis. *Can J Anaesth* 37: 948–950.

Jones BM, Jani P, Bingham RM, Mackersie AM, Hayward R (1992) Complications in paediatric craniofacial surgery: an initial four year experience. *Br J Plast Surg* 45: 225–231.

Kang JK, Lee SW, Baik MW, Son BC, Hong YK, Jung CK, Ryu KH (1998) Perioperative specific management of blood volume loss in craniosynostosis surgery. *Childs Nerv Syst* 14: 297–301.

Kearney RA, Rosales JK, Howes WJ (1989) Craniosynostosis: an assessment of blood loss and transfusion practices. *Can J Anaesth* 36: 473–477.

Kreiborg S, Aduss H, Cohen MM Jr (1999) Cephalometric study of the Apert syndrome in adolescence and adulthood. *J Craniofac Genet Dev Biol* 19: 1–11.

Lauritzen C, Lilja J, Jarlstedt J (1986) Airway obstruction and sleep apnea in children with craniofacial anomalies. *Plast Reconstr Surg* 77: 1–6.

Lefebvre A, Barclay S (1982) Psychosocial impact of craniofacial deformities before and after reconstructive surgery. *Can J Psychiatry* 27: 579–584.

Longatti PL, Paccagnella F, Agostini S, Nieri A, Carteri A (1991) Autologous hemodonation in the corrective surgery of craniostenosis. *Childs Nerv Syst* 7: 40–42.

McGill T (1991) Otolaryngologic aspects of Apert syndrome. *Clin Plast Surg* 18: 309–313.

Meyer P, Renier D, Arnaud E, Jarreau MM, Charron B, Buy E, Buisson C, Barrier G (1993) Blood loss during repair of craniosynostosis. *Br J Anaesth* 71: 854–857.

Mixter RC, David DJ, Perloff WH, Green CG, Pauli RM, Popic PM (1990) Obstructive sleep apnea in Apert's and Pfeiffer's syndromes: more than a craniofacial abnormality. *Plast Reconstr Surg* 86: 457–463.

Moore MH (1993) Upper airway obstruction in the syndromal craniosynostoses. *Br J Plast Surg* 46: 355–362.

Moylan S, Collee G, Mackersie A, Bingham R (1993) Anaesthetic management in paediatric craniofacial surgery. A review of 126 cases. *Paediatr Anaesth* 3: 275–281.

Neil-Dwyer JG, Evans RD, Jones BM, Hayward RD (2001) Tumescent steroid infiltration to reduce postoperative swelling after craniofacial surgery. *Br J Plast Surg* 54: 565–569.

372

Orliaguet GA, Meyer PG, Blanot S, Jarreau MM, Charron B, Cuttaree H, Perie AC, Carli PA, Renier D (1998) Non-invasive aortic blood flow measurement in infants during repair of craniosynostosis. *Br J Anaesth* 81: 696–701.

Palmisano BW, Rusy LM (2002) Anesthesia for plastic surgery. In: Gregory GA, editor. *Pediatric Anaesthesia*. London: Churchill Livingstone.

Parke TJ, Stevens JE, Rice AS, Greenaway CL, Bray RJ, Smith PJ, Waldmann CS, Verghese C (1992) Metabolic acidosis and fatal myocardial failure after propofol infusion in children: five case reports. *BMJ* 305: 613–616.

Polley JW, Berkowitz RA, McDonald TB, Cohen M, Figueroa A, Penney DW (1994) Craniomaxillofacial surgery in the Jehovah's Witness patient. *Plast Reconstr Surg* 93(6): 1258–1263.

Poole MD (1988) Complications in craniofacial surgery. Br J Plast Surg 41: 608–613.

Reich DL, Konstadt SN, Nejat M, Abrams HP, Bucek J (1993) Intraoperative transesophageal echocardiography for the detection of cardiac preload changes induced by transfusion and phlebotomy in pediatric patients. *Anesthesiology* 79: 10–15.

Roche J, Frawley G, Heggie A (2002) Difficult tracheal intubation induced by maxillary distraction devices in craniosynostosis syndromes. *Paediatr Anaesth* 12: 227–234.

Schaller RT Jr, Schaller J, Furman EB (1984) The advantages of hemodilution anesthesia for major liver resection in children. *J Pediatr Surg* 19: 705–710.

Scholtes JL, Thauvoy C, Moulin D, Gribomont BF (1985) Craniofaciosynostosis: anesthetic and perioperative management. Report of 71 operations. *Acta Anaesthesiol Belg* 36: 176–185.

Sher AE (1992) Mechanisms of airway obstruction in Robin sequence: implications for treatment. *Cleft Palate Craniofac J* 29: 224–231.

Sher AE, Shprintzen RJ, Thorpy MJ (1986) Endoscopic observations of obstructive sleep apnea in children with anomalous upper airways: predictive and therapeutic value. *Int J Pediatr Otorhinolaryngol* 11: 135–146.

Shprintzen RJ (1982) Palatal and pharyngeal anomalies in craniofacial syndromes. *Birth Defects Orig Artic Ser* 18: 53–78.

Shprintzen RJ (1992) The implications of the diagnosis of Robin sequence. *Cleft Palate Craniofac J* 29: 205–209.

Tatum SA (1999) Advances in congenital craniofacial surgery. *Facial Plast Surg* 15: 33–43.

Thompson D, Jones B, Hayward R, Harkness W (1994) Assessment and treatment of craniosynostosis. *Br J Hosp Med* 52: 17–24.

Thompson DN, Hayward RD, Harkness WJ, Bingham RM, Jones BM (1995) Lessons from a case of kleeblattschadel. *J Neurosurg* 82: 1071–1074.

Velardi F, Di Chirico A, Di Rocco C (1999) Blood salvage in craniosynostosis surgery. *Childs Nerv Syst* 15: 695–710.

Whitaker LA, Munro IR, Salyer KE, Jackson IT, Ortiz-Monasterio F, Marchac D (1979) Combined report of problems and complications in 793 craniofacial operations. *Plast Reconstr Surg* 64: 198–203.

Wilkinson E, Rieff J, Rekate HL, Beals S (1992) Fluid, blood, and blood product management in the craniofacial patient. *Pediatr Neurosurg* 18: 48–52.

Wolf WJ, Neal MB, Peterson MD (1986) The hemodynamic and cardiovascular effects of isoflurane and halothane anesthesia in children. *Anesthesiology* 64: 328–333.

19
SURGERY

Barry Jones, David Dunaway and Richard Hayward

Introduction

Surgery plays an important part in the management of children with craniosynostosis. Craniofacial osteotomies (bone cuts) may be indicated to correct deformity and to treat functional problems associated with raised intracranial pressure, exorbitism or obstruction of the airways. When premature suture fusion restricts head growth and results in an elevation of intracranial pressure, expansion of the vault may be indicated, while advancement of part or all of the orbito-malar-maxillary complex may protect exposed eyes and enlarge a restricted nasopharyngeal airway.

Deciding on when to carry out a particular procedure may be more problematical than deciding which operation is most appropriate. Where surgery is performed to treat functional impairment, the severity and progression of the pathological process will usually dictate when to intervene. The timing of surgery to correct deformity presents more of a dilemma. There is a natural desire, both among doctors and among parents, to produce the best possible appearance at the earliest possible age so that normal psychological and social development may be facilitated. However, any surgical intervention may affect subsequent growth. Following a cranial vault expansion, this influence may be positive in relieving raised intracranial pressure, but when operations affecting the face precede skeletal maturity the effect more frequently is negative. In addition, surgery cannot prevent the continuing abnormal growth that might be associated with the ongoing effects of whatever primary genetic abnormality has been responsible for the deformity in the first place (see Chapter 3). Injudicious surgical timing can, therefore, compound rather than ameliorate the effects of the primary disease process and it is necessary to temper natural, well-motivated enthusiasm with the experience of long-term case analysis. This presents an obvious problem in that an average senior (consultant) surgical career spans approximately 25 years and the period from birth to facial skeletal maturity is 17 years. Consequently there is only a relatively short period for any surgeon to assess the effects of his or her own decision making and integrate this with technical advances.

Technically the best time to correct a deformity is when growth of the affected part is complete. Growth is not uniform and continues in different parts of the craniofacial skeleton for varying lengths of time at different rates (see Chapter 1). It is therefore reasonable to consider undertaking surgery to the calvarium early in life since its most rapid growth phase, by far, is during the first year, while surgery to finalise the correction of a mandibular deformity should usually be postponed until the age of 17 years or later.

Physical and technical considerations must always be balanced with the general and emotional well-being of the patient as well as their educational and social needs, so that waiting until the completion of growth may not be practical for some because of intervening functional or psychological problems. It is, nevertheless, always important to bear in mind that when surgery, particularly facial surgery, is performed early, it is frequently necessary to repeat or revise the procedure later in order to achieve the best end result.

The aim of this chapter is to provide a brief description of the more common procedures employed to treat the craniofacial disorders most often associated with craniosynostosis and also explain the rationale for their use. It is not intended to duplicate standard surgical texts, nor to argue for one procedure over another. Instead it should be considered an overview of present techniques with a bias towards those procedures in most common use in our unit.

Most craniofacial operations are based around osteotomies, i.e. they involve cutting and repositioning elements of the facial and/or cranial skeleton to restore normal form and function, and it is these that are described in most detail. Very frequently soft tissue procedures are involved also, either simultaneously or subsequent to the skeletal surgery, but they are beyond the scope of this chapter and are mostly described in standard plastic surgery texts.

Craniofacial surgery

The development of modern craniofacial surgery was initiated by the French plastic surgeon Paul Tessier during the 1950s although he did not publish his work until 1967 (Tessier 1967). He had studied in England with Sir Harold Gillies who had published the Le Fort III osteotomy in 1951 (and is reputed to have commented 'Do not do it it's too difficult'). Tessier's interest was sparked when, as a surgeon performing mainly burns and eyelid operations, a young man with what he described as 'terrible facial deformities' arrived in his consulting room. Although he did not know this at the time, the deformities were caused by Crouzon syndrome. Existing techniques were inadequate to produce a worthwhile improvement and so by a careful study of the work of others (such as Gillies) and painstaking anatomical dissection and analysis he sought a solution. The result was the creation of craniofacial surgery as a specialty based on sound principles that permitted safe and effective surgery. These fundamental principles remain:

1   The establishment of a group, or team, of specialists to treat these complex conditions on a relatively frequent basis.
2   Wide exposure of the craniofacial skeleton through cosmetically acceptable incisions minimising visible scars.
3   The use of bone grafts to fill skeletal defects and support bones in a new position so preventing relapse and recurrent deformity.
4   The recognition that large sections of calvarial bone can be removed (split if necessary into inner and outer tables) and successfully replaced as bone grafts.
5   Finally – and crucially – since the anterior cranial fossa floor and the orbital roof are the same structure, a transcranial approach will simultaneously facilitate complex manipulation of the craniofacial skeleton and protection of the brain.

It was the application of these principles that led to the wide adoption during the 1970s of a variety of craniofacial procedures to treat both 'simple' (single suture) and complex (multi-suture and syndrome-associated) forms of craniosynostosis. At first the facial surgery was confined to the Le Fort III procedure and derivatives of it, but with experience the scale of the surgery was expanded to include the monobloc frontofacial advance and the facial bipartition. To these have now been added the knowledge gained since the application of distraction techniques to craniofacial surgery.

THE GENERAL PRINCIPLES OF CRANIOFACIAL SURGERY
These may be considered under the following headings:

- Access (incisions)
- Neurosurgical considerations
- Fixation of osteotomies
- Bone grafts

Access and incisions
In order to carry out craniofacial osteotomies it is necessary to gain access to the skeleton. This may be via a variety of routes, which can be combined as necessary.

Exposure is usually gained through incisions in cosmetically favourable areas that afford the best possible visualisation of osteotomy sites while limiting the undesirable effects of cutaneous scarring. These incisions are often distant from the area to be operated upon. We have found that postoperative swelling can be very significantly reduced, and dissection facilitated by infiltrating the facial and scalp soft tissues with a 'tumescent', weight-related volume of a solution containing Hartman's solution, triamcinolone, hyalase, adrenaline, lignocaine (xylocaine) and bupivicaine (marcaine) (Table 19.1).

The most commonly used incisions are:

- Coronal
- Palpebral (eyelids)
- Intra-oral

TABLE 19.1
'Tumescent' solution for the reduction of peroperative bleeding and postoperative swelling

Drug	Concentration	Dose
HARTMAN'S	–	500 ml
XYLOCAINE	1% with adrenaline 1:200,000	10 ml
MARCAINE	0.25%	20 ml
ADRENALINE	1:1000	1 ml
HYALASE	1:500 iu	1 ml
TRIAMCINOLONE (KENALOG)	40 mg/ml	1.25 ml

Note: 7 ml/kilo (body weight) to be injected along the incision and into all facial areas likely to be affected by postoperative swelling

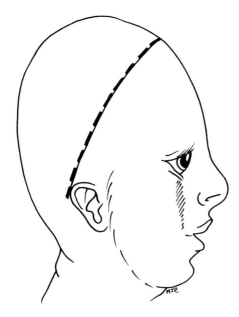

Fig. 19.1 Coronal incision. We now favour this angled 'Alice band' position over a zig-zag as we have found that it leaves a less conspicuous scar.

The coronal incision. This incision extends over the vertex of the scalp, from one ear to the other, following the line of an 'Alice band' (Fig. 19.1). The initial dissection is in the subgaleal plane and is deepened subperiosteally about 1 cm above the orbits to protect the supraorbital and supratrochlear nerves. The frontal skin, muscle and periosteum can be reflected downwards as a flap to expose the forehead and orbits. The incision and dissection may be extended to allow access to the malar body and arch. It is possible to reach the pterygo-maxillary junction and upper buccal sulcus in this way although not under direct vision. A posterior flap may also be raised to expose the remainder of the calvarium when necessary. If an operation is planned which breaches the nasal roof/anterior cranial fossa floor junction, a vascularised pericranial flap is preserved and used later to line the anterior fossa and cover bone grafts.

This incision is well hidden within the hair and so is generally cosmetically acceptable. Although alopecia should not occur around the scar, hair will not grow within it, so if stretching develops it may become noticeable particularly when the hair is wet or thin. In craniofacial surgery the coronal incision is often used to facilitate some sort of cranial or facial advancement, which will inevitably result in skin tension and make stretching of the scar more likely than in such aesthetic surgical procedures as brow or subperiosteal facelifts. As a consequence several modifications have been described. Most popular is an incision zig-zagged laterally so that the fall of the hair will conceal the scar. At Great Ormond Street we have not found this reliable as it results too often in a stretched zig-zagged scar, so we now favour a sinuous incision that starts in the post-auricular region and extends obliquely as it runs upwards and anteriorly, allowing the scar to be masked more effectively by the hair. The wide exposure afforded by the coronal incision makes it the primary approach for craniofacial access. Healing is generally quick and reliable but parasthesiae (tingling, 'pins and needles') and fomication (itching) are common during the first six postoperative months or so. If these symptoms are distressing, antihistamines may be helpful and occasionally Amitryptiline may be required.

Palpebral incisions. The common eyelid incisions (Fig. 19.2) are:

- Subciliary
- Subconjuctival – with or without a lateral canthotomy
- Upper lid incisions

These incisions provide access to the periorbital skeleton and orbit. Exposure is limited and wound extension cannot be readily achieved. The cornea must always be carefully protected to avoid abrasion. The subciliary is the most frequently used approach as it provides good visualisation of the inferior orbital margin, lateral orbital wall and orbital floor and leaves an imperceptible scar. Its major disadvantage lies in the risk of ectropion or scleral show if middle lamella contracture occurs. Canthopexy or canthoplasty should always be considered for support, and a Frost suture (a suture between the lower eyelid and eyebrow) for 48 hours may be helpful.

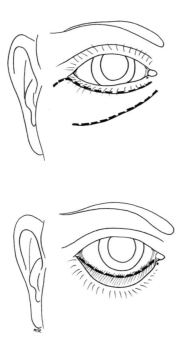

Fig. 19.2 Three eyelid incisions. From above down: subciliary, infraorbital and subconjunctival.

378

The transconjunctival approach provides good visualisation of the orbital floor with no visible scar and a much reduced ectropion risk. The technique is simple to master, and while a plethora of specialised instruments is described to facilitate it they are not necessary. The incision need not be sutured (healing is very fast) and ointments must *not* be put into the eye or paraffin granulomas may result.

Upper lid (supratarsal) incisions are not commonly used in craniofacial surgery but they may improve visualisation of the orbital roof and lachrymal gland, and may facilitate canthopexy.

Intraoral incisions. Intraoral incisions can be made in the upper or lower buccal sulcus. The upper buccal sulcus incision enables access to the maxilla, infraorbital region, malar body and anterior aspect of the malar arch, while the inferior exposes the anterior mandible. When using these approaches it is important to leave a cuff of mucosa on the alveolar aspect of the incision to facilitate suture closure and, in the lower buccal sulcus, to repair very carefully the mentalis musculature so as to avoid lower lip incompetence.

Incisions through or around the palatal mucosa are occasionally required to gain access to the hard palate. Although generally well tolerated and rarely causing functional problems, care must be taken to avoid damaging the teeth or producing palatal fistula through post-operative mucosal breakdown.

Neurosurgical considerations

Protection of the brain, meninges and venous sinuses is crucial in all craniofacial operations. Burr holes are usually used to access the extradural space dura and separate the dura from the overlying bone. They should be sited so as not to be visible as concavities in the overlying skin postoperatively and are best placed beneath the temporalis muscles laterally and relatively high medially but not in the low frontal (forehead) region. They may be usefully filled in with bone dust at the end of the procedure.

Dural lacerations should be carefully avoided and when they do occur they must be meticulously repaired. A postoperative CSF leak adds considerably to surgical morbidity, and a dural defect beneath a calvarial bone defect may lead to a 'growing fracture', particularly in the presence of raised intracranial pressure. When a difficult dural dissection has been predicted preoperatively a prophylactic lumbar drain should be considered. Bleeding from dural venous sinuses can be catastrophic and particular difficulties may be encountered in the region of the torcula and sigmoid/lateral sinus junctions and in children with raised intracranial pressure. It should be remembered that in the dysostosis syndromes there may be abnormal intracranial venous drainage leading to a major proportion of the cerebral circulation draining via per-osseous emissary veins rather than through the sigmoid-jugular complex (see Chapter 8). Interruption of such veins may produce uncontrollable cerebral oedema and when their presence has been predicted it is sensible to consider imaging the venous anatomy preoperatively using (for example) MR (magnetic resonance) venography. The dura should be exposed for as short a time as possible during surgery, over-zealous retraction of the underlying brain must be avoided, and protection from saws and osteotomies ensured by using stainless steel malleable retractors (copper alloy may be damaged by power tools leaving metal filings with the potential to produce sensitivity reactions).

Fixation of osteotomies

In common with most other types of bony surgery, craniofacial osteotomies must be fixed securely to prevent unwanted movement, facilitate bony union and avoid relapse. Such fixation may be either internal or external. Generally, rigid internal fixation of bones in their new positions is preferred, using wires, or specially designed titanium plates and screws, which are inert, mechanically ideal, strong and of low profile. Such hardware rarely causes problems postoperatively though it can make secondary surgery more difficult and thus increase its morbidity.

Occasionally, wires, plates and screws may become palpable through the skin, and when used in the cranial vault of very young children they can, as a result of differential bone growth and absorption, 'migrate' over time through both tables of the skull until the screws eventually rest on the dura. Although this rarely results in serious consequences it is clearly undesirable and, in an attempt to avoid it, dissolving plates and screws made from polylactic or polyglycolic acid polymers have recently been marketed. They are still in a relatively early stage of development but they have proved useful, especially in surgery for infants where stresses are relatively small and long-term problems most likely. Unfortunately, they are much more bulky than their titanium counterparts, less rigid and take a long time to dissolve, although in the future it is hoped that such disadvantages will be overcome.

Bone grafts

Autologous bone grafts are essential to bridge bony gaps created by the advancement or expansion of the craniofacial skeleton (except when this is achieved by distraction osteogenesis).

The common sites for harvest of bone grafts are:

- Calvarium (split or full thickness)
- Hip (inner and outer table of ilium)
- Rib
- Tibia

Calvarium. The calvarium has many advantages as a bone graft donor site for craniofacial surgery: it is in the operating field; in most individuals over the age of 8 years the bone can be split into inner and outer tables allowing one half to be used as a graft and the other to be replaced to fill the donor site; and, in general, membranous bone appears to survive more reliably as a free graft. However, the volume of bone available is limited, and in many dysostosis syndromes it may not be possible to split the bone because it is too thin, relatively brittle and difficult to mould.

Hip. The ilium can provide a considerable volume of malleable, cancellous bone. A scar at the donor site is inevitable, although this should be relatively discreet if carefully positioned beneath the iliac crest. The crest must be reconstructed following the harvesting of the graft to avoid a noticeable defect, but the wing of the ilium can be easily split into inner and outer tables to provide a robust combination of cancellous and cortical bone to fill craniofacial bone defects and reconstruct the nose and malar arches. A major disadvantage of using the hip is postoperative pain, and disability due to difficulty walking may be considerable for a month or so.

Rib. Ribs are too flimsy to make them reliable as a bone graft donor site, and the resulting scar on the chest is always visible. The one useful contribution of this site is as a graft for the nasal dorsum when costal cartilage is included for the nasal tip.

Tibia. The tibia is used infrequently for bone grafting in craniofacial operations, but when much bone is needed and stock is limited it can be very useful as a source of both cancellous and cortical bone. The residual defect is relatively small and no functional defect should result.

The operations most commonly employed in craniosynostosis surgery

CLASSIFICATION
The relevant procedures can be classified according to the region of the skeleton that they address:

1 Cranial vault/forehead/supraorbital
These operations include simple strip craniectomies and more formal vault remodelling such as the fronto-orbital advancement, and various vault expansion procedures.

2 Subcranial
Subcranial procedures are limited to the facial skeleton. They may involve parts or all of the orbito-malar-maxillary complex (the 'midface'), and the mandible. Their discussion will be limited to those midfacial osteotomies most commonly used in the treatment of craniofacial dysostosis:

- Le Fort I, II, III osteotomies to address antero-posterior and vertical deficiencies in the facial skeleton.
- Subcranial hypertelorism corrections.

3 Craniofacial
Craniofacial osteotomies involve surgery to both the cranial and facial skeleton simultaneously. They are demanding and complicated procedures and have a particular risk of complications since they inevitably transgress the barrier between the anterior cranial fossa and the nose, nasopharynx and nasal sinuses.
    They may be further subdivided into:

- Osteotomies to address antero-posterior and vertical anomalies only – the 'monobloc' procedure.
- Osteotomies to address lateral or vertical anomalies of the orbits – such as the orbital box osteotomy.
- Osteotomies which address three-dimensional anomalies of the skull, face and orbits – the facial bipartition.
- Distraction osteogenesis

OPERATIONS ON THE CRANIAL VAULT, FOREHEAD AND UPPER ORBITAL REGION

This group of procedures is designed to alter the morphology of the cranial vault and forehead. They are performed through a coronal incision and may be required for both functional and aesthetic reasons. They are the mainstay of treatment for single suture synostosis and may play an important part in the early management of craniofacial dysostoses (e.g. Crouzon and Apert syndrome) and multisutural craniosynostosis when a reduced intracranial volume is associated with raised intracranial pressure (see Chapter 8). They will be described under the conditions for which they are most commonly used.

Scaphocephaly

Sagittal synostosis results in scaphocephaly (a long narrow cranium). Commonly, there is an associated frontal bossing and temporal hollowing producing a 'peanut head' appearance. Scaphocephaly is usually an isolated synostosis, not associated with functional problems, and correction is undertaken for cosmetic reasons. Occasionally, however, it may be part of a dysostosis syndrome (particularly Crouzon syndrome) that may not have been apparent at the initial presentation.

The first operations described for sagittal synostosis were strip craniectomies involving simply the excision and then discarding of the fused sagittal suture. This procedure relies on future brain growth, unrestricted by the synostosed suture, to normalise the head shape before full reconstitution of the removed bone occurs. It must be performed while the calvarial bones are malleable and a significant amount of brain growth has still to occur – at the latest by the age of 6 months. Its effects, however, are limited, not least because calvarial bone regenerates so rapidly from the osteogenically potent pericranium and dura of the infant head. Recognition of its limitations has resulted in the evolution of more complicated and extensive variants, usually involving wider craniectomies combined with some manoeuvre designed to shorten the antero-posterior dimension of the skull while widening it laterally (a biparietal plication, or – as we now favour – a modified 'pi' procedure – see Fig. 19.3).

If surgery is not carried out within the first six months or so of life the operations required for the correction of scaphocephaly become significantly more extensive since it is no longer possible to harness the moulding effect of a rapidly growing brain on malleable cranial bone. A full reconstruction now involves the removal of all the bones of the calvarium, their reshaping and then their replacement in, it is hoped, an improved configuration. Such an operation inevitably has a significantly higher potential morbidity than surgery performed

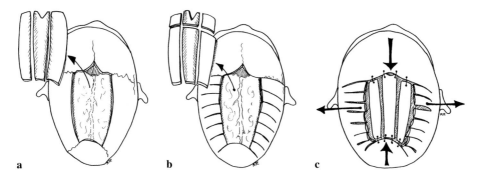

a   b   c

Fig. 19.3 The modified 'pi' procedure for the young (below 6 months) child with sagittal synostosis. (a) Removal of a 7 cm sagittal strip of bone. (b) The sagittal strip is divided up and vertical cuts are made in each parietal bone. (c) The central pieces of bone are replaced after they have been shortened. Pulling on the sutures that hold them to ensure end-to-end bone contact shortens the antero-posterior diameter of the head while allowing the biparietal diameter to expand.

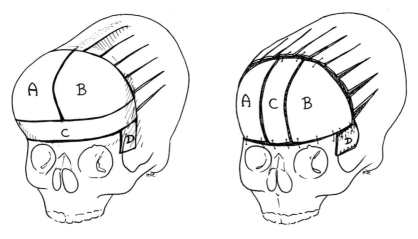

Fig. 19.4 A method for correcting the narrowed and bossed forehead of an older child with sagittal synostosis. The removal of bone segment C takes away much of the angle of protrusion of the forehead, and its curve usually means that it can conveniently be used to widen the forehead by interposing it between segments B and C. The hollowed pterional region D is also expanded.

at an early stage, because of the potential for venous bleeding, particularly in the region of the torcula and around the sigmoid sinuses. For this reason, we may (if the degree of abnormality of the child's head justifies surgery at all) recommend a more limited procedure for children presenting late with scaphocephaly and concentrate on the bossed and narrowed forehead and pterional region while leaving the posterior part of the deformity to be obscured by hair growth (Fig. 19.4).

Trigonocephaly, brachycephaly and anterior plagiocephaly

Trigonocephaly is caused by metopic synostosis and results in vertical ridging of the central forehead, hypotelorism and a triangular shape to the front of the head when it is viewed from above. Anterior plagiocephaly (forehead asymmetry) and brachycephaly (a wide head that is short in the antero-posterior diameter) are usually caused by unicoronal and coronal synostosis respectively. Each of these conditions results in abnormalities of the anterior craniofacial skeleton and to some degree affects the face also, because of the involvement of the anterior skull base. In fact the primary abnormality may well reside in the sphenoid region of the skull base rather than in the more visible vault sutures. This is reflected in the hypotelorism usually associated with metopic synostosis and the facial scoliosis that contributes to the deformity associated with unicoronal synostosis. Although these effects may at first be mild, if a genetic defect is present (the PRO 250 ARG mutation in unicoronal synostosis, for example) they can progress in severity until growth is complete. In fact, an underlying dysostosis syndrome should always be suspected in cases of coronal synostosis.

Surgically, these conditions can be considered together because, although the emphasis of the operation may vary, their correction involves reconstruction of both the forehead and superior parts of the orbits (fronto-orbital remodelling). Mostly the operations needed have to be performed bilaterally but in some cases of unicoronal synostosis producing only a moderate degree of plagiocephaly a unilateral procedure may be sufficient.

Access is via a coronal incision. Having separated the affected areas of the vault from the underlying dura, the frontal bones are usually removed in a single block and set aside for later reshaping and replacement. Traditionally, the supraorbital bar (which measures approximately 1 cm in depth superior to the orbits and includes the anterior aspects of the orbital roofs, root of the nose and varying mounts of the lateral orbital walls) is then removed. It is now reshaped 'on the bench' by making partial thickness cuts in it that allow it to be bent into an improved shape which can be reinforced if necessary by using plates and screws or wires. The reformed bar is then replaced in the optimal position to normalise the anatomical relationship of the supraorbital region with the rest of the craniofacial skeleton (Fig. 19.5).

Fixation may be with wires or plates and screws. It has been recommended that there should be no attachment between the bar and the skull vault (i.e. it should be attached to the face only), so that brain expansion can continue to push it forwards – the so-called 'floating forehead'. We are unconvinced of the validity of this theory and prefer to provide as much stability as possible. The frontal bone block (also reshaped as necessary) is now reattached to the supraorbital bar. We have found commercially produced templates for the new forehead to be too small, leaving the patient with the risk of developing unsightly vertical ridges laterally on each side, and we now favour a larger construct that extends 'round the corner' into the temporal regions and behind the hairline.

An alternative method, having removed the frontal bone block, is to remove the supraorbital bone completely down to the orbital roof, and fashion an entirely new one from a suitably shaped piece of bone taken from elsewhere in the calvarium. The technique has the advantage of achieving symmetry more easily, but can create difficulties in reproducing exactly the normal contours of this topographically complex area.

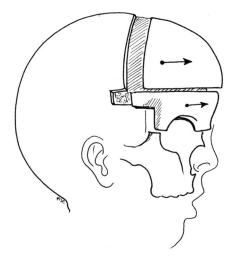

Fig. 19.5 A fronto-orbital reconstruction/advance. The frontal bones and supraorbital ridges are cut out separately and (in this illustration) advanced as shown to correct recession of the forehead and supraorbital regions.

More recently, we have dispensed with the reconstruction of the supraorbital bar as a separate entity altogether. Instead, the frontal bone block is cut into various pieces and then reconstructed with a mixture of rigid (usually wires) and non-rigid (usually absorbable monofilament) suture material to provide a replacement that stretches vertically from the orbital roofs to the vertex and horizontally from one pre-auricular region to the other. At the end of the operation shallow vertical concavities are burred out from the lower border of the new forehead to create an anatomically accurate shape for the superior border of the orbits. (Figs 19.6 and 19.7 demonstrate this approach for unicoronal and metopic synostosis respectively.)

Posterior plagiocephaly, and posterior vault expansion
Flattening of one side (or rarely both sides) of the occipital region may be caused by lambdoid synostosis but is much more commonly 'positional'. Current advice that infants should be nursed supine to avoid sudden infant death syndrome has produced an 'epidemic' of posterior skull vault asymmetries which are not synostotic in origin They can be distinguished clinically from the few rare cases of lambdoid synostosis and should not, generally, be treated surgically (see Chapter 7).

True posterior vault remodelling is rarely indicated for aesthetic purposes since hair usually disguises the problem and separation of bone from dura in the presence of intact sutures makes bleeding from the region of the torcula, sagittal, lateral and sigmoid sinuses a definite hazard. In some instances of multiple suture fusion associated with raised ICP, however, a posterior vault expansion may be preferred to an anterior approach – or may precede it. Once again a coronal incision is used. The posterior quadrant of the skull vault

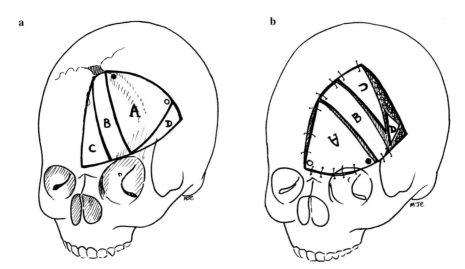

Fig. 19.6 A method for the unilateral correction of left coronal synostosis without restructuring the supraorbital ridge as a separate entity. (a) The frontal block (including the anterior part of the parietal bone) is cut out in one piece to include the supraorbital ridge. It is then divided up as shown. (b) The pieces are replaced as shown. The posterior edge of piece A usually has a contour that makes for a suitable supraorbital ridge, and pieces B, C and D can be positioned (their own curvatures adjusted as necessary) to bring forward the flattened forehead. A concavity (not shown) can then be burred away along the inferior surface of the new frontal bone (A) to recreate the shape of the top of the orbit.

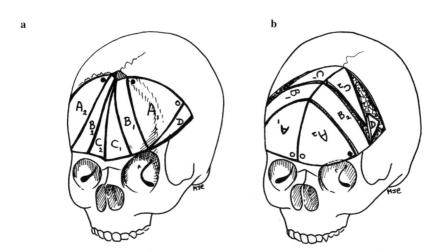

Fig. 19.7 A method for correcting trigonocephaly associated with metopic synostosis. (a) The frontal block of bone (down to and including the supraorbital ridges) is cut out in one piece and then divided in the midline. The posterior edge of segments A_1 and A_2 usually has a contour that makes for a suitable supraorbital ridge. (b) After pieces A_1 and A_2 have been cut out they are replaced as shown to provide the lower part of the new forehead. The remainder of each original frontal bone block is then subdivided as necessary to provide a suitable contour for the remainder of the frontal region.

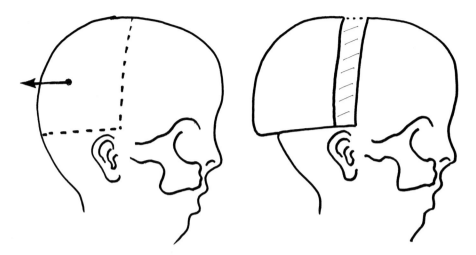

Fig. 19.8 A posterior skull vault expansion. After the posterior quadrant of the skull has been mobilised (if there is premature fusion of the posterior vault sutures the dura will not be stuck to their undersurfaces), it can usually be moved back approximately 1.5–2.0 cm while still allowing the skin incision to be closed (under some tension).

is cut out in one block from vertex to as low down as possible and then transposed posteriorly to expand the intracranial volume as much as is possible while still allowing the skin incision to be closed (Fig. 19.8). Fixation can be with wires, or plates and screws. A posterior vault expansion can be particularly complicated when undertaken in very young children with severe forms of syndromic craniosynostosis. In this situation the dura may be extremely thin and protrude into a honeycomb of defects in the overlying bone, making it difficult to avoid tears.

SUBCRANIAL OSTEOTOMIES

The most commonly performed subcranial osteotomies are designed to alter the antero-posterior and vertical dimensions of the face and correct the disproportions of the upper and lower jaws seen so frequently in the craniofacial dysostoses. They are generally performed to correct cosmetic deformity, but they also have an important role in the management of such functional problems as upper airway obstruction, lack of globe protection (exorbitism) and difficulties with mastication caused by abnormal dental occlusion.

Subcranial osteotomies are described as being at the Le Fort I, II or III level and are named after the fracture patterns produced by craniofacial trauma. The craniofacial surgeon takes advantage of the naturally occurring lines of weakness in the facial skeleton to separate the facial bones into subunits that may then be moved to alter facial proportions. Only the Le Fort I and III osteotomies are commonly used to treat craniofacial dysostoses.

The Le Fort III osteotomy

The Le Fort III (Figs 19.9 and 19.10) osteotomy is a high-level osteotomy that effectively cleaves the facial skeleton from the undersurface of the cranium from which it is suspended. Once this has been achieved, the entire facial skeleton may be advanced. To correct a cosmetic deformity alone, the operation is best carried out at the end of facial growth – around the age of 17 to 18. However it is often performed at an earlier age for functional reasons or to address the psychological concerns that can arise in the late childhood or adolescence of children with facial deformity.

The operation is performed via a coronal incision. Preparation and exposure of the upper facial skeleton are undertaken in a similar fashion to that required for a monobloc osteotomy (see below). Osteotomy cuts using a reciprocating saw are made through the zygomatic arch and the lateral, inferior and medial walls of the orbits. These cuts extend from the region of the zygomatico-frontal suture to the anterior part of the inferior orbital fissure and then across the floor of the orbit. The orbital osteotomy is then completed by dividing the medial orbital wall posterior to the nasolacrimal duct. It is not necessary to divide the medial canthal tendon to achieve this. Once both orbits have been osteotomised the cuts are joined by a further osteotomy across the root of the nose in the region of the

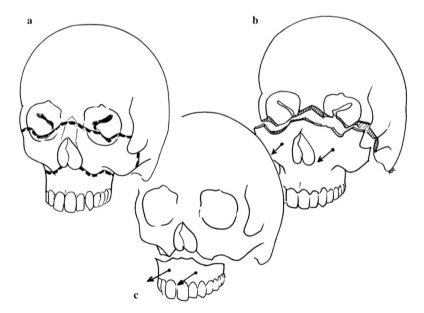

Fig. 19.9 Two Le Fort osteotomies. (a) The upper line shows the osteotomy cuts for the Le Fort III, and the lower for the Le Fort I. (b) The Le Fort III allows the maxilla to be drawn forwards. (c) The Le Fort I allows the tooth-bearing segment of the maxilla to be drawn forward.

In both cases, the mobilised segment can be brought forward in one piece, either immediately after the osteotomy cuts have been made (and held forward with bone grafts, plates and screws, etc.), or slowly over the next two weeks or so, by gradual distraction (when long-term stability will be provided by new bone formation stimulated by the distraction process).

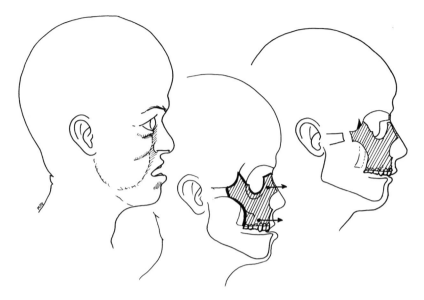

Fig. 19.10 The Le Fort III procedure viewed from the side. The advanced segment will correct recession of the malar areas as well as a class III malocclusion.

nasofrontal suture. The nasal septum is then cleaved from the base of the skull with a broad osteotome and pterygo-maxillary disjunctions performed as described for the monobloc osteotomy below. Once the bone cuts are complete it should be possible to mobilise the face gently forwards, initially by pressure from behind and then, if necessary, using disimpaction forceps.

The entirely mobile facial skeleton can now be guided to its desired position. Temporary intermaxillary fixation (IMF) is then applied using a preformed acrylic wafer. Once the Le Fort III segment has been advanced to its desired position, bone grafts harvested from the ilium or calvarium are fashioned to fit the spaces created at the zygomatic arches, lateral orbital wall, orbital floor and nose. These bone grafts provide the rigid fixation required to maintain the position of the Le Fort III segment and are secured with titanium or resorbable plates and lag screws. At this stage the IMF can be released. Lateral canthopexies are then performed, mobilised soft tissues re-suspended, suction drains inserted and the coronal flap is closed. Nasopharyngeal airways are inserted, together with a nasogastric tube for post-operative feeding. Frost sutures are placed and retained for 24–48 hours to prevent corneal abrasion during the phase of maximal postoperative periorbital swelling. Postoperative care is as for the monobloc osteotomy.

The Le Fort I osteotomy
The Le Fort I osteotomy (Fig. 19.9) is performed at a lower level in the midface. The osteotomy is performed in the maxilla just above the level of the tooth roots. It advances the tooth-bearing part of the maxilla and can also be used to address vertical disproportions

in the lower midface. In adolescents with craniofacial dysostoses the procedure is usually performed to make final adjustments to facial proportions after the generalised retrusion of the craniofacial skeleton has been addressed by either a monobloc or a Le Fort III osteotomy. It can be undertaken either at the same time as these operations or as a separate procedure at a later date.

Alterations at the Le Fort I level are needed in a proportion of craniofacial patients because the degree of facial retrusion varies at different levels in the face, with the more marked retrusion usually present at the dental level. The midface is also often deficient in the vertical dimension in its lower part. This deficiency can be addressed by moving the Le Fort I segment downwards. The Le Fort I osteotomy is also used to correct the alignment of the dental arches to improve dental occlusion. Where this is a primary concern, the procedure may be combined with a mandibular osteotomy (bimaxillary osteotomy). A Le Fort I osteotomy cannot be performed until the permanent dentition has erupted sufficiently to allow the osteotomy cuts to be made above the level of the tooth roots. This does not usually occur until the age of 9 or 10. In practical terms, however, it is rarely desirable to undertake this procedure until the end of facial growth (see Chapter 1).

Careful orthodontic assessment and planning are required to ensure that a satisfactory and stable dental occlusion is achieved after surgery. In the final phase of planning, an acrylic dental wafer is constructed to aid accurate placement of the osteotomy into its ideal position.

The Le Fort I osteotomy is carried out under general anaesthesia with naso-tracheal intubation. The osteotomy is performed through an intraoral incision that extends trans-versely high in the buccal sulcus from the level of the molars on each side. The periosteum is then lifted from the underlying bone to expose the maxilla to above the level of the tooth roots. The piriform fossa is exposed and the periosteum lifted from the nasal floor over its entire length. The osteotomy cuts are performed at the level of the maxillary sinus. The lateral cuts are made with a reciprocating saw and extend from the piriform fossa to the posterior maxilla. The lateral wall of the nasal cavity is then osteotomised at the level of the nasal floor and the nasal septum divided at the same level. Pterygo-maxillary osteotomies are then made through the intraoral incision. Once these cuts have been made, only the posterior wall of the maxillary sinus holds the Le Fort I segment to the facial skeleton. It can now be mobilised by performing a gentle downfracture with digital pressure. Disimpaction forceps may then be used to free and stretch soft tissue attachments.

The mobilised maxilla is then placed in its required position using a preformed acrylic wafer and temporary IMF is applied. Trimming of the maxillary bone may be required to achieve this. Bone grafts may be required to fill any gaps created. The Le Fort I segment is then plated to the maxilla and the IMF is released. The occlusion is checked again and the intraoral incisions are closed with resorbable sutures.

Postoperatively a soft diet is required for six weeks. It is important to pay meticulous attention to oral hygiene. Orthodontic elastic traction may be required to make fine adjust-ments to the occlusion.

Osteotomies to address antero-posterior/vertical anomalies –
the monobloc frontofacial advancement

The monobloc frontofacial osteotomy (Fig. 19.11) combines a transcranial frontal advance and extracranial Le Fort III midfacial advance into a single procedure. It is primarily designed to treat Crouzon syndrome when there is severe exorbitism, angle class III malocclusion and, perhaps, restriction of the nasopharyngeal airway causing respiratory obstruction or apnoea. The operation is surgically challenging and proper preparation and aftercare are critical. It should only be performed in craniofacial centres with considerable experience.

The bony barrier between the anterior cranial fossa floor and the nose is inevitably breached which increases risk, particularly of infection. Meticulous dural closure is essential and, whenever possible, a vascularised seal is introduced at the root of the nose in the form of a bone graft covered with a periosteal/pericranial flap. The intracranial dead space, which results following advancement, is also a concern, since if it is not filled rapidly by an expansion of the brain, blood and CSF and air can accumulate. This process predisposes to infection and prevents revascularisation of the frontal bone flap, possibly resulting in bone necrosis. Herein lies a conundrum for surgical timing – the younger the patient the more rapidly the brain will expand to fill the dead space, but the older the patient the more stable the result is likely to be in terms of facial growth and relapse. In general we believe that there is no indication for this type of surgery in young children for aesthetic reasons alone, since the risks are too great and any benefits will inevitably be lost over time (wholly or in part) to reversion/relapse as further abnormal growth occurs. If there is severe exorbitism with subluxation of the globe, raised intracranial pressure associated with respiratory obstruction,

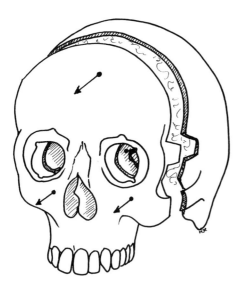

Fig. 19.11 The monobloc procedure. The frontal bones and the maxilla are brought forward in one piece either immediately after the osteotomy cuts have been made (and held forward with bone grafts), or slowly over the next two weeks or so, by gradual distraction (when long-term stability will be provided by new bone formation stimulated by the distraction process).

and difficulties feeding which cannot be adequately managed in other ways, then monobloc advancement should be considered. In such a situation it may now be preferable to achieve the desired advance by distraction osteogenesis rather than immediately at surgery (see below). In the absence of such severe symptoms the operation is best delayed until skeletal maturity is approaching, i.e. 12 years plus.

Monobloc advancement has the advantage over two-stage procedures (a frontal advance followed by a Le Fort III midface advance) of reducing the number of surgical procedures required and providing much greater rigidity in the orbital region for fixation, and thus the potential for a more stable result. The disadvantages have been outlined above. In most cases the amount of advancement required at the orbital and dental level will be different and a greater anterior translocation is needed dentally. If the whole face is advanced by this larger amount, it can leave the patient with enophthalmos which is difficult to correct. Our philosophy, therefore, is to try to normalise both the orbital and frontal configuration as far as possible during the monobloc advance itself, leaving the 'fine tuning' of the dental relationship to maturity, when the relatively minor Le Fort I osteotomy may be all that is required.

The monobloc frontofacial osteotomy is carried out under general anaesthesia with either nasal or oro-tracheal intubation. In the latter case we would favour fixation of the endotracheal tube with a circum-mandibular wire to prevent accidental extubation. Temporary tarsorhaphies are inserted to protect the eyes. Initially bone grafts are harvested (usually from the hip) so that they are available for support and fixation later in the procedure. An approach is made via the upper buccal sulcus and a subperiosteal dissection carried out over the anterior maxilla, malar body, anterior malar arch and inferior orbit. The nasal mucosa is carefully dissected from the piriform aperture in order to maintain its integrity. The hard palate mucosa is freed from the underlying bone, either via two small lateral incisions or a U-shaped anterior palatal incision. A coronal incision is then made and a standard subperiosteal dissection made over the frontal bone towards the orbits. A vascularised pericranial flap should be preserved to seal the anterior cranial fossa at the end of the procedure.

Laterally the dissection continues beneath the temporoparietal fascia until 2 cm above the malar arch when it is deepened beneath the superficial layer of the temporalis fascia to protect the temporal branch of the facial nerve. The periorbita are freed and the nasolacrimal duct and inferior orbital fissure identified. The masseter muscle is completely released from the malar arch – if this release is inadequate, advancement of the face will be severely restricted. The dissection from above will now have been joined laterally with that from below.

Next a bi-frontal craniotomy is performed and the bone flap set aside. Tongue-in-groove osteotomies may be designed posteriorly to support the eventual advance of the face and a supraorbital bandeau may or may not be preserved from which to suspend the face. The dura covering the frontal lobes is dissected posteriorly as far as the cribriform plate and lesser wing of the sphenoid. It is at this point of the dissection that tears in the dura that may lead later to CSF rhinorrhoea may occur.

The osteotomies are now made with a combination of oscillating saws and osteotomes. It is easiest to begin laterally at the inferior orbital fissure, extending upwards through the lateral orbital wall and into the orbital roof/anterior cranial fossa floor. This cut extends medially, in front of the cribriform plate to meet that of the opposite side. The medial orbital wall is sectioned behind the naso-lacrimal duct, continuing into the orbital floor to join with the medial end of the inferior orbital fissure. The nasal septum should be divided from above taking care not to perforate the endotracheal tube. Finally the maxillary tuberosity is sectioned from the pterygoid plates, either from above (our preference) or below. This osteotomy may be difficult to achieve since in many craniodysostotic syndromes a dense bony block exists here.

Once the bone cuts are complete it should be possible to mobilise the face gently forwards, initially by pressure from behind and then, if necessary, using disimpaction forceps. When forward movement is adequate the teeth are placed in a pre-prepared dental wafer and temporary intermaxillary fixation (IMF) is secured with wires. Bone grafts are then contoured and placed in the lateral orbital walls, orbital floor and malar arch to support and maintain the surgical advance. Titanium plates may be needed to fix the grafts, but if possible they are best secured with lag screws alone as 'bone plates'. At this stage the IMF can be released. A bone graft is placed in the anterior cranial fossa floor and covered with the vascularised pericranial flap to seal the intracranial from the nasal space. The advanced facial segment is secured to the supraorbital bandeau if it has been preserved, the frontal bone is replaced or a new one of better contour constructed, and the wounds are closed. Nasopharyngeal airways are inserted, together with a nasogastric tube for postoperative feeding. The tarsorhaphies are replaced with Frost sutures for 48 hours or so to protect the corneas from abrasion.

Postoperatively oral intake is limited to water only for seven days, after which the nasopharyngeal airways are removed. Diet should be relatively soft for three months (though not liquidised) while consolidation of the osteotomies occurs. Elastic traction may be instituted at the dental level to support and continue to configure the dental occlusion. All contact sports should be avoided for at least three months.

Osteotomies to address three-dimensional deformity

*   Facial bipartition (midline faciotomy)
*   Orbital box osteomy

A facial bipartition occurs naturally in a midline (Tessier 0–14) facial cleft. Surgically a midline split can be created as an extension of a monobloc frontofacial advancement (Fig. 19.12). Its most obvious application is in the treatment of orbital hypertelorism and Apert syndrome.

The preliminary surgical procedure is identical to the monobloc, but having made all the osteotomies for that operation a triangular segment of bone, based superiorly, is removed from the root of the nose and a central diastema (gap) created between the upper incisor teeth. This allows the two hemifacial segments to be rotated together, so narrowing the inter-orbital distance and expanding the maxilla. At the same time they may be 'bent' backwards laterally, so creating a natural curve to the upper orbit and brow when these are too flat. The

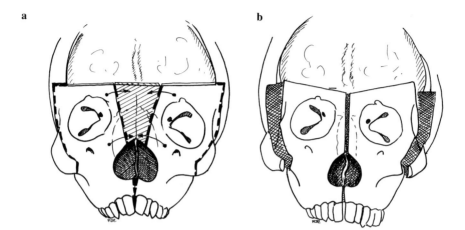

Fig. 19.12 The facial bipartition. (a) After the maxillae and orbits (still connected) have been mobilised, a wedge of bone is removed from the midline, and the central osteotomy cut extended down to between the central incisors. (b) Closure of the gap decreases the distance between the orbits and also corrects any downgoing slant in their previous alignment. This usually produces a gap between the central incisors (not shown here) that will require postoperative orthodontic attention.

medial rotation of the facial halves will, in turn, tend to correct a laterally downgoing slant to the eyes, such as occurs in Apert syndrome.

It is usually necessary to create a new supraorbital bandeau with an appropriate curve and often a new frontal bone also. The degree of maxillary expansion can be controlled with a midline wire. Some expansion is desirable in Apert syndrome but usually needs to be limited as much as possible in the treatment of hypertelorism occurring in the absence of a craniosynostosis-associated syndrome (i.e. frontonasal dysplasia). The amount of inter-orbital narrowing can be calculated from preoperative measurements and fixation is either with a plate or wires. Lateral canthopexy is generally required but medial canthopexy may be avoided if care is taken not to detach the medial canthal ligaments during dissection and mobilisation. This operation provides unparalleled opportunity for manipulation of a deformed facial skeleton and so can produce results which could not be achieved by any other technique. Aftercare is identical to that for monobloc advancement.

Hypertelorism and vertical orbital dystopia may be addressed by the so-called box osteotomy. In this procedure a 360-degree osteotomy is made around one or both orbits, allowing them to be translocated medially, upwards (Fig. 19.13) or downwards, after appropriate manipulation of the surrounding bones. Although this approach has been used extensively for the treatment of hypertelorism (horizontal dystopia) we have generally found it to be suboptimal and favour when possible the facial bipartition, the results of which are more reliable, more stable and more pleasing. The box osteotomy retains a valuable place, however, in the treatment of vertical dystopias and when lateral movement of a single orbit is required. As has been mentioned in Chapter 1, however, it must be remembered that the horizontal osteotomy below the orbit(s) runs between the orbital floor above and the roots of the permanent dentition below. This is a cut that can only be made when the patient is

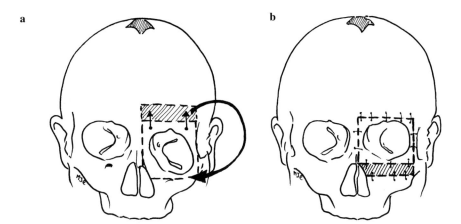

Fig. 19.13 Treating vertical dystopia with a box-type osteotomy to raise the orbit. (a) The anterior rim of the orbit is cut out and a segment removed from the frontal bone above. (b) The front of the orbit is now raised and the removed piece of bone replaced below it. These procedures need a bone graft within the floor of the orbit as well (not shown).

sufficiently old for there to be enough space above the roots to avoid damaging them. Failure to observe this rule will cause permanent damage to the teeth, resulting in at best failure of them to erupt and at worst disordered development of the maxilla.

Distraction osteogenesis

Distraction osteogenesis is the process by which new bone is generated by the gradual distraction of callus between two vascularised bone surfaces. The technique was pioneered by Ilizarov, a Russian surgeon who used distraction osteogenesis to lengthen long bones of the limbs. The bone to be distracted is usually divided by an osteotomy (through the full thickness of the bone) or a corticotomy (through just its cortical surfaces) and stabilised by an internal or external fixation device which can then be used to pull (or push) the bone edges slowly apart. For midface distraction this needs to be anchored to the skull.

The process of clinical distraction osteogenesis can be divided into four phases:

1   An osteotomy or corticotomy to divide the bone to be lengthened.
2   A latent phase in which a callus is allowed to form.
3   A period of active distraction in which the bones are lengthened (separated). This usually takes place at a rate of 1–2 mm a day.
4   A consolidation phase in which the distracted callus is allowed to mature and form rigid bone. The distractor is left on during this phase in order to immobilise the bony segments. In the facial skeleton this phase usually lasts for 6–8 weeks, so the whole process takes a total of 9–12 weeks or so.

In 1992, McCarthy et al published the first clinical reports of distraction in the craniofacial skeleton. They reported experience with gradual distraction of the mandible and have since

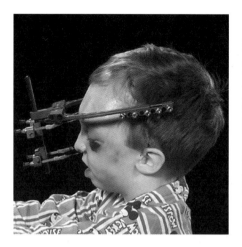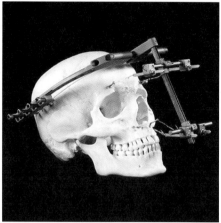

Fig. 19.14 An external distraction frame (RED frame) used in midfacial and craniofacial distraction. The upper part of the frame provides fixation to the skull. Fixation to the facial skeleton is via the plates and wires shown. Various screws on the device are turned daily to provide the distraction force. The device is left *in situ* during the consolidation phase.

published a 10-year review. The process proved very effective and by 1997 reliable techniques and devices had been developed for midfacial distraction, enabling the principle to be applied to craniofacial dysostoses syndromes.

In the management of craniosynostosis, distraction osteogenesis may be used to advance the craniofacial skeleton at the monobloc or Le Fort I, II or III level, and sometimes following a bipartition.

Conventional osteotomies allow accurate placement of bony fragments but have a number of significant disadvantages. The degree of advancement is limited by the elasticity of the soft tissue envelope. Large advancements may require significant volumes of bone graft, which are often unavailable in young children. Titanium plates and screws used in the fixation of these osteotomies may occasionally extrude, or in younger patients may become buried in bone with subsequent facial growth. Many younger patients require further osteotomies in later life and these buried plates and screws create considerable technical difficulties with repeat osteotomies and thus increase operative morbidity.

The process of distraction creates its own bone and therefore bone grafts are not required and there is no need for plates and screws (absorbable or non-absorbable) to hold them. The gradual distraction process overcomes the restrictions imposed by the soft tissue envelope, allowing greater advances than would be possible with conventional 'all in one go' techniques.

The disadvantages of distraction include a longer hospital stay and treatment time with an orthotic device in position, as well as difficulties controlling the exact angle of movement (the vector) during the distraction process.

There are essentially two types of distractor used in midfacial advancement: internal and external.

Internal distractors

These are placed subcutaneously at the time of surgery. They have the advantage of minimal bulk and they are well tolerated. To date, their disadvantages include the need for a more extensive secondary procedure to remove them at the end of treatment (which may be facilitated by the introduction of bio-absorbable materials), and difficulty in adjusting vectors of movement once distraction has begun.

External distractors

These rely on external halo devices similar to those used in the immobilisation of the neck following cervical trauma for cranial fixation. The halo is then connected to the mobilised facial skeleton, usually through a series of rods and wires that can then gradually be shortened to pull the face gently forwards. External distraction devices tend to be bulky, although the use of modern materials means that they are very light. Fine control of distraction vectors is facilitated by having multiple wires or rods that can be shortened or lengthened in whatever proportions are dictated by the patient's needs. They are also easier to remove at the end of treatment than internal devices.

At Great Ormond Street we favour external devices because of their versatility in controlling the direction of movement by using several points of fixation for the application and control of the distraction force to the mobilised segment. This fixation may be either through specially designed titanium plates, which are attached by screws to appropriate points on the craniofacial skeleton (usually the piriform fossa, supraorbital ridge and malar prominences), or through dental splints that apply the distracting force to the maxillary teeth. Once the required facial fixation devices have been placed, the wounds are closed and the external distractor is finally attached. In patients with craniofacial dysostoses, new bone creation occurs very rapidly in many parts of the midfacial skeleton, particularly in the region of the pterygoid plates and medial orbital walls. We therefore use a very short latency period of just 24 hours and then distract at a rate of 1.5 mm a day until the midface has moved the distance required (as judged both clinically and by using three-dimensional CT).

In children, distraction continues until the deformity is moderately over-corrected, to allow for further disordered growth. A six-week consolidation period follows before removal of the distractors.

In our experience, midfacial distraction produces predictable, significant and stable advancements. In our patients advancements of up to 22 mm (which would have been difficult to obtain by conventional means) have been achieved. The technique reliably encourages rapid new bone formation in the pterygoid and medial orbital regions, although the process is considerably slower in the calvarium and the zygomatic arches.

Distraction osteogenesis is a very promising tool for treating midfacial hypoplasia. It has the advantage over conventional techniques that bone grafts are not required, and there is early evidence to suggest that the quality of the bone generated by distraction is superior in preventing postoperative relapse. Simultaneous soft tissue elongation is a potential bonus too, but although in long bones there is good evidence that new soft tissues grow along with the new bone, this has yet to be convincingly demonstrated in the face. Distraction osteogenesis is particularly applicable to the correction of severe facial deformities in children, but there is little evidence yet to document the effects it might have on subsequent growth.

In summary the principal advantages of midfacial distraction osteogenesis are:

- No bone grafts are required.
- No internal fixation devices are needed (relevant to future surgery).
- Larger movements are possible.
- Significant functional improvements may be achieved.

Disadvantages of the technique include:

- Distraction devices are cumbersome and require a second operation to remove them.
- Midfacial distraction osteogenesis often results in a prolonged hospital stay.
- Procedures still involve major surgery and have similar complication rates to conventional osteotomies.

Complications

No discussion of surgical technique would be complete without considering potential complications. Although serious complications following craniofacial procedures are statistically uncommon in experienced hands, because of the nature of the surgery, when they do occur they may be life-threatening. Surgical complications are usually categorised according to when they may occur:

- Operative, early (within the first postoperative week)
- Intermediate (within the first postoperative month)
- Late

OPERATIVE COMPLICATIONS

Major surgical complications include severe bleeding (particularly from dural venous sinuses when the ICP is raised), brain and eye injury, and the acute intracranial hypertension that may be associated with an alteration in the patient's position on the operating table (producing flexion of the neck) or interruption of major emissary veins, raising the intracranial pressure. Inadvertent bony fractures may occur, making stable fixation difficult or impossible. Careful planning and meticulous attention to detail by an experienced team can reduce these serious risks to a minimum but will never eliminate them altogether.

EARLY COMPLICATIONS

The early postoperative period presents a number of potential hazards and the patients require careful management in a dedicated high dependency or intensive care unit where diligent care by well-trained dedicated nursing staff will limit the risks. Of most concern is compromise of the airway. Nursing in a semi-sitting position, the use of nasopharyngeal airways, frequent suction and immediate access to anaesthetic support are essential. While tracheostomy is required for some patients (emergency reintubation can be difficult in patients undergoing midface distraction), it is best avoided whenever possible because of the increased surgical infection risk it may expose the patient to.

Haematoma is a hazard in all surgical procedures, but the potential consequences are particularly serious if it occurs intracranially, and patients must therefore be closely monitored postoperatively so that if there is any suspicion that their ICP is rising an emergency brain scan can be swiftly carried out, and any haematoma promptly evacuated. Swelling of the forehead, eyelids and face occurs with such frequency after craniofacial surgery (its degree reflecting the scale of the operation) that some would probably not classify it as a complication. It does however impede assessment of the papillary reactions postoperatively (when monitoring for intracranial haemorrhage is at its most intense) and, when the child cannot see for perhaps two or three days because of eyelid oedema, it adds significantly to both the patient's distress and the length of their hospital stay. We now use a large volume 'tumescent' solution infiltrated subcutaneously before the operation begins and have found that this can have a dramatic effect in reducing (and sometimes abolishing altogether) postoperative swelling (see earlier in this chapter for its 'formula').

Visual compromise is surprisingly rare, but should be diligently looked for when there has been movement of the orbits and thus of the eyes themselves.

Difficulties in postoperative fluid and electrolyte management may indicate pituitary dysfunction and are most likely to occur following treatment of a congenital midline anomaly such as a frontoethmoidal encephalocoele whose bone defect in the skull base may extend as far back as the pituitary fossa.

CSF leakage, usually via the nose (rhinorrhoea), may become evident at this stage. Management is initially by lumbar puncture or the insertion of an external lumbar drain but in refractory cases an endoscopic procedure to close the defect in the skull base may be required. In our experience it has been a particular problem following midface distraction but it has been suggested that increasing the delay between the osteotomies and the onset of the distraction process itself to six or seven days may reduce the risk.

An extradural collection of air beneath the frontal bone flap (aerocoele) predisposes to infection. Insertion of nasopharyngeal airways when there is a risk of communication between the nose and intracranial space reduces this risk.

Acute infection is rare, but if it does occur needs to be treated vigorously with appropriate intravenous antibiotics. Our prophylactic antibiotic regime for all our craniofacial cases is as follows:

FLUCLOXACILLIN   25 mg/kilo body weight (kbw)
AMIKACIN   10 mg/kbw
METRONIDAZOLE   7.5 mg/kbw

INTERMEDIATE COMPLICATIONS
Infection remains a risk, particularly in the presence of the large intracranial 'dead space' that is the inevitable result of any frontal advance. The duration of this air-filled space depends on its initial volume, the child's intracranial pressure (if previously raised, the dead

399

space will be filled in more quickly), and the underlying craniofacial pathology (the ability of the brain and dura to expand to fill the space is greater in Crouzon syndrome, for example, than in Apert syndrome).

A number of ophthalmic complications may become evident following orbital manipulation. These include diplopia, astigmatism and reduced visual acuity.

Failure of bony fixation may require further intervention.

Alteration of the upper aero-digestive tract may cause speech and feeding difficulties. The most significant of these are velopharyngeal incompetence and aspiration.

LATE COMPLICATIONS

Chronic persistent low-grade infection is usually related to devascularisation (or failure of revascularisation) of bone and may need radical debridement and secondary reconstruction.

Bony relapse in severe dysostotic syndromes is inevitable when surgery is carried out before maturity since the primary genetic defect remains active. This may be considered not as real relapse but rather a failure of further normal growth. True relapse of bony positioning will result from poor bony fixation or inadequate soft tissue release and may necessitate further surgery.

Fixing plates, screws or wires can become palpable through the skin and may require surgical removal.

Occlusal defects can usually be managed by skilled orthodontics but occasionally need surgical adjustment. Damage to tooth roots or dental devascularisation may not become apparent until a late stage and may require prosthetic dental reconstruction.

Soft tissue inadequacies such as temporal hollowing from loss of bulk in the temporalis muscle may need further surgical intervention using either the patient's own bone or a malleable prosthetic substance, but careful soft tissue management at the initial operation will reduce these risks.

REFERENCES

McCarthy JG, Schreiber J, Karp N et al (1992) Lengthening the human mandible by gradual distraction. *Plast Reconstr Surg* 89: 1.

McCarthy JG, Stelnicki EJ, Grayson BH (1999) Distraction osteogenesis of the mandible: a ten year experience. *Semin Orthod* 5: 3.

Tessier P, Guiot G, Rougerie J, Delbet JP, Pastoriza J (1967) Osteotomies cranio-naso-orbitales: hypertelorisme. *Ann Chir Plast* 12: 103.

AFTERWORD
THE EVOLUTION OF A MODERN
CRANIOFACIAL UNIT

Barry Jones

The concept and underlying principles of craniofacial surgery were devised by Paul Tessier during the late 1950s and early 1960s but he did not present them in public until 1968. The surgery required both a craniofacial surgeon (usually based in plastic surgery) and a neuro-surgeon working together to be safely performed. The Hospital for Sick Children, Great Ormond Street (as it was called before trusts were invented) became involved at an early stage when David Mathews, the senior plastic surgeon at the hospital, visited Tessier to learn from him. Tessier was persuaded to perform surgery at Great Ormond Street in 1972 as a preliminary to setting up a unit there. Kenneth Till provided the neurosurgical expertise despite initial reservations on his part since the operations breached many of the accepted tenets of neurosurgical practice! Between 1972 and 1978, when Mathews retired, a good deal of craniofacial surgery was done at GOS, it being the only centre in England (Ian Jackson was developing the Canniesburn unit in Glasgow). The results of a series of 50 hypertelorism corrections were published in 1979.

My own interest in craniofacial surgery was stimulated during a visit to Tessier and Daniel Marchac in Paris in early 1984. Although I had read about these dramatic procedures during my training, this was the first opportunity I had to witness them at first hand. To separate the men and their techniques is impossible, one could not fail to be profoundly influenced by both – Tessier, the pioneer and instigator, a truly great and extraordinary man by any standards, and Marchac, a gentleman, consummate technician and educator, pushing the boundaries of surgery in young children. In February 1985 I was appointed to the staff at GOS and promptly left for Paris on a Royal College of Surgeons travelling scholarship with Marchac, which also allowed me to visit Tessier regularly.

Following David Mathews' retirement, true craniofacial surgery lost some impetus at GOS although the neurosurgeons continued to treat craniosynostosis. I was very fortunate to be welcomed and encouraged by two highly skilled and talented neurosurgeons keen to advance and embrace new techniques, Norman Grant (now retired) and Richard Hayward. This was the nucleus of the current craniofacial unit. In 1987 the Department of Health recognised the significance of craniofacial surgery, and the importance of limiting its prac-tice to a few centres so that experience and expertise could be gained, by designating it a 'supra-regional' service, funded centrally. Three centres were nominated, in London (GOS),

Oxford and Birmingham, to be joined more recently by Liverpool. These four units continue to be funded by what is now the National Specialist Commissioning Advisory Group (NSCAG).

We were always aware that the 'carpentry' of surgery, important and challenging as it was, represented only a part of caring for children with craniofacial deformities and supporting their families. Our unit has developed by liaison with other related specialties and by establishing an active research programme. This has produced internationally recognised contributions on the incidence and causes of raised intracranial pressure in craniosynostosis and its relationship to intracranial volume; an investigation into disturbances of intracranial–extracranial venous drainage in severe craniofacial disorders and the role and treatment of respiratory obstruction in these conditions; pioneering investigations into the genetic basis for craniofacial dysostosis syndromes have helped identify some of the defective amino acid combinations responsible for their occurrence; a number of previously unrecognised ophthalmological defects have been identified and we are now able to photograph and record the appearance of the optic discs, which permits closer monitoring of trends in intracranial pressure without invasive tests; speech, language and developmental disorders have been defined where they were previously unrecognised; dental anomalies have been identified, modifying surgical approaches and benefiting final outcome; technical refinements have improved outcomes in the treatment of both craniosynostosis and dysostosis syndromes and this continues in the field of distraction osteogenesis.

This list of research projects is not exhaustive but it illustrates the contributions of many committed specialists to improving care for children with craniofacial disorders. Our firm belief in the multidisciplinary nature of our specialty is reflected also in the breadth of contributions to this book from the various members of the Great Ormond Street team.

It is to be hoped also that this book will provide further support for the argument – which surprisingly still persists in some quarters – that these complex patients should only be managed under the aegis of a properly staffed, equipped and experienced craniofacial unit, and that failure to do so will only result in affected children being unable to achieve their full functional and social potential.

What constitutes such a unit? The craniofacial unit at Great Ormond Street Hospital for Children consists at present of the following core members, all of whom have contributed to this volume:

Plastic surgery – Barry Jones and David Dunaway
Neurosurgery – Richard Hayward
Orthodontics – Robert Evans
Ophthalmology – Ken Nischal
Psychology – Daniela Hearst
Speech and language – Caroleen Shipster and Valerie Pereira
ENT – Susannah Leighton
Genetics – Louise Wilson
Anaesthetics – Robert Bingham

Clinical Nurse Specialist (craniofacial) – Andrea White
Clinical Nurse Specialist (respiratory)

In addition, NSCAG provide funding for a unit administrator, database manager and clinical fellow.

What sort of workload does the unit have? (The following figures exclude overseas patients and refer only to patients with craniosynostosis-related conditions.)

In 2001, children with the following conditions were referred to us as new cases:

Craniofacial dysostosis – 19
Other craniosynostosis-associated syndromes – 9
Non-syndromic craniosynostosis (predominantly single suture synostosis) – 59

Of these 2001 new referrals, the majority were from the Greater London area or the southeast of England, while 43 were from other parts of the UK.

During 2001 the following operations were performed:

Complex major cases (predominantly facial bipartitions and monobloc frontofacial advances, with or without distraction) – 11
Major cases (mainly fronto-orbital reconstructions and vault expansions) – 56
Intermediate and minor procedures – 72
Intracranial pressure monitoring – 18

In summary, I hope that this brief outline of the history, the present personnel and the workload of the craniofacial unit at Great Ormond Street Hospital for Children NHS Trust will emphasise what is perhaps the main message of this book – that if the interests of the child with either an apparently simple or a more obviously complex form of craniosynostosis are to be properly met, this can only be accomplished in the setting of a multidisciplinary unit to which is regularly referred a critical mass of patients with these unusual but challenging conditions.

INDEX

410

411

415

421